New Developments in Myeloma

Editor

PETER LEIF BERGSAGEL

HEMATOLOGY/ONCOLOGY CLINICS OF NORTH AMERICA

www.hemonc.theclinics.com

Consulting Editors
GEORGE P. CANELLOS
EDWARD J. BENZ JR

April 2024 • Volume 38 • Number 2

ELSEVIER

1600 John F. Kennedy Boulevard • Suite 1800 • Philadelphia, Pennsylvania, 19103-2899

http://www.theclinics.com

HEMATOLOGY/ONCOLOGY CLINICS OF NORTH AMERICA Volume 38, Number 2
April 2024 ISSN 0889-8588, ISBN 13: 978-0-443-13077-9

Editor: Stacy Eastman
Developmental Editor: Shivank Joshi

Hematology/Oncology Clinics (ISSN 0889-8588) is published bimonthly by Elsevier Inc., 360 Park Avenue South, New York, NY 10010-1710. Months of issue are February, April, June, August, October, and December. Business and Editorial Offices: 1600 John F. Kennedy Blvd., Ste. 1800, Philadelphia, PA 19103–2899. Customer Service Office: 3251 Riverport Lane, Maryland Heights, MO 63043. Periodicals postage paid at New York, NY and at additional mailing offices. Subscription prices are $498.00 per year (domestic individuals), $100.00 per year (domestic students/residents), $525.00 per year (Canadian individuals), $100.00 per year (Canadian students/residents), $597.00 per year (international individuals), and $255.00 per year (international students/residents). For institutional access pricing please contact Customer Service via the contact information below. International air speed delivery is included in all *Clinics* subscription prices. All prices are subject to change without notice. **POSTMASTER:** Send address changes to *Hematology/Oncology Clinics of North America*, Elsevier Health Sciences Division, Subscription Customer Service, 3251 Riverport Lane, Maryland Heights, MO 63043. Customer Service (orders, claims, online, change of address): Elsevier Health Sciences Division, Subscription **Customer Service, 3251 Riverport Lane, Maryland Heights, MO 63043. Tel: 1-800-654-2452 (U.S. and Canada); 314-447-8871 (outside U.S. and Canada). Fax: 314-447-8029. E-mail: journalscustomerservice-usa@elsevier.com (for print support); journalsonlinesupport-usa@elsevier.com (for online support)**.

Reprints. For copies of 100 or more, of articles in this publication, please contact the Commercial Reprints Department, Elsevier Inc., 360 Park Avenue South, New York, New York 10010-1710; Tel.: 212-633-3874, Fax: 212-633-3820, E-mail: reprints@elsevier.com.

Hematology/Oncology Clinics of North America is covered in *MEDLINE/PubMed (Index Medicus), EMBASE/ Excerpta Medica, and BIOSIS.*

Contributors

CONSULTING EDITORS

GEORGE P. CANELLOS, MD
William Rosenberg Professor of Medicine, Department of Medical Oncology, Dana-Farber Cancer Institute, Boston, Massachusetts

EDWARD J. BENZ Jr, MD
Professor, Pediatrics, Richard and Susan Smith Professor, Medicine, Professor, Genetics, Harvard Medical School, President and CEO Emeritus, Office of the President, Dana-Farber Cancer Institute, Boston, Massachusetts

EDITOR

PETER LEIF BERGSAGEL, MD, FASCO
Consultant, Department of Medicine, Mayo Clinic Arizona, Phoenix, Arizona; Professor of Medicine, Division of Hematology Oncology, Mayo Clinic, Mayo Clinic College of Medicine, Scottsdale, Arizona

AUTHORS

NADINE ABDALLAH, MD
Division of Hematology, Mayo Clinic, Rochester, Minnesota

NIZAR J. BAHLIS, MD
Arnie Charbonneau Cancer Institute, University of Calgary, Calgary, Alberta, Canada

PETER LEIF BERGSAGEL, MD, FASCO
Consultant, Department of Medicine, Mayo Clinic Arizona, Phoenix, Arizona; Professor of Medicine, Division of Hematology Oncology, Mayo Clinic, Mayo Clinic College of Medicine, Scottsdale, Arizona

AJAI CHARI, MD
University of California, San Francisco, San Francisco, California

XIAOYI CHEN, MD, PhD
Center Blood Cancer, Perlmutter Cancer Center, New York University, New York, New York

MARTA CHESI, PhD
Associate Professor, Department of Medicine, Mayo Clinic, Scottsdale, Arizona

ADAM D. COHEN, MD
Associate Professor, Division of Hematology/Oncology, Department of Medicine, Abramson Cancer Center, University of Pennsylvania, Philadelphia, Pennsylvania

FAITH DAVIES, MD
Center Blood Cancer, Perlmutter Cancer Center, New York University, New York, New York

BENJAMIN A. DERMAN, MD
Section of Hematology/Oncology, University of Chicago, Chicago, Illinois

ANUP JOSEPH DEVASIA, MBBS, MD, DM
Clinical Research Fellow, Myeloma and Plasma Cell Disorders, Division of Medical Oncology and Haematology, Princess Margaret Cancer Centre, Toronto, Ontario, Canada

MADHAV V. DHODAPKAR, MD
Professor, Department of Hematology/Medical Oncology, Emory University, Atlanta, Georgia

MEGAN TIEN DU, MS
Department of Medicine, Mayo Clinic, Scottsdale, Arizona

HERMANN EINSELE, MD
Professor, Department of Internal Medicine II, University Hospital of Würzburg, Würzburg, Germany

RAFAEL FONSECA, MD
Division of Hematology and Medical Oncology, Mayo Clinic in Arizona, Phoenix, Arizona

ALFRED L. GARFALL, MD
Associate Professor, Division of Hematology/Oncology, Department of Medicine, Abramson Cancer Center, University of Pennsylvania, Philadelphia, Pennsylvania

MORIE A. GERTZ, MD, MACP
Professor of the Art of Medicine, Mayo Clinic, Rochester, Minnesota

ZAINUL S. HASANALI, MD, PhD
Instructor, Division of Hematology/Oncology, Department of Medicine, Abramson Cancer Center, University of Pennsylvania, Philadelphia, Pennsylvania

KLAUS MARTIN KORTUEM, MD
Professor, Department of Internal Medicine II, University Hospital of Würzburg, Würzburg, Germany

ANUPAMA D. KUMAR, MD
University of California, San Francisco, San Francisco, California

SHAJI K. KUMAR, MD
Division of Hematology, Mayo Clinic, Rochester, Minnesota

GUIDO SEBASTIAN LANCMAN, MD
Clinical Associate, Division of Medical Oncology and Haematology, Princess Margaret Cancer Centre, Toronto, Ontario, Canada

HOLLY LEE, MD, MSc
Arnie Charbonneau Cancer Institute, University of Calgary, Calgary, Alberta, Canada

FRANCESCO MAURA, MD
University of Miami, Miami, Florida

CONSTANTINE S. MITSIADES, MD, PhD
Department of Medical Oncology, Dana-Farber Cancer Institute, Harvard Medical School, Boston, Massachusetts; Broad Institute of Massachusetts Institute of Technology (MIT) and Harvard, Cambridge, Massachusetts; Ludwig Center at Harvard, Boston, Massachusetts

GARETH MORGAN, MB BCh, PhD
Center Blood Cancer, Perlmutter Cancer Center, New York University, New York, New York

PAOLA NERI, MD, PhD
Arnie Charbonneau Cancer Institute, University of Calgary, Calgary, Alberta, Canada

MARC S. RAAB, MD
Department of Internal Medicine V, Heidelberg University Clinic Hospital, Heidelberg, Germany

S. VINCENT RAJKUMAR, MD
Edward W. and Betty Knight Scripps Professor of Medicine, Division of Hematology, Mayo Clinic, Rochester, Minnesota

LEO RASCHE, MD
Department of Internal Medicine 2, University Hospital of Würzburg, Mildred Scheel Early Career Center (MSNZ), Würzburg, Germany

BEATRICE RAZZO, MD
Fellow, Division of Hematology/Oncology, Department of Medicine, Abramson Cancer Center, University of Pennsylvania, Philadelphia, Pennsylvania

CAROLINA SCHINKE, MD
Myeloma Center, University of Arkansas for Medical Sciences, Little Rock, Arkansas

EDWARD A. STADTMAUER, MD
Professor, Division of Hematology/Oncology, Department of Medicine, Abramson Cancer Center, University of Pennsylvania, Philadelphia, Pennsylvania

ALEXANDER KEITH STEWART, MBChB
Professor, Division of Medical Oncology and Haematology, Princess Margaret Cancer Centre, Toronto, Ontario, Canada

SANDRA P. SUSANIBAR-ADANIYA, MD
Assistant Professor, Division of Hematology/Oncology, Department of Medicine, Abramson Cancer Center, University of Pennsylvania, Philadelphia, Pennsylvania

NIELS W.C.J. VAN DE DONK, MD, PhD
Department of Hematology, Amsterdam UMC, Vrije Universiteit Amsterdam, Cancer Center Amsterdam, Cancer Biology and Immunology, Amsterdam, The Netherlands

GAURAV VARMA, MD
Center Blood Cancer, Perlmutter Cancer Center, New York University, New York, New York

NIELS WEINHOLD, PhD
Department of Internal Medicine V, Heidelberg University Clinic Hospital, Heidelberg, Germany

XIANGHUI XIAO, MD
Department of Internal Medicine II, University Hospital of Würzburg, Würzburg, Germany

XIANG ZHOU, MD
Department of Internal Medicine II, University Hospital of Würzburg, Würzburg, Germany

SONJA ZWEEGMAN, MD, PhD
Department of Hematology, Amsterdam UMC, Vrije Universiteit Amsterdam, Cancer Center Amsterdam, Cancer Biology and Immunology, Amsterdam, The Netherlands

Contents

Multiple myeloma is a malignancy of bone-marrow-localized, isotype-switched plasma cells that secrete a monoclonal immunoglobulin and cause hyperCalcemia, Anemia, Renal failure, and lytic Bone disease. It is preceded, often for decades, by a relatively stable monoclonal gammopathy lacking these clinical and malignant features. Both conditions are characterized by the presence of types of immunoglobulin heavy gene translocations that dysregulate a cyclin D family gene on 11q13 (*CCND1*), 6p21 (*CCND3*), or 12q11 (*CCND2*), a maf family gene on 16q23 (*MAF*), 20q11 (*MAFB*), or 8q24 (*MAFA*), or *NSD2/FGFR3* on 4p16, or the presence of hyperdiploidy. Subsequent loss of function of tumor suppressor genes and mutations activating *MYC*, RAS, NFkB, and cell cycle pathways are associated with the progression to malignant disease.

This research indicates that monoclonal gammopathy of undetermined significance (MGUS) and myeloma may stem from chronic immune activation and inflammation, causing immune dysfunction and spatial immune exclusion. As the conditions progress, a shift toward myeloma involves ongoing immune impairment, affecting both innate and adaptive immunity. Intriguingly, even in advanced myeloma stages, susceptibility to immune effector cells persists. This insight highlights the intricate interplay between immune responses and the development of these conditions, paving the way for potential therapeutic interventions targeting immune modulation in the management of MGUS and myeloma.

Smoldering multiple myeloma (SMM) is an intermediate clinical stage in the spectrum of monoclonal plasma cell disorders. It represents a heterogeneous clinically defined condition in which some patients (approximately 50%) have monoclonal gammopathy of undetermined significance (pre-malignancy), and some (approximately 50%) have multiple myeloma (biologic malignancy). Using specific prognostic factors, patients with SMM, in whom malignant transformation has already likely occurred, can be

Cereblon-targeting ligase degraders in myeloma: Mechanisms of action and resistance

Holly Lee, Paola Neri, and Nizar J. Bahlis

Cereblon-targeting degraders, including immunomodulatory imide drugs lenalidomide and pomalidomide alongside cereblon E3 ligase modulators like iberdomide and mezigdomide, have demonstrated significant anti-myeloma effects. These drugs play a crucial role in diverse therapeutic approaches for multiple myeloma (MM), emphasizing their therapeutic importance across various disease stages. Despite their evident efficacy, approximately 5% to 10% of MM patients exhibit primary resistance to lenalidomide, and resistance commonly develops over time. Understanding the intricate mechanisms of action and resistance to this drug class becomes imperative for refining and advancing novel therapeutic combinations.

Proteasome Inhibitors in Multiple Myeloma: Biological Insights on Mechanisms of Action or Resistance Informed by Functional Genomics

Constantine S. Mitsiades

During the last 20 years, proteasome inhibitors have been a cornerstone for the therapeutic management of multiple myeloma (MM). This review highlights how MM research has evolved over time in terms of our understanding of the mechanistic basis for the pronounced clinical activity of proteasome inhibitors in MM, compared with the limited clinical applications of this drug class outside the setting of plasma cell dyscrasias.

Monoclonal Antibodies in the Treatment of Multiple Myeloma

Niels W.C.J. van de Donk and Sonja Zweegman

The incorporation of monoclonal antibodies into backbone regimens has substantially improved the clinical outcomes of patients with newly diagnosed and relapsed/refractory multiple myeloma (MM). Although the SLAMF7-targeting antibody elotuzumab has no single-agent activity, there is clinical synergy between elotuzumab and immunomodulatory drugs in patients with relapsed/refractory disease. Daratumumab and isatuximab are CD38-targeting antibodies which have single-agent activity and a favorable safety profile, which make these agents an attractive component of combination regimens. Monoclonal antibodies may cause infusion-related reactions, but with subcutaneous administration these are less frequently observed. All therapeutic antibodies may interfere with assessment of complete response. Next-generation Fc-engineered monoclonal antibodies are in development with the potential to further improve the outcome of patients with MM.

Bispecific Antibodies in the Treatment of Multiple Myeloma

Xiang Zhou, Xianghui Xiao, Klaus Martin Kortuem, and Hermann Einsele

The treatment of multiple myeloma (MM) is evolving rapidly. In recent years, T-cell-based novel immunotherapies emerged as new treatment

strategies for patients with relapsed/refractory MM, including highly effective new options like chimeric antigen receptor (CAR)-modified
T cells and bispecific antibodies (bsAbs). Currently, B-cell maturation
antigen is the most commonly used target antigen for CAR T-cell and
bsAb therapies in MM. Results from different clinical trials have demonstrated promising efficacy and acceptable safety profile of bsAb in
RRMM.

Chimeric antigen receptor T cells (CARTs) represent another powerful way
to leverage the immune system to fight malignancy. Indeed, in multiple
myeloma, the high response rate and duration of response to B cell maturation antigen-targeted therapies in later lines of disease has led to 2 Food
and Drug Administration (FDA) drug approvals and opened the door to the
development of this drug class. This review aims to provide an update on
the 2 FDA-approved products, summarize the data for the most promising
next-generation multiple myeloma CARTs, and outline current challenges
in the field and potential solutions.

No therapy in multiple myeloma has been as extensively investigated as
stem cell transplantation following high-dose chemotherapy. A search of
the national library of medicine in February 2023 revealed over 27,000 publications covering stem cell transplantation. No other treatment for multiple
myeloma has been so vigorously investigated. However, given the rapid
advances seen in the treatment of multiple myeloma, it is legitimate to
ask whether the technique first introduced in 1983 by Thomas McIlwain
still has relevance. In 1984,Barlogie introduced infusional vincristine, doxorubicin, and dexamethasone and in 1986 published a first series on high-
dose therapy with autologous marrow-derived stem cells. At this point, the
only available therapies were melphalan, prednisone, other intensive steroids such as methylprednisolone, and interferon. Cyclophosphamide
was used both orally and parenterally. VBMCP was introduced as a combination therapy at Memorial Hospital subsequently shown not to be superior to melphalan and prednisone.

Consolidation therapy consists of short-term therapy after stem cell transplant in multiple myeloma. Key consolidation trials have shown mixed results on whether consolidation should be included after transplant, leading
to varied clinical practice. Maintenance therapy consists of long-term, typically fixed-duration or indefinite, therapy. Standard-risk patients typically
receive single-agent therapy, whereas high-risk may benefit from doublet
therapy and beyond. Adverse events and quality of life concerns should be
considered, as optimal duration of maintenance therapy continues to be
studied.

Treatment options have expanded rapidly and widely in the past two decades for patients with multiple myeloma. Triplet novel agent-based induction regimens have been accepted as the standard practice wordwide over the last decade both for transplant-eligible and non-eligible patients. The addition of anti-CD38 monoclonal antibodies as part of quadruplet regimens has led to even deeper and longer-lasting responses. The impressive results shown by the quadruplets havebeen practice-changing where accessible in recent years. Chimeric antigen receptor T cell therapy and bispecific antibodies are being tested in the upfront setting and have the potential to once again shift the paradigm of treatment of newly diagnosed MM.

Multiple myeloma is characterized by a highly heterogeneous disease distribution within the bone marrow-containing skeletal system. In this review, we introduce the molecular mechanisms underlying clonal heterogeneity and the spatio-temporal evolution of myeloma. We discuss the clinical impact of clonal heterogeneity, which is thought to be one of the biggest obstacles to overcome therapy resistance and to achieve cure.

Measurable (minimal) residual disease (MRD) has already proven to be one of the most important prognostic factors in multiple myeloma (MM). Each improvement in the depth of MRD testing has led to superior discrimination of outcomes, and sustained MRD negativity seems to be paramount to durable responses. Peripheral blood assays to assess for MRD are still under investigation but hold promise as complementary tools to bone marrow MRD assays such as next-generation sequencing and flow cytometry. Herein, the authors explore the evidence and potential benefits and drawbacks of MRD-adapted clinical decision-making in MM.

Improving the outcome of high-risk myeloma (HRMM) is a key therapeutic aim for the next decade. To achieve this aim, it is necessary to understand in detail the genetic drivers underlying this clinical behavior and to target its biology therapeutically. Advances have already been made, with a focus on consensus guidance and the application of novel immunotherapeutic approaches. Cases of HRMM are likely to have impaired prognosis even with novel strategies. However, if disease eradication and minimal disease states are achieved, then cure may be possible.

Despite improved treatments, most patients with multiple myeloma (MM) will experience relapse. Several novel agents have demonstrated activity and tolerability in early phase clinical trials. Venetoclax is a B-cell lymphoma 2 (Bcl-2) inhibitor with activity in patients with t(11;14) and/or Bcl-2 expression. Iberdomide and mezigdomide are cereblon E3 ligase modulators with higher potency, immunomodulatory, and antiproliferative activity compared with lenalidomide and pomalidomide. They have shown promising activity in heavily pretreated patients. Modakafusp alfa is an immunocytokine that targets interferons to CD38+ cells. It has demonstrated single agent activity in relapsed/refractory MM in the phase 1 setting.

Immunocompetent mouse models of multiple myeloma (MM) are particularly needed in the era of T cell redirected therapy to understand drivers of sensitivity and resistance, optimize responses, and prevent toxicities. Three mouse models have been extensively characterized: the Balb/c plasmacytomas, the 5TMM, and the Vk*MYC. In the last year, additional models have been generated, which, for the first time, capture primary MM initiating events, like MMSET/NSD2 or cyclin D1 dysregulation. However, the long latency needed for tumor development and the lack of transplantable lines limit their utilization. Future studies should focus on modeling hyperdiploid MM.

HEMATOLOGY/ONCOLOGY CLINICS OF NORTH AMERICA

SERIES OF RELATED INTEREST

Surgical Oncology Clinics
https://www.surgonc.theclinics.com
Advances in Oncology
https://www.advances-oncology.com

THE CLINICS ARE AVAILABLE ONLINE!
Access your subscription at:
www.theclinics.com

Preface

Extraordinary Progress in the Treatment of Multiple Myeloma: Is a Cure on the Horizon?

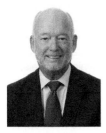

Peter Leif Bergsagel, MD, FASCO
Editor

My father, Daniel Bergsagel, reported on the activity of melphalan in the treatment of multiple myeloma (MM) in 1962, and melphalan and prednisone (MP) remained the standard of care for more than 40 years. This frustrated him, and he would tell me that to make progress we needed better drugs, and a better understanding of disease pathogenesis. Now we have both. The last major study to use MP as a control arm (VISTA) reported in 2010 a median progression-free survival (PFS) of 17 months and overall survival (OS) of 44 months. The period of therapeutic stagnation with MP contrasts dramatically with the rapid advances that have occurred starting approximately 25 years ago with the widespread adoption of high-dose melphalan with autologous hematopoietic stem cell transplantation and the introduction of thalidomide analogs and proteasome inhibitors. The progress became such that median OS was no longer a practical endpoint for discriminating between therapeutic approaches. The standard of care for about a decade used these newer modalities: lenalidomide, bortezomib and dexamethasone induction, stem cell transplant, and lenalidomide maintenance. In 2021, the DETERMINATION study reported a median PFS of 68 months and 5-year OS of 81% for newly diagnosed patients treated with this approach. The final major advance for the treatment of newly diagnosed MM was the introduction of a CD38 monoclonal antibody. At this point even median PFS was no longer a practical endpoint. In December 2023, the PERSEUS study reported that patients in whom daratumumab was added to induction, consolidation, and maintenance had a 4-year PFS of 84% and undetectable minimal residual disease (MRD) in 75% of patients, introducing the next standard of care. To continue to make rapid advances, we need surrogate endpoints for clinical

Hematol Oncol Clin N Am 38 (2024) xiii–xv
https://doi.org/10.1016/j.hoc.2023.12.015

trials with a more rapid readout than median PFS, of which MRD is the leading candidate. Luckily, it is clear that we will continue to make therapeutic advances, and incredibly, it seems likely to be at an even more rapid pace than the last decade. This is because the last couple of years have seen the FDA approval of two revolutionary approaches harnessing T cells: Chimeric Antigen Receptor T cells (ide-cel and cilta-cel) and T-cell engaging bispecific antibodies (teclistamab, elranatamab, and talquetamab). These agents are inducing unprecedented responses in relapsed, refractory MM and are being introduced into earlier disease stages.

The precursor stages of MM, monoclonal gammopathy of undetermined significance and smoldering MM, are very common conditions, affecting 5% and 0.5% of the adult population, respectively. Considerable work studying tumor genetics and microenvironment is helping to dissect which of these patients are at high risk of progression and may be candidates for early preventive or therapeutic interventions. Given that these patients are asymptomatic, it is important to design clinical trials that are safe and have suitable surrogate endpoints. Trial design can be informed by faithful preclinical models, such as the Vk*MYC genetically engineered immunocompetent mouse model of MM, that progresses over 1 year from a low-level monoclonal gammopathy to a symptomatic MM. Studies examining diet, microbiome, immunotherapies, and small molecules can all be evaluated first in mice to provide proof of concept. There are two main approaches to intervention in smoldering MM, prevention, which seeks to use nontoxic methods to delay the progression to symptomatic MM, and cure, which seeks to use all available means to eradicate all traces of disease. So far, it is clear that we can delay progression, but no evidence that we are able to cure the disease.

I see two main challenges for the future: achieving durable disease control in patients with high-risk MM (HRMM) and preventing late relapse in patients with undetectable MRD. The identifiable causes of HRMM include complete inactivation of tumor suppressor genes (TP53, RB1, CDKN2C) common to many cancers. While this presents a daunting challenge, the unique plasma cell biology suggests there may be a MM-specific synthetic lethality. It is important to rigorously define HRMM and identify patients in real-time so that they may be offered enrollment in specially designed clinical trials. Finally, the late relapses that occur in patients that have gone for years with undetectable MRD are vexing. Understanding the nature of the MM cell that escapes therapy and detection is a key question for researchers in the field and critical for obtaining cure. We are unlikely to cure MM with empiric therapy alone.

In conclusion, after 40 years with little progress, the last quarter century has witnessed accelerating advances in MM therapy. Although a cure remains elusive, ever fewer patients are dying of MM.

DISCLOSURE

Dr P.L. Bergsagel reports research funding from Pfizer, Celgene, Sanofi, Novartis; consulting for Janssen, Cellcentric, Omeros, Oncopeptides, Salarius; licensing fees for intellectual property related to human CRBN transgenic mice, and Vk*MYC transgenic mice.

Peter Leif Bergsagel, MD, FASCO
Department of Medicine
Mayo Clinic Arizona
5881 East Mayo Boulevard
Phoenix, AZ, USA

Mayo Clinic College of Medicine
Scottsdale, AZ, USA

E-mail address:
Bergsagel.leif@mayo.edu

Dedication

Remembering the Contributions of W. Michael Kuehl, MD
October 25, 1939–April 24, 2023

We dedicate this issue of *Hematology/Oncology Clinics of North America* to the memory of Dr Michael Kuehl (**Fig. 1**). Multiple myeloma research has seen tremendous progress over the last quarter century, a period that coincides, not incidentally, with Dr Kuehl's entry into the field. His foundational work provides the basis for our current understanding of the molecular pathogenesis of multiple myeloma.

Dr Kuehl graduated from Harvard Medical School in 1965 and pursued postdoctoral studies at the National Heart Lung and Blood Institute and Albert Einstein College of Medicine. Under the mentorship of Dr Matt Scharff, he studied the mechanism of immunoglobulin production[1] and somatic cell hybridization with mouse myeloma.[2] He joined the faculty of the University of Virginia Medical School in 1974 where he continued his studies of B-cell development and immunoglobulin production.[3] He returned to the NIH in 1980, learning molecular biology in the laboratory of Dr Phil Leder,[4] joining with Dr John Minna in 1982 to establish the molecular biology unit in the NCI–Navy Medical Oncology Branch, moving finally to the Genetics Branch in 1999. At the NIH he continued his studies of B-cell differentiation[5] and biology of mouse myeloma.[6,7]

I entered his laboratory in 1988, a medical oncology fellow with no laboratory experience. Under his patient mentorship I learned molecular biology while studying the genetics of mouse myeloma. I was keen to transition to the study of human myeloma; however, Mike felt strongly that it was crucial to first obtain and validate a panel of human myeloma cell lines to be used for analysis. We set about acquiring and extensively validating human myeloma cell lines from all over the world, an endeavor that took years, and to some extent continues to this day, and has generated an invaluable and unparalleled resource for the scientific community.

In those days before digital distractions there was more time for reading the scientific literature, for discussion, and for reflection. As Mike was known for his intellectual curiosity and eagerness to get to the bottom of each question, our daily, seemingly endless discussions generated the central hypotheses that chromosome translocations to the immunoglobulin heavy chain locus must occur in human myeloma, must be mediated by isotype switch recombination, and for some reason may not be evident from conventional metaphase karyotypes. We developed a Southern blot assay to identify illegitimate class switch recombination events, applied it to our panel of validated human myeloma cell lines, constructed and screened genomic bacteriophage libraries to clone these potential breakpoints, and used somatic cell hybrids to map the genomic locations involved in the chromosomal translocations. Thanks to Mike's profound knowledge of molecular biology, this all happened very rapidly: the idea for the assay occurred on December 5, 1994 at the Annual Society of Hematology meeting in Nashville, and on February 14, 1995, the result of the somatic cell hybrid mapping identified 16q23 as the breakpoint. Remarkably, we had already identified MAF as the target gene at 16q23, based on our earlier work using subtractive cDNA libraries to identify genes selectively expressed in human myeloma cell lines.[8] We

Hematol Oncol Clin N Am 38 (2024) xvii–xix
https://doi.org/10.1016/j.hoc.2024.01.002
0889-8588/24/© 2024 Published by Elsevier Inc.

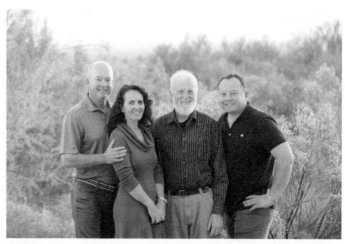

Fig. 1. Dr Michael Kuehl alongside his mentees, Drs Leif Bergsagel, Marta Chesi (*left*), and Rafael Fonseca (*right*).

eventually proceeded to identify recurrent immunoglobulin heavy chain gene chromosome translocations to 11q13, 6p21, 4p16, 16q23, 20q11 and formed the conceptual framework for our current model for the molecular pathogenesis of multiple myeloma.[9]

While identifying these novel translocations, Mike remained fascinated by the role of MYC in human myeloma. He was puzzled by the fact that MYC is almost universally activated by immunoglobulin class switch translocations in murine myeloma, but despite intense scrutiny, the homologous t(8;14) translocations were only rarely identified in patients with myeloma, although diverse rearrangements of MYC were almost universal in human myeloma cell lines. We concluded that MYC translocations were a very late event associated with the establishment of human myeloma lines.[10] Nevertheless, with his characteristic tenacity, Mike would periodically return to MYC over the years, reexamining its role as technology improved. It was with some pleasure that twenty-five years after having concluded that MYC translocations were rare in patients with myeloma, in 2020 we published that cryptic MYC rearrangements are present in half of newly diagnosed patients with myeloma and are likely responsible for the transition of a benign to a malignant plasma cell neoplasm.[11]

His scientific contributions earned him the prestigious Waldenström Lifetime Achievement Award from the International Myeloma Workshop in 2011. It gave him immense satisfaction to see the clinical impact of his work for patients with multiple myeloma. Mike was known for his generosity with the resources from his laboratory, sharing the genomic probes for FISH, and the human myeloma cell lines with multiple investigators. He was also renowned for sharing his critical insights at seminars and meetings and as a peer reviewer. He had an infectious joy for science—and life in general—that he communicated to all that had the pleasure to interact with him. Mike fostered the growth of many in the scientific community. His mentorship extended to numerous researchers and clinicians, including Drs Ethan Dimitrovsky, Tim Bender, Leif Bergsagel, Marta Chesi, Rafael Fonseca, and Adriana Zingone, alongside his long-time assistant Leslie Brents. His intellectual rigor, boundless curiosity, and commitment to scientific inquiry were complemented by his personal attributes: his wit, affable nature, and balance between scientific pursuit and family life.

Mike's contributions to science will certainly live on. The basic structure of the molecular classification of multiple myeloma that he developed will not change, although no doubt it will continue to be refined. I am confident that the many people he trained and interacted with will do their best to carry on what Mike taught us: to live a life of purpose, intellectual curiosity, and most importantly, joy.

Peter Leif Bergsagel, MD
Department of Medicine
Mayo Clinic Arizona
Phoenix, AZ, USA

Mayo Clinic College of Medicine
Mayo Clinic Arizona
13400 East Shea Boulevard
Scottsdale, AZ 85259, USA

E-mail address:
Bergsagel.leif@mayo.edu

REFERENCES

1. Kuehl WM, Kaplan BA, Scharff MD. Characterization of light chain and light chain constant region fragment mRNAs in MPC 11 mouse myeloma cells and variants. Cell 1975;5(2):139–47.
2. Margulies DH, Kuehl WM, Scharff MD. Somatic cell hybridization of mouse myeloma cells. Cell 1976;8(3):405–15.
3. Riley SC, Brock EJ, Kuehl WM. Induction of light chain expression in a pre-B cell line by fusion to myeloma cells. Nature 1981;289(5800):804–6.
4. Emorine L, Kuehl M, Weir L, et al. A conserved sequence in the immunoglobulin J kappa-C kappa intron: possible enhancer element. Nature 1983;304(5925):447–9.
5. Bender TP, Kuehl WM. Murine myb protooncogene mRNA: cDNA sequence and evidence for 5' heterogeneity. Proc Natl Acad Sci U S A 1986;83(10):3204–8.
6. Timblin C, Bergsagel PL, Kuehl WM. Identification of consensus genes expressed in plasmacytomas but not B lymphomas. Curr Top Microbiol Immunol 1990;166:141–7.
7. Bergsagel PL, Victor-Kobrin C, Brents LA, et al. Genes expressed selectively in plasmacytomas: markers of differentiation and transformation. Curr Top Microbiol Immunol 1992;182:223–8.
8. Bergsagel PL, Brents LA, Trepel JB, et al. Genes expressed selectively in murine and human plasma cell neoplasms. Curr Top Microbiol Immunol 1995;194:57–61.
9. Bergsagel PL, Chesi M, Nardini E, et al. Promiscuous translocations into immunoglobulin heavy chain switch regions in multiple myeloma. Proc Natl Acad Sci U S A 1996;93(24):13931–6.
10. Kuehl WM, Brents LA, Chesi M, et al. Selective expression of one c-myc allele in two human myeloma cell lines. Cancer Res 1996;56(19):4370–3.
11. Misund K, Keane N, Stein CK, et al. MYC dysregulation in the progression of multiple myeloma. Leukemia 2020;34(1):322–6.

Molecular Pathogenesis of Multiple Myeloma
Clinical Implications

Francesco Maura, MD[a],*, Peter Leif Bergsagel, MD[b],*

KEYWORDS

- Multiple myeloma (MM) • Smoldering multiple myeloma (SMM)
- Monoclonal gammopathy of undetermined significance (MGUS) • Plasma cell (PC)
- Hyperdiploidy • MYC • RAS • NFkB

KEY POINTS

- Primary genetic events divide multiple myeloma into 5 subgroups based on the presence of 1 of 3 types of recurrent immunoglobulin heavy chain gene translocations, hyperdiploidy, or of neither of these.
- The primary and initiating genetic events are present in pre-malignant monoclonal gammopathy and precede overt malignancy by several decades.
- Myeloma-defining secondary genetic events include activation of the MYC, RAS, NFkB, cell cycle pathways, and inactivation of tumor suppressor genes.
- Current therapies target vulnerabilities inherent in the plasma cell phenotype, while therapies targeting genetic mutations have not been yet successful.

INTRODUCTION

Multiple myeloma (MM) is a malignancy of long-lived, bone marrow-localized, plasma cells (PC) that have undergone immunoglobulin gene somatic hypermutation and isotype switch recombination in the germinal center. Its clinical presentation is characterized by hyperCalcemia, Renal failure, Anemia, and lytic Bone disease directly caused by either the tumor PC proliferation or their monoclonal proteins.[1] Errors during the process of isotype switch recombination contribute to the development of immunoglobulin heavy chain gene chromosomal translocations, which together with hyperdiploidy represents the initiating events being present in the earliest stages, including monoclonal gammopathy of undetermined significance (MGUS), and persist throughout all stages of PC neoplasia (**Fig. 1**).[2,3] Multiple secondary genetic events are accumulated and selected over time leading to the development of symptomatic

[a] University of Miami, 1120 Northwest 14th Street, Miami, FL 33136, USA; [b] Mayo Clinic Arizona, 13400 East Shea Boulevard, Scottsdale, AZ 85259, USA
* Corresponding authors.
E-mail addresses: fxm557@med.miami.edu (F.M.); Bergsagel.leif@mayo.edu (P.L.B.)

Hematol Oncol Clin N Am 38 (2024) 267–279
https://doi.org/10.1016/j.hoc.2023.12.010
0889-8588/24/© 2024 Elsevier Inc. All rights reserved.

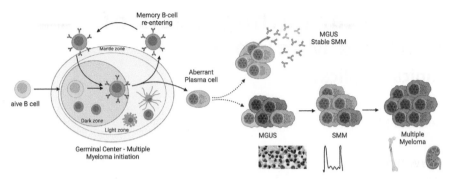

Fig. 1. Initiation of plasma cell (PC) neoplasms in the germinal center. The initial genetics events (chromosome translocations and hyperdiploidy) occur in the germinal center B-cell and are present in all stages of plasma cell neoplasms. Subsequent genetic events cause the progression from monoclonal gammopathy of undetermined significance (to smoldering myeloma and multiple myeloma (MM).Figure was generated using biorender.

MM requiring treatment and contributing to considerable intra-tumor and spatial heterogeneity.[4] Although the various genetic mutations are not the target of current therapies, they provide a framework for disease classification and risk stratification for myeloma precursor conditions progression and early treatment.

MULTIPLE MYELOMA IS PRECEDED BY AN ASYMPTOMATIC MONOCLONAL GAMMOPATHY

MM is consistently preceded by the asymptomatic expansion of clonal PC, termed either "monoclonal gammopathy of undetermined significance (MGUS)" or "smoldering myeloma (SMM)." While, according to the Icelandic iStopp national screening study, these 2 conditions are found in 5% and 0.5% of the adult population over the age of 40, only a small fraction will ultimately progress to MM. In fact, the risk of progression to MM is between 0.2% and 2% per year for MGUS[5] and approximately 10-fold higher for SMM.[6] The incidence of MM per 100,000 (2015–2019) was 7 in the US population, 8.6 in men, 5.7 in women, and 14.3 among African Americans.[7] The increased incidence in Blacks is felt to be due to genetic as opposed to environmental factors as a similarly high incidence of MGUS and MM is seen in Black Africans.[8,9] MM is almost always preceded by MGUS by many years[10–12] and based on sequence analysis the initial genetic lesions occurred decades before symptomatic disease.[13]

IMMUNOGLOBULIN HEAVY CHAIN GENE TRANSLOCATIONS AND HYPERDIPLOIDY ARE PRIMARY GENETIC EVENTS

Every cancer is developed through a clonal and genomic competition of multiple clones originated by a single cell that acquired the initiating event. Since the nineties,[2] we know a catalog of initiating events that occurred as translocations between the immunoglobulin heavy chain gene (IGH) and distinct genomic drivers: CCND1/CCND2/CCND3, MAF/MAFB/MAFA, and NSD2/FGFR3. The initiating role of these translocations in MM pathogenesis is supported by different lines of evidence: 1) they have the strongest impact on gene expression in MM; 2) they are always present in each phase of MM evolution: from MGUS to end stage MM; 3) Based on their structure and mechanisms, they represent very distinct genomic events not observed in any other tumor. Although fluorescence in situ hybridization (FISH) has been the major technique used, there are now a variety of sequencing approaches that can now be used to detect these abnormalities (**Fig. 2**). Later, the authors summarize the key clinical and biological features associated to these key events.

Translocations of a Cyclin D Family Gene

Approximately 20% of patients with MM have a 14q32 translocation which dysregulates a cyclin D gene, most commonly cyclin D1 at 11q13,[14] sometimes cyclin D3 at 6p21,[15] and rarely cyclin D2 at 12p13.[1] The translocations result in high-level, "spiked" expression of the cyclin D gene, but do not result in a highly proliferative tumor. MM with cyclin translocations can be divided in 2 main groups: the first is characterized by low genomic complexity compared to other subtypes of MM, more likely to have mutations of CCND1, or a recurrent mutation of *IRF4* and K123 R, and less frequently have rearrangements of MYC (20%).[16] The second group is enriched for complex genomic features including 1q, high APOBEC mutational signatures, chromothripsis, multiple aneuploidies, and biallelic inactivation of tumor suppressor genes. The t(11;14) is more frequent in African Americans, where it is associated with a germline polymorphism CCND1 c.870 G risk allele.[17] It is also more frequent in MGUS (30%)[18] and amyloidosis (40%)[19] then in MM. It has been associated with a more lymphoplasmacytic morphology, and more frequent expression of B cell markers (eg, CD20).[20] Interestingly and in line with its genomic bimodal distribution, by unsupervised gene expression analysis, patients with t(11;14) MM fall into 2 distinct subtypes with a remarkably different clinical course: one-third are labeled CD-1 without, and two-thirds CD-2 with, CD20 expression.[21] The CD-1 is enriched for genomic complexity, while CD-2 has mostly a simple gneomic profile. Of all of the molecular subtypes, CD-1 had the highest (96%), and CD-2 the lowest (45%) rate of complete response following total therapy,[22] and with 10 years median follow-up, CD-1 had the highest PFS-estimated cure fraction (35%) and CD-2 among the lowest (14%).[23] This clinical heterogeneity reflects a distinct pattern of genomic complexity, in which high genomic complexity associates with shorter survival. MM cell lines with t(11;14) show a high dependency on BCL2, and are particularly sensitive to the BCL2 inhibitor venetoclax.[24] In a clinical trial of relapsed refractory MM, the response rate to single agent

	FISH	Targeted Sequencing	Whole exome sequencing	RNA sequencing	Whole genome sequencing
Canonical IGH translocations	✓✓	✓✓	✗	✓✓	✓✓✓
Mutations in driver genes	✗	✓✓✓	✓✓✓	✓	✓✓
Copy number changes	✗	✓✓	✓	✗	✓✓✓
Mutational signatures	✗	✗	✓	✗	✓✓✓
Structural variants	✗	✓	✗	✓	✓✓✓

Fig. 2. Advantages and disadvantages of different platforms for the detection of genetic abnormalities in MM.

venetoclax was 40% in patients with t(11;14) versus 6% in those without.[25] Although the data are not available at this time, it seems likely that the subset of t(11;14) patients that respond to venetoclax will be enriched in the CD-2 subtype that has a more B-cell phenotype, hopefully improving their relatively poor long-term outcome.

Translocations of a MAF Family Gene

Approximately 6% of patients with MM have a translocation that dysregulates a MAF family gene, most commonly *MAF* on 16q23, sometimes *MAFB* on 20q11, and rarely *MAFA* on 8q24.[1,26] The translocations result in ectopic, high-level expression of the respective MAF family gene. This subgroup is frequently associated with adverse secondary genetic events such as gain1q, del1p, del17p[16] and there is some controversy as to whether the presence of t(14;16) and t(14;20), which are included in the International Myeloma Working Group definition of high-risk myeloma, are independent prognostic factors.[27] Importantly, patients with *MAF/MAFB* translocations are often characterized by high APOBEC mutational burden detectable only by whole exome or genome sequencing and known to be one of the worst prognostic markers for outcomes in MM.[28,29] Unlike other molecular subgroups of patients treated in Total Therapy clinical trials at the University of Arkansas, the MAF subgroup did not appear to benefit much from either the addition of thalidomide in Total Therapy 2, or of bortezomib in Total Therapy 3.[30] A possible explanation for the latter observation is that MAF proteins are ubiquitinated and subsequently degraded by the proteasome so that therapy with proteasome inhibitors results in increased levels of MAF proteins.[31] MAF is a transcription factor that directly transactivates a high-level expression of CCND2 and integrin beta-7, enhancing adhesion to bone marrow stroma and stimulating vascular endothelial growth factor (VEGF) production.[32]

Translocations of NSD2/FGFR3

Approximately 15% of patients with MM have a t(4;14) (p16;q32) IgH translocation in the switch regions which associate the JH and Iu exons, and the Eu intronic enhancer on der 4 with coding exons of NSD2, a histone H3 lysine 36 dimethylase.[33–36] The resulting hybrid transcripts encode for either a full length (two-thirds of t(4;14)), or amino-truncated (one-third of t(4;14)) NSD2 protein resulting in a global increase in H3K36 dimethylation and altered gene expression[36] Two independent studies have reported that the presence of an amino-truncating breakpoint is an independent adverse prognostic factor with overall survival of 29 months as compare to 59 to 75 months for non-truncating t(4;14) breakpoints.[37,38] These results suggest that aberrant NSD2 protein contributes to the pathogenesis of MM, and a role for an enzymatic inhibitor of its demethylase activity in the treatment of t(4;14) MM. A phase I clinical trial of KTX-001 (NCT05651932) is testing this hypothesis.

In about 80% of patients with t(4;14), there is also the reciprocal translocation that juxtaposes the powerful 3′ IgH enhancer on der14 to FGFR3, a receptor tyrosine kinase expressed on the cell surface. A quarter of the patients that ectopically express FGFR3 also have an activating mutation indicating a critical role for the tyrosine kinase activity of FGFR3 in MM progression[39] Clinical trials using FGFR3 tyrosine kinase inhibitors dovitinib[40] and erdafitinib (NCT02952573) have not reported clinical responses in patients with t(4;14) MM. Preclinical studies suggest that kinase inhibition will only be effective in the presence of FGFR3 activating mutations, which has not been an eligibility criteria in the clinical trials. An intriguing case has been reported of a patient with a subclone containing an activating mutation of FGFR3 that was completely eliminated by treatment with erdafitinib, suggesting some promise of this approach if applied to carefully selected patients with clonal activating mutations of FGFR3.[41] In addition, about 10% of patients with t(4;14) have mutations of the serine/threonine kinase PRKD2 which are much less common in other patients with MM. It is unclear if these are activating or inactivating mutations. Patients with t(4;14) have been historically associated with poor outcomes, and this is often driven by a complex combination of additional genomic hits preferentially acquired by tumor cells harboring this translocations such as 1q gain, 13q deletion, and non hotspot DIS3 mutation. Finally, at a level somewhat lower than MAF MM, t(4;14) MM ectopically express CCND2.

Hyperdiploidy

Around half of individuals with MM and myeloma precursor conditions exhibit a distinct cytogenetic profile characterized by multiple large trisomies, frequently involving odd-numbered chromosomes (such as 3, 5, 7, 9, 11, 15, 19, and 21). The tumors are hyperdiploid, most frequently with between 49 and 56 chromosomes, and are enriched in patients lacking IGH translocations.[42] Those hyperdiploid patients with trisomy 11 tend to ectopically express CCND1, while those hyperdiploid patients with disomy 11 express CCND2. The ectopic expression of a cyclin D gene associated with all of the primary genetic subtypes of MM, together with the high frequency of biallelic RB1 deletion in those patients that do not express any cyclin D gene, highlight the nearly uniform dysregulation of the cyclin D/RB pathway as a unifying event in the pathogenesis of MM. Analogous to those with Cyclin D translocations, hyperdiploid MM can be classified into 2 principal groups: one displaying complexity and the other simplicity, with the latter enriched for mutations in the mitogen–activated protein kinase (MAPK) pathway (BRAF, NRAS, KRAS). Furthermore, hyperdiploidy may also encompass other non-odd-numbered chromosomes, like 1q, 6p, and 8q; however, the biological and prognostic implications of these events remain to be fully elucidated.

Additionally, hyperdiploid cases are enriched for translocations of MYC (>50%) of which one-third involve a heavy or light chain immunoglobulin locus, and two-thirds involve other PC super-enhancer loci such as TENT5C, BMP6/TXNDC5, and FOXO3.[43] Intriguingly, patients with Ig lambda translocations are associated with poorer outcomes.[44] While hyperdiploidy is often a clonal event maintained throughout various phases, temporal assessments and mathematical modeling suggest that additional trisomies and large gains on odd-numbered chromosomes can be acquired subsequent to the initiating event.[13] Remarkably, these estimates indicate that hyperdiploidy can emerge up to 30 to 40 years before diagnosis, predominantly during the second and third decades of life.

Patients Without Translocations or Hyperdiploidy

Approximately 10% of MM cases lack both hyperdiploidy and IGH translocations. Despite their negative results with routine FISH probes used in clinical practice, these patients exhibit numerous genomic alterations that become apparent through more comprehensive methods like whole exome and genome sequencing. They are characterized by frequent monosomy 13, 14, and 16, and a variety of mutations that activate the nuclear factor kappa-light-chain-enhancer of activated B cells (NFkB) pathway including TRAF3 inactivation and translocations of MAP3K14.[16] Moreover, when exploring additional genomic drivers, these patients can be categorized into 2 primary groups: the first group demonstrates a relatively simpler genomic profile with a lower frequency of events, while the second group is enriched for complex genomic alterations.

SECONDARY GENETIC EVENTS CAUSE THE PROGRESSION TO SYMPTOMATIC MULTIPLE MYELOMA

IGH translocations and hyperdiploidy alone are insufficient to drive the complete transformation of a B-cell into MM. Throughout the genomic evolution from a germinal center B-cell to MM, a series of additional secondary events are acquired. The advent of next-generation sequencing has provided an unprecedented glimpse into the intricate complexity of MM at a granular level. Numerous oncogenes and tumor suppressor genes undergo multiple somatic events, including single nucleotide variants, structural variants, and focal/large copy number variants. Despite the remarkable complexity and heterogeneity, a substantial portion of these somatic events, acquired during the progression of MM, contribute to the regulation of 4 key pathways: MYC, RAS, NFkB, and the cell cycle. A concise summary of these events is provided later.

MYC (MYC, MAX)

The most frequent alteration events in MM revolve around somatic events directly or indirectly involving MYC, which are detectable in up to 50% of patients. MYC can undergo upregulation through various mechanisms, including translocations with immunoglobulin genes or non-immunoglobulin superenhancers, as well as through focal structural variants like duplications and chromothripsis events. Moreover, MYC can also be affected by focal amplifications, single nucleotide variants, and deletions and inversions that relocate MYC near the superenhancers of NSMCE2, roughly 2 Mb upstream. While the precise prognostic impact of MYC alterations in newly diagnosed MM (NDMM) remains to be fully clarified, their identification in the context of SMM serves as a potent and accurate prognostic marker for predicting progression to active MM. About 4% of patients have biallelic inactivation of MAX, MYC's obligate heterodimerization partner that is required for MYC's transcriptional and oncogenic activities. As in small cell lung cancer and oligodendroglial tumors, MAX inactivation is mutually exclusive with mutations that activate MYC, and in fact is associated with a very low level of MYC transcription. While the mechanism remains to be elucidated, the data suggest MAX inactivation allows an alternate way of activating the MYC transcriptional pathway.[45]

RAS (NRAS, KRAS, BRAF, FGFR3, PTPN11, NF1)

Mutations affecting the RAS pathway are prevalent in nearly 50% of MM cases, with NRAS, KRAS, and BRAF being the genes most frequently affected. Although KRAS mutations are equally distributed across various key biological subgroups, NRAS mutations are notably enriched in patients exhibiting a simpler genomic profile (eg, hyperdiploid and CCND1 translocated patients).[16] While these genetic events may not currently hold significant prognostic value for NDMM, they have demonstrated a robust predictive capacity for the progression of SMM into active MM.[46] Additionally, they represent a promising potential therapeutic target, with several case reports of responses to targeting BRAF, and a phase 2 clinical trial of dabrafenib plus trametinib in BRAF-mutated MM reporting 2 of 10 patients with a partial response.[47] Disappointingly, it appears that when a single mutated gene in the RAS pathway is targeted, subclonal heterogeneity (see below) allows for the rapid selection of a subclone harboring another mutation in the pathway.[48] Recently, it has been reported that RAS mutations activate MTORC1 in MM, suggesting a possible role for combined inhibition MTOR plus MEK/ERK in the treatment of RAS-mutant MM.[49]

NFkB (TRAF2, TRAF3, BIRC2, BIRC3, CYLD, MAP3K14, NFKB1, NFKB2)

The NFκB pathway plays a crucial role in both normal PC and MM. In the bone marrow, BAFF and APRIL secreted by myeloid and stromal cells are ligands for B cell maturation antigen (BCMA) on the surface of PC, activating the NFkB pathway. The authors postulate that high level gamma-secretase–mediated shedding of soluble BCMA from PC binds these critical survival factors in the surrounding PC niche, preventing their use by encroaching PC clones. This presents a limitation to MM growth and expansion which is overcome by stimulating the environment to increase the supply of these ligands, or by the acquisition of various activating mutations downstream of BCMA (**Fig. 3**). Frequently, genes like TRAF2, TRAF3, BIRC2, BIRC3, and CYLD are implicated through substantial deletions, followed by a second-hit event involving focal structural variants or mutations. Additionally, approximately 1% of MM cases show gain-of-function structural variants affecting MAP3K14. Altogether these mutations are present in about 20% of NDMM, and 50% of cell lines capable of in vitro growth.[50]

Glucocorticoids and proteasome inhibitors, mainstays in the treatment of MM, function in part by inhibiting the NFkB pathway. Glucocorticoids trans-repress NFkB-induced transcription by tethering to the transcription machinery orchestrated by CBP/EP300 at NFkB DNA binding sites (that partially overlap with glucocorticoid response elements).[51,52] Proteasome inhibitors inhibit the NFkB pathway by blocking the ubiquitin-proteasome–mediated degradation of negative regulators of the NFkB pathway (IkB, cIAP1, cIAP2, TRAF2, TRAF3) as well as processing of NFKB2 p100 to the active p52.[50,53] This has important clinical implications revealed in a randomized controlled trial of lenalidomide and dexamethasone with or without ixazomib in patients with relapsed refractory MM. This trial reported an improvement in progression free survival (PFS) (HR 0.74, $P = .01$), but not overall survival (OS), with the addition of ixazomib.[54] It appears, however, that most of the PFS benefit from the addition of ixazomib was seen in the 15% of patients with mutations of TRAF2, TRAF3, and BIRC2/3 where the hazard ratio was 0.23 ($P = .0005$) versus 0.83 ($P = .39$) in those without mutations.[55] These data suggest a therapeutic role for more specific inhibitors of the NFkB pathway in MM, particularly an inhibitor (eg, TRC694) of the NFkB-Inducing Kinase MAP3K14, which is activated downstream of most mutations.[56] The critical role

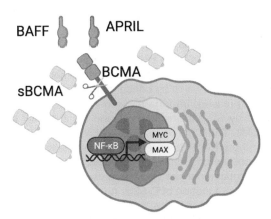

Fig. 3. Soluble B cell maturation antigen (BCMA) protects the PC niche. The BCMA ligands BAFF and APRIL represent limiting growth factors for PC survival. By shedding sBCMA, a PC traps BAFF and APRIL and prevents other PC from encroaching on its niche. For a malignant PC to expand the niche, it needs to increase the supply of BAFF and APRIL, or contitutively activate NFKB and/or MYC.

of NFkB signaling downstream of BCMA likely explains the relatively infrequent mutation of BCMA as a mechanism of resistance to BCMA-chimeric antigen receptor(CAR)-T therapy in MM. Recently, mutations, including those in the CART/ T-cell engagers (TCE) BCMA binding site, have been reported as recurrent mechanisms of resistance to immunotherapies. Intriguingly, these mutations do not affect BCMA expression or its signaling, underscoring the critical role of BCMA for MM cells.[57] It also suggests that the presence of NFkB mutations may allow the MM cell to more easily dispense with BCMA as a general mechanism of resistance to BCMA-targeted therapies.[57] This intricate interplay of genetic alterations highlights the significance of NFκB in the context of MM.

Cell cycle (TP53, RB1, CDKN2C)

Biallelic inactivation of TP53 (4%), RB1 (4%), and CDKN2C (2%) in NDMM significantly perturbs the cell cycle and apoptotic pathways within myeloma cells and has a strong prognostic impact. Biallelic loss of TP53 and RB1 has been associated with particularly unfavorable outcomes. The CDKN2A gene encodes for 2 proteins with unique first exons, but a shared second exon translated in alternate reading frames: p16INK4a binds to CDK4/6 to inhibit cyclin D1 activation of these kinases, while p14ARF forms stable complexes with MDM2 to activate TP53. By reverse transcription-polymerase chain reaction (RT-PCR), Mike Kuehl and colleagues reported no detectable transcription of the first exon of p16INK4a in human MM,[58] and more recently our analysis of RNAseq data from the CoMMpass project found that all of the RNA transcribed from the CDKN2A gene is predicted to encode p14ARF not p16INK4a (Bergsagel, 2023, unpublished). There is minimal transcription (median TPM 0.5), and only rare mutations of CDKN2B and no mutations of CDKN2D. As a result, of the 4 INK4 proteins, only inactivation of p18INK4c encoded by CDKN2C is an important driver of MM pathogenesis.

Copy number abnormalities: 1p loss, 1q gain, monosomy 13, 17p loss

Copy number abnormalities (CNA) involving 1p, 1q, 13, and 17p are prognostically important in SMM and MM, although there remains some uncertainty about the driver genes involved. On 1p, as noted earlier, biallelic inactivation of CDKN2C at 1p32 has the strongest prognostic impact, although RPL5 and EVI5 at 1p22, and TENT5C (FAM46 C) at 1p12 have also been implicated.[59] Gain of 1q in over 30% of NDMM leads to MCL1 overexpression, which can clearly drive MM progression, based on studies in transgenic mice over-expressing related proteins BCL2 and BCL-xL in B cells crossed to MM-prone mice.[60,61] Other candidate genes on 1q (eg, CKS1B)[62] have been shown to be critical dependencies, but not to accelerate disease when-over-expressed. Importantly, most of these genes are involved by focal gains mediated by SV and their expression cumulatively increases with the number of extra copies. Three genes have been implicated on 13: DIS3, RB1, and miR15a/16 to 1. DIS3 on 13q21 is an exosome-associated ribonuclease that is a common essential gene across almost all cell lines examined in the Dependency Map (http://depmap.org) and consistently, the pattern of mutation and deletion suggest that complete loss of function of DIS3 is not tolerated: About half of the mutations involve 1 of 3 hotspot codons, and are never associated with Loss of Heterozygosity.[18] Although the DIS3 homozygous knockout mouse is embryonic lethal, no phenotype was ascribed to heterozygous mice.[63] As noted earlier, biallelic inactivation of RB1 is rare, and there is no evidence for a role of RB1 haploinsufficiency in MM progression.[18] In contrast, one gene that has been shown to accelerate MM progression when haploinsufficient is miR15a/16 to 1.[18] In a cohort of intensively-treated NDMM, deletion of 17p with p53 mutation was associated with a PFS of 18m, versus 27m with del17p and wildtype p53, and 44m for those without del17p.[64] It is not known if the patients with del17p and wildtype p53 eventually progressed because they eventually inactivated the wildtype copy, suggesting that isolated del17p is high risk because it predisposes to biallelic p53 inactivation. Alternatively, it suggests the presence of another gene on 17p which is haploinsufficient. These genetic events collectively underscore their crucial roles in influencing myeloma pathogenesis and clinical outcomes.

IMPACT OF INTRATUMOR SUBCLONAL HETEROGENEITY ON DISEASE PROGRESSION AND DRUG RESISTANCE

The life history of MM is marked by intricate evolution, where various clones vie competing dominance. Over time, these distinct clones acquire additional somatic alterations that confer advantages in terms of proliferation, anti-apoptosis, and evasion from immune responses. This leads to their expansion and positive selection. Notably, multiple rounds of positive selection occur in each patient, aligning with the punctuated evolution observed in other types of tumors. This spontaneous Darwinian evolution serves as the driving force propelling the progression from MGUS to SMM and eventually to active MM over the course of decades. Conversely, recent genomic insights have demonstrated that within the context of treatment, the evolution and selection of minor subclones can take place within weeks to months. The selective pressure exerted by therapeutic interventions creates a bottleneck where only the most resilient and adept clones survive, thus accelerating the evolutionary process. Understanding this intricate dynamic is paramount for identifying resistance mechanisms and optimizing treatment approaches. Notably, this inherent heterogeneity within MM extends beyond the confines of the bone marrow, as distinct clones populate various anatomic sites. This seeding process can be initiated by a single surviving tumor cell and has been observed to accelerate post-treatment, possibly due to a combination of immunosuppression and heightened disease aggressiveness. Grasping and capturing both the clonal and spatial heterogeneity is imperative for comprehensive profiling of MM's biology, and in turn, enhancing our treatment strategies.

SUMMARY

Although there have been dramatic advances in our ability to molecularly classify and risk-stratify patients with SMM and MM using next-generation sequencing, we are still far from fully understanding the MM genomic history and heterogeneity. The clinical and data complexity we are facing is one of the main reasons why these technologies have not yet entered routine clinical practice. This is likely to change over the next decade as sequencing costs plummet and analytical pipelines improve. From where we stand today, it seems unlikely that therapies will directly target the mutations identified and the goal of the molecular analysis will be to provide a genetic definition of MM that requires treatment, and a risk stratified approach both for the follow-up of those patients that do not require immediate treatment, and a graded treatment approach for those that do.

CLINICS CARE POINTS

- FISH for the identification of t(4;14), t(11;14), t(14;16), t(14;20), 1q21, and 17p13 in bone marrow PC should be a part of the standard work-up for patients with MM.

- FISH for the identification of t(4;14), t(14;16), 1q21, and 13q in bone marrow PC should be a part of the standard work-up for patients with SMM.
- FISH is not required for the work-up of patients with monoclonal gammopathy of undetermined significance.
- Intratumor heterogeneity has limited the impact of molecularly-targeted therapy.
- In the future, RNAseq and whole genome sequencing are likely to provide better disease classification and risk stratification.

DISCLOSURE

None.

FUNDING

FM is supported by Leukemai and Lymphoma Society and International Myeloma Fundation. PLB is supported by NIH P50CA186781.

REFERENCES

1. Kuehl WM, Bergsagel PL. Molecular pathogenesis of multiple myeloma and its premalignant precursor. J Clin Invest 2012;122(10):3456–63.
2. Bergsagel PL, Chesi M, Nardini E, et al. Promiscuous translocations into immunoglobulin heavy chain switch regions in multiple myeloma. Proc Natl Acad Sci U S A 1996;93(24):13931–6.
3. Fonseca R, Barlogie B, Bataille R, et al. Genetics and cytogenetics of multiple myeloma: a workshop report. Cancer Res 2004;64(4):1546–58.
4. Keats JJ, Chesi M, Egan JB, et al. Clonal competition with alternating dominance in multiple myeloma. Blood 2012;120(5):1067–76.
5. Kyle RA, Larson DR, Therneau TM, et al. Long-Term Follow-up of Monoclonal Gammopathy of Undetermined Significance. N Engl J Med 2018;378(3):241–9.
6. Kyle RA, Remstein ED, Therneau TM, et al. Clinical course and prognosis of smoldering (asymptomatic) multiple myeloma. N Engl J Med 2007;356(25):2582–90.
7. ACS. Cancer Statistics Center. 2023; Available at: https://cancerstatisticscenter. cancer.org/#!/cancer-site/Myeloma. Accessed June 19, 2023.
8. Greenberg AJ, Vachon CM, Rajkumar SV. Disparities in the prevalence, pathogenesis and progression of monoclonal gammopathy of undetermined significance and multiple myeloma between blacks and whites. Leukemia 2012;26(4):609–14.
9. Landgren O, Graubard BI, Katzmann JA, et al. Racial disparities in the prevalence of monoclonal gammopathies: a population-based study of 12,482 persons from the National Health and Nutritional Examination Survey. Leukemia 2014; 28(7):1537–42.
10. Landgren O, Kyle RA, Pfeiffer RM, et al. Monoclonal gammopathy of undetermined significance (MGUS) consistently precedes multiple myeloma: a prospective study. Blood 2009;113(22):5412–7.
11. Weiss BM, Abadie J, Verma P, et al. A monoclonal gammopathy precedes multiple myeloma in most patients. Blood 2009;113(22):5418–22.
12. Murray DL, Puig N, Kristinsson S, et al. Mass spectrometry for the evaluation of monoclonal proteins in multiple myeloma and related disorders: an International Myeloma Working Group Mass Spectrometry Committee Report. Blood Cancer J 2021;11(2):24.

13. Rustad EH, Yellapantula V, Leongamornlert D, et al. Timing the initiation of multiple myeloma. Nat Commun 2020;11(1):1917.
14. Chesi M, Bergsagel PL, Brents LA, et al. Dysregulation of cyclin D1 by translocation into an IgH gamma switch region in two multiple myeloma cell lines. Blood 1996;88(2):674–81.
15. Shaughnessy J Jr, Gabrea A, Qi Y, et al. Cyclin D3 at 6p21 is dysregulated by recurrent chromosomal translocations to immunoglobulin loci in multiple myeloma. Blood 2001;98(1):217–23.
16. de Leval L, Alizadeh AA, Bergsagel PL, et al. Genomic profiling for clinical decision making in lymphoid neoplasms. Blood 2022;140(21):2193–227.
17. Baughn LB, Li Z, Pearce K, et al. The CCND1 c.870G risk allele is enriched in individuals of African ancestry with plasma cell dyscrasias. Blood Cancer J 2020; 10(3):39.
18. Chesi M, Stein CK, Garbitt VM, et al. Monosomic loss of MIR15A/MIR16-1 is a driver of multiple myeloma proliferation and disease progression. Blood Cancer Discov 2020;1(1):68–81.
19. Bryce AH, Ketterling RP, Gertz MA, et al. Translocation t(11;14) and survival of patients with light chain (AL) amyloidosis. Haematologica 2009;94(3):380–6.
20. Fonseca R, Blood EA, Oken MM, et al. Myeloma and the t(11;14)(q13;q32); evidence for a biologically defined unique subset of patients. Blood 2002;99(10): 3735–41.
21. Zhan F, Huang Y, Colla S, et al. The molecular classification of multiple myeloma. Blood 2006;108(6):2020–8.
22. Nair B, van Rhee F, Shaughnessy JD Jr, et al. Superior results of Total Therapy 3 (2003-33) in gene expression profiling-defined low-risk multiple myeloma confirmed in subsequent trial 2006-66 with VRD maintenance. Blood 2010; 115(21):4168–73.
23. van Rhee F, Zangari M, Schinke CD, et al. Long-term outcome of total therapy regimens: impact of molecular subgroups. Blood 2019;134:3309.
24. Touzeau C, Dousset C, Le Gouill S, et al. The Bcl-2 specific BH3 mimetic ABT-199: a promising targeted therapy for t(11;14) multiple myeloma. Leukemia 2014;28(1):210–2.
25. Kumar S, Kaufman JL, Gasparetto C, et al. Efficacy of venetoclax as targeted therapy for relapsed/refractory t(11;14) multiple myeloma. Blood 2017;130(22): 2401–9.
26. Chesi M, Bergsagel PL, Shonukan OO, et al. Frequent dysregulation of the c-maf proto-oncogene at 16q23 by translocation to an Ig locus in multiple myeloma. Blood 1998;91(12):4457–63.
27. Avet-Loiseau H, Malard F, Campion L, et al. Translocation t(14;16) and multiple myeloma: is it really an independent prognostic factor? Blood 2011;117(6): 2009–11.
28. Walker BA, Wardell CP, Murison A, et al. APOBEC family mutational signatures are associated with poor prognosis translocations in multiple myeloma. Nat Commun 2015;6:6997.
29. Maura F, Petljak M, Lionetti M, et al. Biological and prognostic impact of APOBEC-induced mutations in the spectrum of plasma cell dyscrasias and multiple myeloma cell lines. Leukemia 2018;32(4):1044–8.
30. Weinhold N, Heuck CJ, Rosenthal A, et al. Clinical value of molecular subtyping multiple myeloma using gene expression profiling. Leukemia 2016;30(2):423–30.
31. Qiang YW, Ye S, Chen Y, et al. MAF protein mediates innate resistance to proteasome inhibition therapy in multiple myeloma. Blood 2016;128(25):2919–30.

32. Hurt EM, Wiestner A, Rosenwald A, et al. Overexpression of c-maf is a frequent oncogenic event in multiple myeloma that promotes proliferation and pathological interactions with bone marrow stroma. Cancer Cell 2004;5(2):191–9.

33. Chesi M, Nardini E, Brents LA, et al. Frequent translocation t(4;14)(p16.3;q32.3) in multiple myeloma is associated with increased expression and activating mutations of fibroblast growth factor receptor 3. Nat Genet 1997;16(3):260–4.

34. Chesi M, Nardini E, Lim RS, et al. The t(4;14) translocation in myeloma dysregulates both FGFR3 and a novel gene, MMSET, resulting in IgH/MMSET hybrid transcripts. Blood 1998;92(9):3025–34.

35. Kuo AJ, Cheung P, Chen K, et al. NSD2 links dimethylation of histone H3 at lysine 36 to oncogenic programming. Mol Cell 2011;44(4):609–20.

36. Martinez-Garcia E, Popovic R, Min DJ, et al. The MMSET histone methyl transferase switches global histone methylation and alters gene expression in t(4;14) multiple myeloma cells. Blood 2011;117(1):211–20.

37. Li F, Zhai YP, Lai T, et al. MB4-2/MB4-3 transcripts of IGH-MMSET fusion gene in t(4;14)(pos) multiple myeloma indicate poor prognosis. Oncotarget 2017;8(31): 51608–20.

38. Stong N, Ortiz-Estevez M, Towfic F, et al. The location of the t(4;14) translocation breakpoint within the NSD2 gene identifies a subset of patients with high-risk NDMM. Blood 2023;141(13):1574–83.

39. Benard B, Christofferson A, Legendre C, et al. FGFR3 mutations are an adverse prognostic factor in patients with t (4; 14)(p16; q32) multiple myeloma: an Mmrf commpass analysis. Blood 2017;130:3027.

40. Scheid C, Reece D, Beksac M, et al. Phase 2 study of dovitinib in patients with relapsed or refractory multiple myeloma with or without t(4;14) translocation. Eur J Haematol 2015;95(4):316–24.

41. Croucher DC, Devasia AJ, Abelman DD, et al. Single-cell profiling of multiple myeloma reveals molecular response to FGFR3 inhibitor despite clinical progression. Cold Spring Harb Mol Case Stud 2023;9(2).

42. Fonseca R, Bergsagel PL, Drach J, et al. International Myeloma Working Group molecular classification of multiple myeloma: spotlight review. Leukemia 2009; 23(12):2210–21.

43. Misund K, Keane N, Stein CK, et al. MYC dysregulation in the progression of multiple myeloma. Leukemia 2020;34(1):322–6.

44. Barwick BG, Neri P, Bahlis NJ, et al. Multiple myeloma immunoglobulin lambda translocations portend poor prognosis. Nat Commun 2019;10(1):1911.

45. Kalkat M, De Melo J, Hickman KA, et al. MYC Deregulation in Primary Human Cancers. Genes 2017;8(6).

46. Boyle EM, Deshpande S, Tytarenko R, et al. The molecular make up of smoldering myeloma highlights the evolutionary pathways leading to multiple myeloma. Nat Commun 2021;12(1):293.

47. Subbiah V, Kreitman RJ, Wainberg ZA, et al. Dabrafenib plus trametinib in BRAFV600E-mutated rare cancers: the phase 2 ROAR trial. Nat Med 2023; 29(5):1103–12.

48. Le Calvez B, Le Bris Y, Herbreteau G, et al. RAS mutation leading to acquired resistance to dabrafenib and trametinib therapy in a multiple myeloma patient harboring BRAF mutation. EJHaem 2020;1(1):318–22.

49. Yang Y, Bolomsky A, Oellerich T, et al. Oncogenic RAS commandeers amino acid sensing machinery to aberrantly activate mTORC1 in multiple myeloma. Nat Commun 2022;13(1):5469.

50. Keats JJ, Fonseca R, Chesi M, et al. Promiscuous mutations activate the nonca-nonical NF-kappaB pathway in multiple myeloma. Cancer Cell 2007;12(2):131–44.
51. De Bosscher K, Vanden Berghe W, Vermeulen L, et al. Glucocorticoids repress NF-kappaB-driven genes by disturbing the interaction of p65 with the basal tran-scription machinery, irrespective of coactivator levels in the cell. Proc Natl Acad Sci U S A 2000;97(8):3919–24.
52. Uhlenhaut NH, Barish GD, Yu RT, et al. Insights into negative regulation by the glucocorticoid receptor from genome-wide profiling of inflammatory cistromes. Mol Cell 2013;49(1):158–71.
53. Palombella VJ, Conner EM, Fuseler JW, et al. Role of the proteasome and NF-kappaB in streptococcal cell wall-induced polyarthritis. Proc Natl Acad Sci U S A 1998;95(26):15671–6.
54. Richardson PG, Kumar SK, Masszi T, et al. Final Overall Survival Analysis of the TOURMALINE-MM1 Phase III Trial of Ixazomib, Lenalidomide, and Dexametha-sone in Patients With Relapsed or Refractory Multiple Myeloma. J Clin Oncol 2021;39(22):2430–42.
55. Dash AB, Zhang J, Shen L, et al. Clinical benefit of ixazomib plus lenalidomide-dexamethasone in myeloma patients with non-canonical NF-kappaB pathway activation. Eur J Haematol 2020;105(3):274–85.
56. Morgan D, Garg M, Tergaonkar V, et al. Pharmacological significance of the non-canonical NF-kappaB pathway in tumorigenesis. Biochim Biophys Acta Rev Can-cer 2020;1874(2):188449.
57. Lee H, Ahn S, Maity R, et al. Mechanisms of antigen escape from BCMA- or GPRC5D-targeted immunotherapies in multiple myeloma. Nat Med 2023;29(9):2295–306.
58. Dib A, Peterson TR, Raducha-Grace L, et al. Paradoxical expression of INK4c in proliferative multiple myeloma tumors: bi-allelic deletion vs increased expression. Cell Div 2006;1:23.
59. Walker BA, Leone PE, Chiecchio L, et al. A compendium of myeloma-associated chromosomal copy number abnormalities and their prognostic value. Blood 2010;116(15):e56–65.
60. Chesi M, Robbiani DF, Sebag M, et al. AID-dependent activation of a MYC trans-gene induces multiple myeloma in a conditional mouse model of post-germinal center malignancies. Cancer Cell 2008;13(2):167–80.
61. Linden M, Kirchhof N, Carlson C, et al. Targeted overexpression of Bcl-XL in B-lymphoid cells results in lymphoproliferative disease and plasma cell malig-nancies. Blood 2004;103(7):2779–86.
62. Zhan F, Colla S, Wu X, et al. CKS1B, overexpressed in aggressive disease, reg-ulates multiple myeloma growth and survival through SKP2- and p27Kip1-dependent and -independent mechanisms. Blood 2007;109(11):4995–5001.
63. Wu D, Dean J. RNA exosome ribonuclease DIS3 degrades Pou6f1 to promote mouse pre-implantation cell differentiation. Cell Rep 2023;42(2):112047.
64. Corre J, Perrot A, Caillot D, et al. del(17p) without TP53 mutation confers a poor prognosis in intensively treated newly diagnosed patients with multiple myeloma. Blood 2021;137(9):1192–5.

Immune-Pathogenesis of Myeloma

Madhav V. Dhodapkar, MD

KEYWORDS

- Multiple myeloma • Monoclonal gammopathy of undetermined significance (MGUS)
- Immune • T cells

KEY POINTS

- Increasing body of evidence suggests that monoclonal gammopathy of undetermined significance (MGUS) and myeloma originate in the setting of chronic immune activation and inflammation, leading to immune dysfunction and spatial immune exclusion.
- Transition to myeloma is associated with progressive immune paresis involving both innate and adaptive immunity but even advanced myeloma remains susceptible to immune effector cells.

INTRODUCTION

Multiple myeloma (MM) is a common hematologic malignancy involving progressive growth of malignant plasma cells, predominantly in the bone marrow.[1] It is now well established that MM is universally preceded by precursor stages clinically termed as monoclonal gammopathy of undetermined significance (MGUS) and smoldering myeloma (SMM).[2,3] With recent application of more sensitive techniques and large-scale screening efforts, it has become apparent that both MGUS and SMM are more common than previously thought.[4,5] Interestingly, the presence of MGUS is associated with an increased risk of all-cause mortality, which is only partly explained by the risk of development of MM.[4] However the precise reasons as to why some individuals develop MGUS or may eventually progress to MM remains to be fully clarified. During the past 2 decades, the role of immune system in shaping the evolution of tumors has been recognized and immune-based approaches now form a major component of modern cancer therapy.[6] In addition to the genetic/epigenetic changes in tumor cells, interactions between MM cells and nonmalignant cells in the tumor microenvironment (TME) play a key role in regulating the growth of MM cells.[7] MM itself is a malignancy of an immune cell (plasma cell [PC]), and therefore, as such it is not surprising that interactions with other immune cells can alter the growth and survival of MM tumor cells. Tumor-microenvironment cross talk has now become a major

Department of Hematology/Medical Oncology, Emory University, Winship Cancer Institute, 1365 Clifton Road, Atlanta, GA 30332, USA
E-mail address: madhav.v.dhodapkar@emory.edu

Hematol Oncol Clin N Am 38 (2024) 281–291
https://doi.org/10.1016/j.hoc.2023.12.011
0889-8588/24/© 2023 Elsevier Inc. All rights reserved.

focus of novel therapies in MM.[8,9] In this review, I will discuss how early alterations in immune cells may contribute to the pathogenesis of myeloma (**Table 1**).

IMMUNE RECOGNITION OF PREMALIGNANCY

Studies of the bone marrow TME in MGUS provided one of the earliest examples of the presence of preneoplasia-specific T cells in humans.[10,11] Seminal studies in mouse models established the capacity of the immune system to impact the early growth of tumors, with these interactions characterized by the 3 Es: elimination, equilibrium, and escape.[12] MGUS-specific T cells in the bone marrow were shown to be specific for each individual patient and consist of both CD4+ and CD8+ T cells.[13,14] The genetic basis for patient-specific immune response against MGUS is also supported by the appreciation that MGUS lesions already carry many of the genetic changes detected in MM tumor cells,[15] and there are relatively few shared mutations between patients with MM. In addition to changes in T cells, the TME in MGUS also consists of alterations in innate immune cells, with enrichment of distinct subsets of innate lymphoid cells.[16] Recent studies using mass cytometry and single cell transcriptomics have shown that bone marrow in MGUS is already characterized by broad transcriptional and immuno-phenotypic alterations in immune cells including T, B, natural killer (NK), and myeloid cells.[17–19] Together, these data suggest the presence of altered or dysfunctional profiles in T, B, or NK cells and inflammatory profiles in myeloid cells, beginning as early as MGUS. Inflammatory changes are not restricted to myeloid cells and also observed within the stromal compartment.[20] Further analyses of T cells have revealed distinct alterations in T cell subsets with a decline in T cell factor-1 (TCF1)+ stem-like T cells, along with an increase in terminal effector T cells during the transition from MGUS to MM.[17] Prospective data relating to antigen-specific T cell responses are limited but in a prospective observational trial, T cells against SOX2, an embryonal stem cell-associated antigen, were associated with a reduced risk of progression to clinical MM.[21] Studies in preclinical models such as V-kappa myc mice have provided evidence for immune surveillance depending on both T as well as NK cells.[22] In this model, tumor immunity was enhanced by CD137 engagement[23] and impaired by interleukin (IL)-18–mediated effects.[24] In another model, regulatory T cells (Tregs) were implicated in suppressing tumor immunity.[25] The concept that tumor-extrinsic features in TME may determine the growth of MM tumors in vivo is also illustrated in studies using humanized mice.[26] Although MGUS cells typically exhibit dormant and clinically stable growth

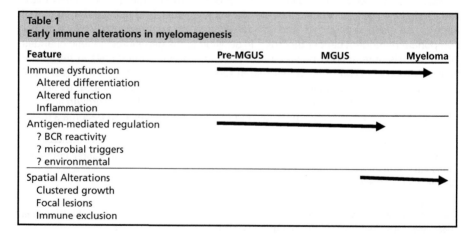

Table 1
Early immune alterations in myelomagenesis

Feature	Pre-MGUS	MGUS	Myeloma

Immune dysfunction
  Altered differentiation
  Altered function
  Inflammation			

Antigen-mediated regulation
  ? BCR reactivity
  ? microbial triggers
  ? environmental			

Spatial Alterations
  Clustered growth
  Focal lesions
  Immune exclusion			

patterns in patients, MGUS tumor cells exhibit progressive growth in these mice on adoptive transfer.[26] Dormancy on MGUS cells may also depend on specific interactions with bone cells in specialized niches.[27]

The concept of immune recognition of precursor lesions has inspired attempts to modulate immunity to prevent clinical MM. Two randomized trials[28,29] have now shown that early application of immune-modulatory drugs such as lenalidomide, which are known to engage both innate and adaptive immunity,[30–32] can lead to reduction in the risk of developing clinical MM. Properties of immune cells at baseline correlated with response to combination therapies in SMM.[30] The concept that immune dysfunction and inflammation-associated signaling is an early feature in MGUS suggests the possibility that interrupting these pathways may promote immune surveillance and could be considered earlier in disease evolution.[7,33]

ROLE OF SPATIAL ARCHITECTURE IN MULTIPLE MYELOMA IMMUNOPATHOGENESIS

One key limitation of most of the existing studies is that analysis of the bone marrow microenvironment is based largely on the evaluation of marrow aspirates and does not fully consider the spatial aspects of immune response in patients with MM/MGUS. This is particularly relevant because multifocal growth of tumors as well as formation of lytic bone lesions due to focal bone destruction are among the defining features of clinical myeloma. Spatial aspects of immune response are now increasingly appreciated as being critical for the biology of tumor–immune interactions. Application of high-dimensional tools to study MM/MGUS biopsies has led to several new insights relating to spatial immunology in MM.[34] MM (but not MGUS) tumor cells exhibit a propensity to grow as tumor clusters both in patients as well as on adoptive transfer in humanized mice, suggesting that this is an intrinsic feature of MM tumor biology. This growth pattern however creates the potential for regions of T cell exclusion, which can be observed in MM biopsies.[34] The biology of MM clusters therefore resembles that of immune-excluded solid tumors. Entry of T cells into MM clusters depends on costimulation (particularly CD2/CD58 axis) and target recognition, mediated by antigen-presenting dendritic cells in tumor proximity. Although these studies provide a mechanistic basis for T-cell redirection in MM, they also illustrate that spatial aspect of host response is likely to be a critical determinant of tumor–immune interactions. For example, regions that exclude T cells may serve as privileged or high-risk sites that may provide a nidus for genomic evolution of distinct subclones. Understanding the regulation of this biology and developing tools to overcome immune exclusion may therefore be critical for immune-prevention of MM. Spatial aspects of immune biology may also be relevant from the perspective of focal lesions, which have already emerged as a myeloma-defining feature in the clinic.

ROLE OF CHRONIC B CELL ACTIVATION

Several lines of evidence support the hypothesis that MGUS and MM originate in the setting of preexisting chronic B cell changes. Some (but not all) epidemiologic studies have suggested an increased risk of MGUS in the setting of autoimmune or allergic conditions.[35] Malignant plasma cells (PCs) from patients with MM show evidence of mutational signatures of cytidine deaminases (such as activation-induced cytidine deaminase [AID] or apolipoprotein B mRNA-editing enzyme catalytic polypeptide [APOBEC]), typically associated with B cell activation, starting as early as third decade of life.[36,37] In fact, the expression of AID in MM can be directly induced by dendritic cell (DC)-mediated interactions.[38] In defined genetic disorders such as Gaucher disease (GD), which lead to the accumulation of immunogenic lipids and chronic inflammation, the risk of MM is increased both in human disease as well as mouse models.[39] In this setting, the PC clone emerges in the setting of underlying polyclonal activation, which often precedes the clonal malignancy. More direct evidence linking the underlying B cell activation to gammopathy has emerged from the finding that the clonal immunoglobulin (Ig) can recognize the underlying immunogenic lipid.[40,41] This concept is also consistent with earlier studies in mouse models, both for the induction of pristane-induced plasmacytomas in Balb-C mice[42] as well as induction of antigen-specific clonal PCs following immunization of v-kappa myc mice.[43] Reactivity to lysolipids in the setting of patients with GD seems to be polyreactive (against multiple lipids) and accordingly a feature of autoreactive or polyreactive B cell receptors.[41] The concept that polyclonal or oligoclonal B cell activation may precede at least some cases of MGUS has begun to emerge from other clinical studies as well.[44] In the setting of GD, both the dominant PC clone as well as some of the associated polyclonal compartments may share the antigenic reactivity. This has now been demonstrated more directly in model systems wherein injection of the putative antigen leads to increased growth of both clonal and polyclonal PCs in vivo.[41] Consistent with this, pharmacologic reduction of underlying antigen leads to the reduction of both polyclonal and monoclonal gammopathy in GD mice and patients.[40,45,46] Therefore, at least in early stages, the plasma cell clones may remain responsive to underlying antigenic triggers.

UNDERSTANDING PREMONOCLONAL GAMMOPATHY OF UNDETERMINED SIGNIFICANCE

As noted earlier, recent application of more sensitive methods to detect clonal Igs has led to the discovery that MGUS may be even more frequent than previously anticipated.[4] Some of these clones may exist in the backdrop of oligoclonality and may well fluctuate above/below limits of detection. Although the clinical significance and malignant potential of such clones remains to be fully defined, such findings raise questions about the mechanisms that underlie the development of these small clones in the first place. The model emerging from these insights is that of MGUS originating in the context of preexisting immune alterations, that we term pre-MGUS. Based on the insights about chronic immune activation as discussed above, it is of interest to gain deeper insights into the nature of triggers that may drive such B/plasma cells. Such studies may require detailed evaluation of candidate B-cell receptors, as well as interrogation of prior or ongoing environmental or host-derived antigenic exposures. Polyreactive B cell receptor (BCRs) in particular may also be more susceptible to stimulation by diverse stimuli including those derived from microbiome.[47] Such BCRs have also been implicated in extrafollicular (EF) and autoimmune responses and exhibit considerable racial differences with enrichment in Black populations.[48] Whether patients with MM exhibit greater susceptibility to such responses in not known. However, in a recent study, spike-specific B cells elicited following severe acute respiratory syndrome coronavirus 2 (SARS CoV-2) vaccination in MM exhibited propensity toward EF responses.[49] Possible role of microbial signals in myeloma-genesis has also been implicated in murine MM models, implicating a role for gut Th17 cells in promoting tumor growth.[50] B cell repertoire may theoretically also be altered by exposure to B-targeting pathogens (such as Epstein Barr virus) and racial or social factors that may in turn affect the risk of gammopathy.[51,52] Further studies are also needed to better understand how signals associated with or leading to chronic inflammation may drive the development of early PC clones because interruption of such triggers may yield novel strategies for immune prevention. Emergence of inflammatory phenotypes may also be linked to genomic alterations in hematopoietic progenitors, as recently shown for IgM gammopathy and Waldenstrom macroglobulinemia.[53,54]

DIVERSE MECHANISMS UNDERLIE IMMUNE PARESIS IN MULTIPLE MYELOMA

Earlier studies have documented the presence of altered function and phenotypes in several immune cells and correlated these changes with outcome.[7] These include changes in all major immune cell types such as B, T, NK, NKT, regulatory T (Tregs), DCs, and myeloid cells including myeloid-derived suppressor cells (MDSCs). One of the most prominent changes in immune cells relates to decline in normal B/plasma cell function, manifest clinically as hypogammaglobulinemia or reduction in uninvolved Igs. These changes often worsen with therapy, particularly those targeting CD38 or B cell maturation antigen (BCMA), and have contributed to both poor responses to vaccines and enhanced susceptibility to infections, as most recently demonstrated during the SARS CoV-2 pandemic.[49,55]

Immune alterations in MM include both quantitative as well as qualitative changes in immune cells. For example, T cells in patients with MM increasingly exhibit features of T cell dysfunction and terminal differentiation.[56,57] This is associated with attrition of a population of stem-like memory or precursor exhausted T cells marked by the expression of TCF1.[17] Altered polarization of T cells has also been documented, with reduced Th1 type signaling and instead, increased Th17 cells,[58,59] which correlated with the presence of MM bone disease. T cells within MM marrow likely consist of both tumor-specific T cells (including neoantigen-specific T cells) and bystander T cells.[60] Although the expression of immune checkpoints such as programmed death-1 (PD1) has been documented in MM, strategies to block PD1 have been largely underwhelming, even when tried in earlier setting.[61,62] Alternate immune inhibitory receptors such as lymphocyte aactivation gene-3 (Lag-3) and T cell immunoreceptor wth Ig and ITIM domains (TIGIT) have been implicated in MM and being actively pursued in the clinic.[63–65] Recent MM mouse models have suggested reconsideration of PD1 blockade to prevent evolution to MM.[25] In addition to T cell intrinsic mechanisms, several T-cell extrinsic mechanisms including "immune suppressive cytokines" (such as IL-6, IL-10, transforming growth factor-beta [TGF-beta], and IL-18),[24,66–68] or cells capable of mediating immune suppression (such as Tregs, MDSCs,[69–73] mesenchymal stem cells, cancer-associated fibroblasts, and osteoclasts)[20,74] have been implicated in mediating immune suppression. In some situations, the underlying mechanisms may be linked or overlapping. For example, inflammatory stromal phenotypes have been linked to T cell exhaustion and immune escape.[20,75] Biology of myeloid cells in MM is complex, with both tumor-promoting and tumor-inhibitory effects documented. Several studies have documented systemic alterations in myeloid-derived suppressor cells in MM,[76–80] which may represent important targets to enhance tumor immunity. In addition to adaptive immunity, changes in innate immunity such as NK or natural killer T (NKT) cells may also be important targets for MM immunity and therapy.[81,82] Considered together, these studies paint a complex picture wherein several mechanisms may contribute to immune paresis observed in patients.

It is important to note however that in spite of these features, MM tumor cells remain susceptible to lysis by both innate and adaptive immune cells.[83–85] The concept that endogenous immune effector T cells can mediate tumor regression has now been translated to the clinic, with the demonstration of clinical tumor regression following bispecific antibodies.[8,86] Such data also illustrate the importance of in-situ activation/engagement of T cells, as well as the need to better understand spatial aspects of immune response.[34] Recent application of single cell methods has also illustrated considerable interpatient heterogeneity in terms of immune TME in MM.[17,19] In this regard, immune profile in each patient with MM or MGUS is likely unique. Thus, as with tumor genetics, immune pathogenesis in MM may also follow diverse pathways.

NONIMMUNOLOGIC CONTRIBUTIONS OF IMMUNE CELLS IN MULTIPLE MYELOMA

MM is a malignancy involving an immune cell (ie, plasma cell). Therefore, it is not surprising that studies have documented direct interactions between MM tumor cells and other immune cells that directly affect MM pathogenesis. For example, interactions between both myeloid or plasmacytoid DCs and MM cells can promote tumor growth, in part, by engaging Baff-mediated signals.[87,88] The presence of Baff-expressing myeloid cells has also been implicated in resistance to chimeric antigen receptor T (CART) cells in MM.[89] Interactions between DCs and tumors can also lead to the activation of cytidine deaminases within MM cells and may contribute to genomic instability.[38] DCs or macrophages in the tumor bed may also contribute more directly to the development of MM bone disease via tumor-induced cell fusion events that lead to the formation of osteoclasts.[90]

SUMMARY AND FUTURE DIRECTIONS

In the past decade, it has become increasingly clear that the immune system has a major impact on the growth and evolution of MM tumors and is a potent approach to therapy. Immune-based therapies seem poised to transform the current landscape for clinical management, both for therapy and prevention of MM. Optimal application and sequencing of these therapies will likely depend on the immune pathogenesis and state of immune cells in individual patients. There also remains an unmet need to better understand the cross talk between MM immunology and genetics, integrating the advances in molecular and immune pathogenesis. Understanding the early events in MGUS pathogenesis may also lead to novel approaches for the prevention of myeloma.

CLINICS CARE POINTS

- MGUS originates in the setting of underlying immune dysfunction and chronic immune activation.
- Modulation of immunity in patients with precursor states may prevent th development of myeloma.

ACKNOWLEDGMENTS

M.V. Dhodapkar is supported in part by funds from LLS, United States Specialized Center for Research, NIH R35 CA197603, U54 CA260563, MMRF and Paula and Rodger Riney Foundation.

DISCLOSURE

M.V. Dhodapkar: Advisory Board: Janssen, Sanofi, Lava Therapeutics. There are no conflicts related to specific content of this review.

REFERENCES

1. Kumar SK, Rajkumar V, Kyle RA, et al. Multiple myeloma. Nat Rev Dis Primers 2017;3:17046.

2. Landgren O, Kyle RA, Pfeiffer RM, et al. Monoclonal gammopathy of undetermined significance (MGUS) consistently precedes multiple myeloma: a prospective study. Blood 2009;113(22):5412–7.
3. Dhodapkar MV. MGUS to myeloma: a mysterious gammopathy of underexplored significance. Blood 2016;128(23):2599–606.
4. El-Khoury H, Lee DJ, Alberge JB, et al. Prevalence of monoclonal gammopathies and clinical outcomes in a high-risk US population screened by mass spectrometry: a multicentre cohort study. Lancet Haematol 2022;9(5):e340–9.
5. Rognvaldsson S, Love TJ, Thorsteinsdottir S, et al. Iceland screens, treats, or prevents multiple myeloma (iStopMM): a population-based screening study for monoclonal gammopathy of undetermined significance and randomized controlled trial of follow-up strategies. Blood Cancer J 2021;11(5):94.
6. Vesely MD, Kershaw MH, Schreiber RD, et al. Natural innate and adaptive immunity to cancer. Annu Rev Immunol 2011;29:235–71.
7. Dhodapkar MV. The immune system in multiple myeloma and precursor states: lessons and implications for immunotherapy and interception. Am J Hematol 2023;98 Suppl 2(Suppl 2):S4–12.
8. Cohen AD, Raje N, Fowler JA, et al. How to Train Your T Cells: Overcoming Immune Dysfunction in Multiple Myeloma. Clin Cancer Res 2020;26(7):1541–54.
9. Shah N, Aiello J, Avigan DE, et al. The Society for Immunotherapy of Cancer consensus statement on immunotherapy for the treatment of multiple myeloma. Journal for immunotherapy of cancer 2020;8(2):e000734.
10. Dhodapkar MV, Krasovsky J, Osman K, et al. Vigorous premalignancy specific effector T cell response in the bone marrow of patients with preneoplastic gammopathy. J Exp Med 2003;198:1753–7.
11. Finn OJ. Premalignant lesions as targets for cancer vaccines. J Exp Med 2003; 198(11):1623–6.
12. Smyth MJ, Dunn GP, Schreiber RD. Cancer immunosurveillance and immunoediting: the roles of immunity in suppressing tumor development and shaping tumor immunogenicity. Adv Immunol 2006;90:1–50.
13. Dhodapkar MV, Krasovsky J, Osman K, et al. Vigorous premalignancy-specific effector T cell response in the bone marrow of patients with monoclonal gammopathy. J Exp Med 2003;198(11):1753–7.
14. Spisek R, Kukreja A, Chen LC, et al. Frequent and specific immunity to the embryonal stem cell-associated antigen SOX2 in patients with monoclonal gammopathy. J Exp Med 2007;204(4):831–40.
15. Maura F, Landgren O, Morgan GJ. Designing Evolutionary Based Interception Strategies to Block the Transition from Precursor Phases to Multiple Myeloma. Clin Cancer Res 2021;27(1):15–23.
16. Kini Bailur J, Mehta S, Zhang L, et al. Changes in bone marrow innate lymphoid cell subsets in monoclonal gammopathy: target for IMiD therapy. Blood Adv 2017;1(25):2343–7.
17. Bailur JK, McCachren SS, Doxie DB, et al. Early alterations in stem-like/resident T cells, innate and myeloid cells in the bone marrow in preneoplastic gammopathy. JCI Insight 2019;5(11):e127807.
18. Boiarsky R, Haradhvala NJ, Alberge JB, et al. Single cell characterization of myeloma and its precursor conditions reveals transcriptional signatures of early tumorigenesis. Nat Commun 2022;13(1):7040.
19. Zavidij O, Haradhvala NJ, Mouhieddine TH, et al. Single-cell RNA sequencing reveals compromised immune microenvironment in precursor stages of multiple myeloma. Nature Cancer 2020;1(5):493–506.

20. de Jong MME, Kellermayer Z, Papazian N, et al. The multiple myeloma microenvironment is defined by an inflammatory stromal cell landscape. Nat Immunol 2021;22(6):769–80.
21. Dhodapkar MV, Sexton R, Das R, et al. Prospective analysis of antigen-specific immunity, stem-cell antigens, and immune checkpoints in monoclonal gammopathy. Blood 2015;126(22):2475–8.
22. Guillerey C, Ferrari de Andrade L, Vuckovic S, et al. Immunosurveillance and therapy of multiple myeloma are CD226 dependent. J Clin Invest 2015;125(7):2904.
23. Guillerey C, Ferrari de Andrade L, Vuckovic S, et al. Immunosurveillance and therapy of multiple myeloma are CD226 dependent. J Clin Invest 2015;125(5):2077–89.
24. Nakamura K, Kassem S, Cleynen A, et al. Dysregulated IL-18 Is a Key Driver of Immunosuppression and a Possible Therapeutic Target in the Multiple Myeloma Microenvironment. Cancer Cell 2018;33(4):634–648 e5.
25. Larrayoz M, Garcia-Barchino MJ, Celay J, et al. Preclinical models for prediction of immunotherapy outcomes and immune evasion mechanisms in genetically heterogeneous multiple myeloma. Nat Med 2023;29(3):632–45.
26. Das R, Strowig T, Verma R, et al. Microenvironment-dependent growth of preneoplastic and malignant plasma cells in humanized mice. Nat Med 2016;22(11):1351–7.
27. Khoo WH, Ledergor G, Weiner A, et al. A niche-dependent myeloid transcriptome signature defines dormant myeloma cells. Blood 2019;134(1):30–43.
28. Mateos MV, Hernandez MT, Giraldo P, et al. Lenalidomide plus dexamethasone versus observation in patients with high-risk smouldering multiple myeloma (QuiRedex): long-term follow-up a randomised, controlled, phase 3 trial. Lancet Oncol 2016;17(8):1127–36.
29. Lonial S, Jacobus S, Fonseca R, et al. Randomized Trial of Lenalidomide Versus Observation in Smoldering Multiple Myeloma. J Clin Oncol 2020;38(11):1126–37.
30. Sklavenitis-Pistofidis R, Aranha MP, Redd RA, et al. Immune biomarkers of response to immunotherapy in patients with high-risk smoldering myeloma. Cancer Cell 2022;40(11):1358–13573 e8.
31. Paiva B, Mateos MV, Sanchez-Abarca LI, et al. Immune status of high-risk smoldering multiple myeloma patients and its therapeutic modulation under LenDex: a longitudinal analysis. Blood 2016;127(9):1151–62.
32. Sehgal K, Das R, Zhang L, et al. Clinical and pharmacodynamic analysis of pomalidomide dosing strategies in myeloma: impact of immune activation and cereblon targets. Blood 2015;125(26):4042–51.
33. Dhodapkar MV, Dhodapkar KM. Moving Immunoprevention Beyond Virally Mediated Malignancies: Do We Need to Link It to Early Detection? Front Immunol 2019;10:2385.
34. Robinson M, Villa NY, Jaye D, et al. Regulation of antigen-specific T-cell infiltration and spatial architecture in myeloma and premalignancy. J Clin Invest 2023;133(15):e167629.
35. McShane CM, Murray LJ, Landgren O, et al. Prior autoimmune disease and risk of monoclonal gammopathy of undetermined significance and multiple myeloma: a systematic review. Cancer Epidemiol Biomarkers Prev 2014;23(2):332–42.
36. Rustad EH, Yellapantula V, Leongamornlert D, et al. Timing the initiation of multiple myeloma. Nat Commun 2020;11(1):1917.
37. Maura F, Rustad EH, Yellapantula V, et al. Role of AID in the temporal pattern of acquisition of driver mutations in multiple myeloma. Leukemia 2020;34(5):1476–80.

38. Koduru S, Wong E, Strowig T, et al. Dendritic cell-mediated activation-induced cytidine deaminase (AID)-dependent induction of genomic instability in human myeloma. Blood 2012;119(10):2302–9.
39. Weinreb NJ, Mistry PK, Rosenbloom BE, et al. MGUS, lymphoplasmacytic malignancies, and Gaucher disease: the significance of the clinical association. Blood 2018;131(22):2500–1.
40. Nair S, Branagan AR, Liu J, et al. Clonal Immunoglobulin against Lysolipids in the Origin of Myeloma. N Engl J Med 2016;374(6):555–61.
41. Nair S, Sng J, Boddupalli CS, et al. Antigen-mediated regulation in monoclonal gammopathies and myeloma. JCI Insight 2018;3(8):e98259.
42. Claflin JL, Rudikoff S, Potter M, et al. Structural, functional, and idiotypic characteristics of a phosphorylcholine-binding IgA myeloma protein of C57BL/ka allotype. J Exp Med 1975;141(3):608–19.
43. Chesi M, Robbiani DF, Sebag M, et al. AID-dependent activation of a MYC transgene induces multiple myeloma in a conditional mouse model of post-germinal center malignancies. Cancer Cell 2008;13(2):167–80.
44. Kumar S, Larson DR, Dispenzieri A, et al. Polyclonal serum free light chain elevation is associated with increased risk of monoclonal gammopathies. Blood Cancer J 2019;9(6):49.
45. Nair S, Bar N, Xu ML, et al. Glucosylsphingosine but not Saposin C, is the target antigen in Gaucher disease-associated gammopathy. Mol Genet Metab 2020;129(4):286–91.
46. Pavlova EV, Archer J, S ZW, et al. Inhibition of UDP-glucosylceramide synthase in mice prevents Gaucher disease-associated B-cell malignancy. J Pathol 2015;235(1):113–24.
47. Chen JW, Rice TA, Bannock JM, et al. Autoreactivity in naive human fetal B cells is associated with commensal bacteria recognition. Science 2020;369(6501):320–5.
48. Myles A, Sanz I, Cancro MP. T-bet(+) B cells: A common denominator in protective and autoreactive antibody responses? Curr Opin Immunol 2019;57:40–5.
49. Azeem MI, Nooka AK, Shanmugasundaram U, et al. Impaired SARS-CoV-2 Variant Neutralization and CD8+ T-cell Responses Following 3 Doses of mRNA Vaccines in Myeloma: Correlation with Breakthrough Infections. Blood Cancer Discov 2023;4(2):106–17.
50. Calcinotto A, Brevi A, Chesi M, et al. Microbiota driven interleukin 17 producing cells and eosinophils synergize to accelerate multiple myeloma progression. Nat Commun 2018;9(1):4832.
51. Dhodapkar MV, Sexton R, Hoering A, et al. Race-Dependent Differences in Risk, Genomics, and Epstein-Barr Virus Exposure in Monoclonal Gammopathies: Results of SWOG S0120. Clin Cancer Res 2020;26(22):5814–9.
52. Bosseboeuf A, Feron D, Tallet A, et al. Monoclonal IgG in MGUS and multiple myeloma targets infectious pathogens. JCI Insight 2017;2(19):e95367.
53. Kaushal A, Nooka AK, Carr AR, et al. Aberrant Extrafollicular B Cells, Immune Dysfunction, Myeloid Inflammation, and MyD88-Mutant Progenitors Precede Waldenstrom Macroglobulinemia. Blood Cancer Discov 2021;2(6):600–15.
54. Rodriguez S, Celay J, Goicoechea I, et al. Preneoplastic somatic mutations including MYD88(L265P) in lymphoplasmacytic lymphoma. Sci Adv 2022;8(3):eabl4644.
55. Nooka AK, Shanmugasundaram U, Cheedarla N, et al. Determinants of Neutralizing Antibody Response After SARS CoV-2 Vaccination in Patients With Myeloma. J Clin Oncol 2022;JCO2102257.

56. Chung DJ, Pronschinske KB, Shyer JA, et al. T-cell Exhaustion in Multiple Myeloma Relapse after Autotransplant: Optimal Timing of Immunotherapy. Cancer Immunol Res 2016;4(1):61–71.

57. Joshua DE, Vuckovic S, Favaloro J, et al. Treg and Oligoclonal Expansion of Terminal Effector CD8(+) T Cell as Key Players in Multiple Myeloma. Front Immunol 2021;12:620596.

58. Dhodapkar KM, Barbuto S, Matthews P, et al. Dendritic cells mediate the induction of polyfunctional human IL17-producing cells (Th17-1 cells) enriched in the bone marrow of patients with myeloma. Blood 2008;112(7):2878–85.

59. Prabhala RH, Pelluru D, Fulciniti M, et al. Elevated IL-17 produced by TH17 cells promotes myeloma cell growth and inhibits immune function in multiple myeloma. Blood 2010;115(26):5385–92.

60. Perumal D, Imai N, Lagana A, et al. Mutation-derived Neoantigen-specific T-cell Responses in Multiple Myeloma. Clin Cancer Res 2020;26(2):450–64.

61. Bar N, Costa F, Das R, et al. Differential effects of PD-L1 versus PD-1 blockade on myeloid inflammation in human cancer. JCI Insight 2020;5(12):e129353.

62. Costa F, Das R, Kini Bailur J, et al. Checkpoint Inhibition in Myeloma: Opportunities and Challenges. Front Immunol 2018;9:2204.

63. Andrews LP, Yano H, Vignali DAA. Inhibitory receptors and ligands beyond PD-1, PD-L1 and CTLA-4: breakthroughs or backups. Nat Immunol 2019;20(11): 1425–34.

64. Guillerey C, Harjunpaa H, Carrie N, et al. TIGIT immune checkpoint blockade restores CD8(+) T cell immunity against multiple myeloma. Blood 2018;132(16): 1689–94.

65. Minnie SA, Kuns RD, Gartlan KH, et al. Myeloma escape after stem cell transplantation is a consequence of T cell exhaustion and is reversed by TIGIT inhibition. Blood 2018;132(16):1675–88.

66. Akhmetzyanova I, Aaron T, Galbo P, et al. Tissue-resident macrophages promote early dissemination of multiple myeloma via IL-6 and TNFalpha. Blood Adv 2021; 5(18):3592–608.

67. Hayashi T, Hideshima T, Nguyen AN, et al. Transforming growth factor beta receptor I kinase inhibitor down-regulates cytokine secretion and multiple myeloma cell growth in the bone marrow microenvironment. Clin Cancer Res 2004;10(22): 7540–6.

68. Wang S, Yang J, Qian J, et al. Tumor evasion of the immune system: inhibiting p38 MAPK signaling restores the function of dendritic cells in multiple myeloma. Blood 2006;107(6):2432–9.

69. Brimnes MK, Vangsted AJ, Knudsen LM, et al. Increased Level of both CD4+FOXP3+ Regulatory T Cells and CD14+HLA-DR−/low Myeloid-Derived Suppressor Cells and Decreased Level of Dendritic Cells in Patients with Multiple Myeloma 2010;72(6):540–7.

70. Guillerey C, Nakamura K, Vuckovic S, et al. Immune responses in multiple myeloma: role of the natural immune surveillance and potential of immunotherapies. Cell Mol Life Sci 2016;73(8):1569–89.

71. Alrasheed N, Lee L, Ghorani E, et al. Marrow-Infiltrating Regulatory T Cells Correlate with the Presence of Dysfunctional CD4(+)PD-1(+) Cells and Inferior Survival in Patients with Newly Diagnosed Multiple Myeloma. Clin Cancer Res 2020; 26(13):3443–54.

72. Prabhala RH, Neri P, Bae JE, et al. Dysfunctional T regulatory cells in multiple myeloma. Blood 2006;107(1):301–4.

73. Tai YT, Lin L, Xing L, et al. APRIL signaling via TACI mediates immunosuppression by T regulatory cells in multiple myeloma: therapeutic implications. Leukemia 2019;33(2):426–38.
74. Tai YT, Cho SF, Anderson KC. Osteoclast Immunosuppressive Effects in Multiple Myeloma: Role of Programmed Cell Death Ligand 1. Front Immunol 2018;9:1822.
75. Wu X, Wang Y, Xu J, et al. MM-BMSCs induce naive CD4+ T lymphocytes dysfunction through fibroblast activation protein alpha. Oncotarget 2017;8(32): 52614–28.
76. Ramachandran IR, Martner A, Pisklakova A, et al. Myeloid-Derived Suppressor Cells Regulate Growth of Multiple Myeloma by Inhibiting T Cells in. Bone Marrow 2013;190(7):3815–23.
77. Gorgun GT, Whitehill G, Anderson JL, et al. Tumor-promoting immune-suppressive myeloid-derived suppressor cells in the multiple myeloma microenvironment in humans. Blood 2013;121(15):2975–87.
78. Serafini P, Meckel K, Kelso M, et al. Phosphodiesterase-5 inhibition augments endogenous antitumor immunity by reducing myeloid-derived suppressor cell function. J Exp Med 2006;203(12):2691–702.
79. Asimakopoulos F, Hope C, Johnson MG, et al. Extracellular matrix and the myeloid-in-myeloma compartment: balancing tolerogenic and immunogenic inflammation in the myeloma niche. J Leukoc Biol 2017;102(2):265–75.
80. Hope C, Foulcer S, Jagodinsky J, et al. Immunoregulatory roles of versican proteolysis in the myeloma microenvironment. Blood 2016;128(5):680–5.
81. Jinushi M, Vanneman M, Munshi NC, et al. MHC class I chain-related protein A antibodies and shedding are associated with the progression of multiple myeloma. Proc Natl Acad Sci 2008;105(4):1285–90.
82. Neparidze N, Dhodapkar MV. Harnessing CD1d-restricted T cells toward antitumor immunity in humans. Ann N Y Acad Sci 2009;1174:61–7.
83. Dhodapkar MV, Krasovsky J, Olson K. T cells from the tumor microenvironment of patients with progressive myeloma can generate strong tumor specific cytolytic responses to autologous tumor loaded dendritic cells. Proc Natl Acad Sci USA 2002;99:13009–13.
84. Dhodapkar MV, Geller MD, Chang DH, et al. A reversible defect in natural killer T cell function characterizes the progression of premalignant to malignant multiple myeloma. J Exp Med 2003;197(12):1667–76.
85. Noonan K, Matsui W, Serafini P, et al. Activated marrow infiltrating lymphocytes effectively target plasma cells and their clonogenic precursors. Cancer Res 2005;65(5):2026–34.
86. Lancman G, Sastow DL, Cho HJ, et al. Bispecific Antibodies in Multiple Myeloma: Present and Future. Blood Cancer Discov 2021;2(5):423–33.
87. Kukreja A, Hutchinson A, Dhodapkar KM, et al. Enhancement of clonogenicity of human multiple myeloma by dendritic cells. J Exp Med 2006;203(8):1859–65.
88. Chauhan D, Singh AV, Brahmandam M, et al. Functional interaction of plasmacytoid dendritic cells with multiple myeloma cells: a therapeutic target. Cancer Cell 2009;16(4):309–23.
89. Dhodapkar KM, Cohen AD, Kaushal A, et al. Changes in Bone Marrow Tumor and Immune Cells Correlate with Durability of Remissions Following BCMA CAR T Therapy in Myeloma. Blood Cancer Discov 2022;3(6):490–501.
90. Kukreja A, Radfar S, Sun BH, et al. Dominant role of CD47-thrombospondin-1 interactions in myeloma-induced fusion of human dendritic cells: implications for bone disease. Blood 2009;114(16):3413–21.

Smoldering Multiple Myeloma

Observation Versus Control Versus Cure

S. Vincent Rajkumar, MD[a],*, P. Leif Bergsagel, MD[b],
Shaji Kumar, MD[a]

KEYWORDS

- Myeloma • Therapy • Prognosis • Smoldering myeloma

KEY POINTS

- Smoldering multiple myeloma is a clonal plasma cell proliferative disorder that has a 10% per year risk of progression to myeloma in the first 5 years following diagnosis.
- Smoldering multiple myeloma can be risk-stratified using common laboratory and imaging variables into high-risk versus low-/intermediate-risk subtypes.
- Patients with high-risk smoldering multiple myeloma are candidates for early intervention.

INTRODUCTION

Monoclonal gammopathy of undetermined significance (MGUS), smoldering multiple myeloma (SMM), and multiple myeloma (MM) are part of a spectrum of clonal plasma cell proliferative disorders.[1] MGUS is a classic premalignancy and does not require intervention, whereas MM, at the other end of the spectrum, is a clear malignancy that is fatal without therapy. SMM is an asymptomatic, intermediate, clinically defined entity comprising a heterogeneous mix of patients, approximately two-thirds with MGUS (premalignancy) and one-third with MM (malignancy). Because of significant overlap in cytogenetic and molecular features, it is not easy to differentiate patients with SMM who have MGUS versus patients with MM using clinical or laboratory tests. Several risk-stratification models have been developed to identify the subset of patients with SMM in whom malignant transformation has likely occurred (high-risk SMM) to enable appropriate counseling and patient care. Although observation is

Authorship contribution statement: All of the authors collectively conceived the paper, researched the literature, and wrote the article.

[a] Division of Hematology, Mayo Clinic, 200 First Street, SW, Rochester, MN 55905, USA;
[b] Division of Hematology Oncology, Mayo Clinic, 13400 East Shea Boulevard, Scottsdale, AZ 85259, USA
* Corresponding author. Division of Hematology, Mayo Clinic, 200 First Street Southwest, Rochester, MN 55905.
E-mail address: rajkumar.vincent@mayo.edu

the standard of care in low-/intermediate-risk SMM, which is enriched for patients likely in the MGUS (premalignant) stage, early intervention studies have targeted high-risk SMM in an attempt to delay progression (control) or to eradicate the clone (cure). In this article, diagnostic criteria, risk-stratification models, and the various approaches to manage SMM (observation, control, and cure) are discussed.

DIAGNOSTIC CRITERIA AND CLINICAL FEATURES

MGUS, SMM, and MM are differentiated from each other using the criteria listed in **Table 1**.[2] MGUS presents in 5% of the general population over the age of 50,[3–5] with a 1% per year risk of progression to malignancy.[6,7] SMM is present in approximately 0.5% of the population above the age of 40 years[8] and is associated with a risk of progression to symptomatic malignancy of approximately 10% per year for the first 5 years following diagnosis, 3% per year over the next 5 years, and 1.5% per year thereafter.[9] Although both disorders are asymptomatic, it is important to keep the categories separate for clinical reasons because the risk of progression of SMM is 10 times higher than MGUS in the first 5 years following diagnosis.[10] This affects patient counseling and follow-up as well as the intensity of intervention strategies. In MGUS, the lifetime risk of progression to MM is only approximately 10% after adjusting for competing causes of death, whereas the risk of progression in SMM is 50% within 2 years in the high-risk SMM subset. Intervention strategies in which the risk of progression is very low (MGUS) should differ markedly from ones in which the risk is considerable.

Although SMM is asymptomatic, as with MGUS, related paraprotein clinical disorders, such as monoclonal gammopathy–associated peripheral neuropathy or monoclonal gammopathy–associated renal disorders, can occur and coexist.[11,12] Similarly, as with MGUS, symptoms secondary to these paraprotein-related disorders do not qualify as myeloma defining events even though myeloma-like treatments may be used to control them. MM is a malignancy diagnosed using the criteria listed in **Table 1**. During follow-up of SMM, progression to MM (malignancy) must be differentiated from and treated differently than progression or association with paraprotein-related disorders that occur independent of malignant transformation based solely on the nature of the M protein.

Baseline laboratory studies in SMM should include complete blood count, serum creatinine, serum calcium, whole-body low-dose computed tomography (CT) or PET-CT, serum protein electrophoresis, serum immunofixation (IFE), 24-hour urine protein electrophoresis, urine IFE, and serum free light chain (FLC) assay.[13] Bone marrow examination with fluorescent in situ hybridization studies to detect high-risk cytogenetic abnormalities (del 17p, t(4;14), gain 1q, del 13) and plasma cell immunophenotyping by multiparametric flow cytometry is needed. If no myeloma defining events are present on the above evaluation, patients with suspected high-risk SMM should also preferably have an MRI of the spine and pelvis (or whole-body MRI) to ensure that focal myeloma defining lesions are not missed.[14]

RISK STRATIFICATION

The goal of risk stratification is to differentiate patients with SMM in whom the underlying clonal plasma cell population has already undergone malignant transformation (high-risk SMM) from those in whom the underlying clone is premalignant (low-/intermediate-risk SMM). High-risk SMM has a 50% risk of progression to MM in 2 years and requires consideration of early intervention strategies, whereas low-/intermediate-risk SMM has a risk of progression of approximately 5% per year and is mostly

Table 1
International Myeloma Working Group diagnostic criteria for monoclonal gammopathy of undetermined significance, smoldering multiple myeloma, and multiple myeloma and related plasma cell disorders

Disorder	Disease Definition
IgM monoclonal gammopathy of undetermined significance (IgM MGUS)	All 3 criteria must be met: • Serum IgM monoclonal protein <3 g/dL • Bone marrow lymphoplasmacytic infiltration <10% • No evidence of anemia, constitutional symptoms, hyperviscosity, lymphadenopathy, or hepatosplenomegaly that can be attributed to the underlying lymphoproliferative disorder
Non-IgM monoclonal gammopathy of undetermined significance (MGUS)	All 3 criteria must be met: • Serum monoclonal protein (non-IgM type) <3 g/dL • Clonal bone marrow plasma cells <10%[a] • Absence of end-organ damage, such as hypercalcemia, renal insufficiency, anemia, and bone lesions (CRAB) that can be attributed to the plasma cell proliferative disorder
Light-chain MGUS	All criteria must be met: • Abnormal FLC ratio (<0.26 or >1.65) • Increased level of the appropriate involved light chain (increased kappa FLC in patients with ratio >1.65 and increased lambda FLC in patients with ratio <0.26) • No immunoglobulin heavy-chain expression on immunofixation • Absence of end-organ damage that can be attributed to the plasma cell proliferative disorder • Clonal bone marrow plasma cells <10% Urinary monoclonal protein <500 mg/24 h
Smoldering multiple myeloma	Both criteria must be met: • Serum monoclonal protein (IgG or IgA) ≥3 g/dL, or urinary monoclonal protein ≥500 mg per 24 h and/or clonal bone marrow plasma cells 10%–60% • Absence of myeloma defining events or amyloidosis

Multiple myeloma	Both criteria must be met:
	• Clonal bone marrow plasma cells ≥10% or biopsy-proven bony or extramedullary plasmacytoma
	• Any one or more of the following myeloma defining events:
	  ○ Evidence of end-organ damage that can be attributed to the underlying plasma cell proliferative disorder, specifically:
	    ■ Hypercalcemia: serum calcium >0.25 mmol/L (>1 mg/dL) higher than the upper limit of normal or >2.75 mmol/L (>11 mg/dL)
	    ■ Renal insufficiency: creatinine clearance <40 mL per minute or serum creatinine >177 μmol/L (>2 mg/dL)
	    ■ Anemia: hemoglobin value of >2 g/dL below the lower limit of normal, or a hemoglobin value <10 g/dL
	    ■ Bone lesions: one or more osteolytic lesions on skeletal radiography, CT, or PET-CT

(continued on next page)

Table 1 (continued)	
Disorder	**Disease Definition**
	○ Clonal bone marrow plasma cell percentage ≥60% ○ Involved: uninvolved serum FLC ratio ≥100 (involved FLC level must be ≥100 mg/L and urine monoclonal protein level at least 200 mg per 24 h on urine protein electrophoresis) ○ >1 focal lesions on MRI studies (at least 5 mm in size)

[a] A bone marrow can be deferred in patients with low-risk MGUS (IgG type, M protein <1.5 g/dL, normal FLC ratio), in patients with uncomplicated suspected IgM MGUS <1.5 g/dL, and in patients with serum FLC ratio <8, in whom there are no clinical features concerning for myeloma, macroglobulinemia, or amyloidosis.

Modified from Rajkumar SV, Dimopoulos MA, Palumbo A, et al. International Myeloma Working Group updated criteria for the diagnosis of multiple myeloma. Lancet Oncol 2014;15:e538-e548.

managed with observation alone. Several prognostic factors have been identified, and these variables have been used in combination to create multiple risk-stratification models for clinical use.[9,15–22]

The earliest prognostic markers identified were the size and type of monoclonal protein, and the extent of bone marrow involvement.[9] Numerous prognostic factors have since been identified, and these include simple blood-based biomarkers as well as imaging studies and bone marrow abnormalities. A reduction in the level of uninvolved immunoglobulins is associated with increased risk of progression.[9,15] The serum FLC ratio is also particularly valuable and has been incorporated into risk-stratification models.[16] Imaging provides valuable information on prognosis at baseline and during follow-up. Thus, the presence of one focal nonosteolytic lesion or presence of diffuse (nonfocal) abnormalities on MRI is associated with an increased risk of progression to MM and suggests the need for more close follow-up and repeat imaging in 3 to 6 months.[23] Similarly increased uptake on PET-CT without bone destruction indicates a higher risk of progression.[24]

Bone marrow immunophenotyping with multiparametric flow cytometry can be used to distinguish and quantitate bone marrow plasma cells with malignant potential (aberrant) from normal plasma cells.[25] The median time to progression is significantly shorter when the proportion of aberrance bone marrow plasma cells is ≥95%. Cytogenetic abnormalities detected on bone marrow examination of clonal plasma cells, t(4;14), del(17p), and gain(1q) are associated with a higher risk of progression.[18,19,26]

Multiple risk-stratification models have been developed over the years, and the main goal with these models is to identify patients with the highest risk of progression for early intervention.[9,15–22] Essentially, these models attempt to identify patients in whom malignant transformation has already occurred, and they do so with a combination of either laboratory and imaging variables, genomics, or both. In clinical practice, one needs to accurately identify patients with at least a 50% risk of progression within 2 years, because they are most likely to benefit from early intervention. The Mayo 2018 criteria, also referred to as the 20-2-20 criteria, use 3 high-risk factors: serum FLC ratio >20, serum M protein level >2 g/dL, bone marrow clonal plasma cells >20%.[27] The presence of 2 or 3 of these factors is considered high-risk SMM (**Box 1**) and have been validated in a separate cohort by the International Myeloma Working Group (IMWG; see **Box 1**).[10] However, the IMWG validation study provides a scoring system for more accurate estimation of prognosis and is preferable if data on the variables are available at the point of care.

Box 1
Risk stratification of smoldering multiple myeloma

Mayo 2018 Criteria (20-2-20 criteria)
  High-risk SMM (2-year risk of progression 50%)
    Any 2 to 3 of the following high-risk factors:
      Serum monoclonal protein >2 g/dL
      Serum free light chain ratio (involved/uninvolved) >20
      Bone marrow plasma cells >20%
  Intermediate-risk SMM
    Any 1 high-risk factor
  Low-risk SMM
    No high-risk factor

International Myeloma Working Group Scoring System for SMM
  Risk factor scores
    Serum free light chain involved/uninvolved ratio
      0 to 10: 0
      11 to 25: 2
      26 to 40: 3
      >40: 5
    Serum monoclonal protein level (g/dL)
      0 to 1.5: 0
      1.6 to 2.9: 3
      $\geq$3: 4
    Bone marrow plasma cell percentage
      0 to 15: 0
      16 to 20: 2
      21 to 30: 3
      31 to 40: 5
      >40: 6
    High-risk FISH abnormalities (del 17p, gain 1q, t(4;14), or del 1).
      Absent: 0
      Present: 2
  Risk stratification using IMWG score
  High-risk SMM (2-year risk of progression, 75%)
    Score >12
  High- to intermediate-risk SMM (2-year risk of progression, 50%)
    Score 9 to 12
  Low- to intermediate-risk SMM (2-year risk of progression, 25%)
    Score 5 to 8
  Low-risk SMM (2-year risk of progression, 5%)
    Score 1 to 4

Abbreviation: FISH, fluorescent in situ hybridization.

Derived from Lakshman A, et al. Risk stratification of smoldering multiple myeloma incorporating revised IMWG diagnostic criteria. Blood Cancer J 2018;8:59; and Mateos MV, et al. International Myeloma Working Group risk stratification model for smoldering multiple myeloma (SMM). Blood Cancer J 2020;10:102.

Besides baseline prognostic factors, a change in one or more of the above parameters over time is of critical importance.[28] In one study, an evolving change in monoclonal protein (0.5 g/dL increase in M protein) along with an evolving change in hemoglobin (0.5 g/dL decrease in hemoglobin) over a 12-month period was associated with high risk of progression.[29] Among patients with bone marrow plasma cells $\geq$20%, evolving M protein and evolving hemoglobin were independent predictors of progression; the 2-year progression rate was 90.5% in patients who had both an evolving M protein and an evolving hemoglobin. Importantly, a recent study has found the Mayo 2018 high-risk criteria can be used in follow-up, and patients who are initially diagnosed as low-risk SMM can be later reclassified based on changes in M protein, serum FLC ratio, and/or bone marrow involvement.

Current risk-stratification models are not perfect, but they are readily available around the world. However, it is important to continue to develop better models. One caveat now is that none of the models are very sensitive, and so only a proportion of patients at high risk are identified by each model. By combining models, more patients can probably be captured at risk, and the estimate on the risk of progression will be more precise. In the future, modern genomic sequencing methods may be able to separate patients who need immediate intervention from those who can be followed. However, these studies are not standardized and are not widely available, with methods and techniques varying across laboratories. Furthermore, even patients who are considered not to have malignancy by genomic methods can always have a malignant transformation at some point in the future, and hence, such studies can neither fully reassure a patient nor do they negate the need for follow-up even in patients not considered to have malignant transformation.

APPROACH TO TREATMENT
Observation

Observation without therapy every 3 to 4 months is the standard of care for patients with low- and intermediate-risk SMM. After 5 years, the interval between follow-up visits can be extended. In general, serum M protein, serum FLC levels, complete blood count, serum calcium, and serum creatinine should be monitored.[30] Bone imaging and bone marrow biopsies are recommended if clinical suspicion for progression occurs. If during follow-up, patients with low-risk SMM have increases in M protein, bone marrow plasma cells, serum FLC levels, or changes in other relevant parameters that meet high-risk criteria, then they should be managed according to the high-risk SMM pathway.[29] In patients with MRI showing diffuse infiltration, solitary focal lesion, or equivocal lesions, follow-up radiographic examination in 3 to 6 months is recommended.[23]

In high-risk SMM, some investigators continue to recommend observation alone instead of early intervention. However, there are many problems with this approach. First, it may not be possible to intervene in time before serious end-organ damage even with close follow-up. Second, as discussed in later discussion, early intervention in high-risk SMM is associated with 90% reduction in risk of progression with concurrent end-organ damage. Third, the treatment duration and intensity are not indefinite, and there are no data from current trials to suggest any adverse effect on response to future lines of therapy or overall survival. In fact, overall survival benefit has been seen with early intervention in the Spanish trial. Observation alone was reasonable before availability of effective therapy, before evidence from randomized trial, and before good risk-stratification models to identify the subset of SMM most likely to benefit from intervention. This is not the case anymore, and hence, the authors do not prefer observation alone for high-risk SMM. If a decision is made not to offer treatment to patients with newly diagnosed high-risk SMM, patients should have a clear discussion on the pros and cons. In many parts of the world, lenalidomide is inexpensive, and cost is not a barrier to initiation of therapy.

Control

The authors' current approach to management of SMM mirrors the control approach and is provided in **Fig. 1**.[30] This approach has been tested in randomized trials and provides important clinical benefit.[31,32] The control approach consists of limited

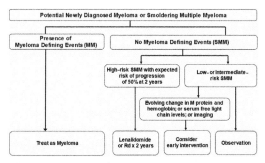

Fig. 1. Approach to the management of SMM.

duration intervention and is only recommended for patients with newly diagnosed high-risk SMM who have a 50% risk of progression by reliable risk-stratification models. The authors recommend therapy with either lenalidomide or lenalidomide plus dexamethasone (Rd) for 2 years, or enrollment in a clinical trial testing early therapy. This recommendation is based on 2 randomized trials with lenalidomide in high-risk SMM showing benefit. In the Spanish randomized trial, time to progression to MM with end-organ damage was significantly longer in patients treated with Rd compared with observation (median time to progression not reached vs 21 months; P<.001).[25,31] Overall survival was also longer, 3-year survival rate 94% versus 80%, respectively (P = .03). Importantly, early intervention with Rd did not affect the impact of subsequent therapy after progression or survival after progression, arguing against any long-term deleterious effect of early intervention. In the randomized trial conducted by the Eastern Cooperative Oncology Group (ECOG), early therapy with lenalidomide prolonged time to symptomatic MM with end-organ damage in patients with high-risk SMM.[33] Among patients meeting Mayo 2018 high-risk criteria, both the Spanish trial and the ECOG trial found a striking 90% reduction in time to end-organ damage. Between lenalidomide and Rd, the choice should be made considering the patient's age, comorbidities, and tolerance to dexamethasone. Patients with high-risk SMM who are treated with lenalidomide or Rd should have peripheral blood stem cells collected for cryopreservation after approximately 4 to 6 cycles of therapy.[34,35] Besides lenalidomide, other myeloma agents are also being tested in high-risk SMM, including daratumumab. A randomized trial of daratumumab versus observation (NCT03301220) has completed accrual and is awaiting analysis.

Can SMM be better controlled using a triple regimen as is used in the treatment of MM rather than lenalidomide alone or Rd? This is an important question and is the subject of randomized trials. A randomized trial testing daratumumab, lenalidomide, dexamethasone versus Rd is ongoing (NCT03937635), and the authors are awaiting its results. Another randomized trial is testing isatuximab, lenalidomide, dexamethasone versus Rd (NCT04270409). These trials are not meant to cure SMM but provide better disease control and prolong time to end-organ damage and improve overall survival. Addition of a third drug carries other risks, and hence the need to wait for long-term data from randomized trials before recommending such therapy in asymptomatic patients. Nevertheless, there is a small subset of patients with high-risk SMM in whom the risk of progression in 2 years approaches that used to revise the diagnostic criteria for MM, and in such patients, careful consideration to MM-like therapy may not be unreasonable.

The role of bisphosphonates to delay bone events in SMM is not fully settled. In a randomized trial, a reduction in skeletal-related events (SRE) has been seen with pamidronate (once a month for 12 months) compared with observation.[36] However, no improvement in time to progression or survival was seen. In another randomized trial, a reduction in SREs was noted with zoledronic acid (once a month for 12 months), 56% versus 78%, respectively (P = .04).[37] The authors recommend once-yearly bisphosphonate similar to that used for the treatment of osteoporosis for patients with SMM who have osteopenia or osteoporosis.

Cure

It is possible that MM is not a curable disease because the intervention is started too late, when the disease is already advanced. One hypothesis is that MM can be cured if intense therapy is used at the early asymptomatic high-risk SMM stage when the clonal cells are not cytogenetically advanced and are more susceptible to therapy. Patients with high-risk SMM are good candidates for clinical trials testing intensive therapy with curative intent.[38] Two such trials, CESAR and ASCENT (NCT02415413, NCT03289299), have completed accrual and await long-term analysis to determine if a plateau exists and to see if early aggressive intervention at the SMM stage can be curative. The cure approach is of academic interest but is still investigational and is not recommended outside of clinical trials.

FUTURE DIRECTIONS

Results of randomized trials testing whether a standard myeloma therapeutic triplet will be superior to prophylactic doublet therapy with Rd in patients with high-risk SMM are awaited. Also, long-term results of cure trials are awaited to determine if such an intense approach may be of value in selected patients. Importantly, the authors are pursuing continuous development of risk-stratification models, including genomics, to identify patients more accurately for intervention.

CLINICS CARE POINTS

- Following diagnosis of smoldering multiple myeloma, patients should be risk-stratified to identify patients with high-risk disease needing early intervention.
- The best defined early intervention is lenalidomide or lenalidomide plus dexamethasone for 2 years.
- Patients with smoldering multiple myeloma should be considered for enrollment in clinical trials testing early intervention.

ACKNOWLEDGMENTS

This work was supported in part by grants CA 168762 and CA186781 from the National Cancer Institute, United States, Rockville, MD, USA, and the Marvin Family Grant.

DISCLOSURE

No significant conflicts of interests to disclose. Dr S.V. Rajkumar reports grants from NIH, United States outside the submitted work. Dr S. Kumar reports consultancy from BMS/Celgene, Takeda, United States, and Janssen, United States, and research funding from BMS, United States/Celgene, Takeda, Novartis, Switzerland, AbbVie, Janssen, and Amgen, United States. Dr L. Bergsagel reports grants from the NCI, United States, research funding from Pfizer, United States, consultancy for Pfizer, and AbbVie.

REFERENCES

1. Rajkumar SV. Multiple myeloma: 2020 update on diagnosis, risk-stratification and management. Am J Hematol 2020;95:548–67.
2. Rajkumar SV, Dimopoulos MA, Palumbo A, et al. International Myeloma Working Group updated criteria for the diagnosis of multiple myeloma. Lancet Oncol 2014;15:e538–48.
3. Kyle RA, Therneau TM, Rajkumar SV, et al. Prevalence of monoclonal gammopathy of undetermined significance. N Engl J Med 2006;354:1362–9.
4. Dispenzieri A, Katzmann JA, Kyle RA, et al. Prevalence and risk of progression of light-chain monoclonal gammopathy of undetermined significance: a retrospective population-based cohort study. Lancet 2010;375:1721–8.
5. Murray D, Kumar SK, Kyle RA, et al. Detection and prevalence of monoclonal gammopathy of undetermined significance: a study utilizing mass spectrometry-based monoclonal immunoglobulin rapid accurate mass measurement. Blood Cancer J 2019;9:102.
6. Kyle RA, Therneau TM, Rajkumar SV, et al. A long-term study of prognosis of monoclonal gammopathy of undetermined significance. N Engl J Med 2002; 346:564–9.
7. Kyle RA, Larson DR, Therneau TM, et al. Long-term follow-up of monoclonal gammopathy of undetermined significance. N Engl J Med 2018;378:241–9.
8. Thorsteinsdottir S, Gislason GK, Aspelund T, et al. Prevalence of smoldering multiple myeloma: results from the Iceland screens, treats, or prevents multiple myeloma (iStopMM) study. Blood 2021;138:151.
9. Kyle RA, Remstein ED, Therneau TM, et al. Clinical course and prognosis of smoldering (asymptomatic) multiple myeloma. N Engl J Med 2007;356:2582–90.
10. Mateos MV, Kumar S, Dimopoulos MA, et al. International Myeloma Working Group risk stratification model for smoldering multiple myeloma (SMM). Blood Cancer J 2020;10:102.
11. Chaudhry HM, Mauermann ML, Rajkumar SV. Monoclonal gammopathy-associated peripheral neuropathy: diagnosis and management. Mayo Clin Proc 2017;92:838–50.
12. Sethi S, Rajkumar SV. Monoclonal gammopathy-associated proliferative glomerulonephritis. Mayo Clin Proc 2013;88:1284–93.
13. Kyle RA, Durie BGM, Rajkumar SV, et al, International Myeloma Working Group. Monoclonal gammopathy of undetermined significance (MGUS) and smoldering (asymptomatic) multiple myeloma: IMWG consensus perspectives risk factors for progression and guidelines for monitoring and management. Leukemia 2010;24: 1121–7.
14. Hillengass J, Usmani S, Rajkumar SV, et al. International Myeloma Working Group consensus recommendations on imaging in monoclonal plasma cell disorders. Lancet Oncol 2019;20:e302–12.
15. Perez-Persona E, Vidriales MB, Mateo G, et al. New criteria to identify risk of progression in monoclonal gammopathy of uncertain significance and smoldering multiple myeloma based on multiparameter flow cytometry analysis of bone marrow plasma cells. Blood 2007;110:2586–92.
16. Dispenzieri A, Kyle RA, Katzmann JA, et al. Immunoglobulin free light chain ratio is an independent risk factor for progression of smoldering (asymptomatic) multiple myeloma. Blood 2008;111:785–9.
17. Rosinol L, Blade J, Esteve J, et al. Smoldering multiple myeloma: natural history and recognition of an evolving type. Br J Haematol 2003;123:631–6.

18. Rajkumar SV, Gupta V, Fonseca R, et al. Impact of primary molecular cytogenetic abnormalities and risk of progression in smoldering multiple myeloma. Leukemia 2013;27:1738–44.

19. Neben K, Jauch A, Hielscher T, et al. Progression in smoldering myeloma is independently determined by the chromosomal abnormalities del(17p), t(4;14), gain 1q, hyperdiploidy, and tumor load. J Clin Oncol 2013;31:4325–32.

20. Dhodapkar MV, Sexton R, Waheed S, et al. Clinical, genomic, and imaging predictors of myeloma progression from asymptomatic monoclonal gammopathies (SWOG S0120). Blood 2014;123:78–85.

21. Bianchi G, Kyle RA, Larson DR, et al. High levels of peripheral blood circulating plasma cells as a specific risk factor for progression of smoldering multiple myeloma. Leukemia 2013;27:680–5.

22. Hillengass J, Fechtner K, Weber MA, et al. Prognostic significance of focal lesions in whole-body magnetic resonance imaging in patients with asymptomatic multiple myeloma. J Clin Oncol 2010;28:1606–10.

23. Merz M, Hielscher T, Wagner B, et al. Predictive value of longitudinal whole-body magnetic resonance imaging in patients with smoldering multiple myeloma. Leukemia 2014;28:1902–8.

24. Zamagni E, Nanni C, Gay F, et al. 18F-FDG PET/CT focal, but not osteolytic, lesions predict the progression of smoldering myeloma to active disease. Leukemia 2016;30:417–22.

25. Mateos M-V, Hernández M-T, Giraldo P, et al. Lenalidomide plus Dexamethasone for High-Risk Smoldering Multiple Myeloma. N Engl J Med 2013;369:438–47.

26. Lakshman A, Paul S, Rajkumar SV, et al. Prognostic significance of interphase FISH in monoclonal gammopathy of undetermined significance. Leukemia 2018;32(8):1811–5.

27. Lakshman A, Rajkumar SV, Buadi FK, et al. Risk stratification of smoldering multiple myeloma incorporating revised IMWG diagnostic criteria. Blood Cancer J 2018;8:59.

28. Fernandez de Larrea C, Isola I, Pereira A, et al. Evolving M-protein pattern in patients with smoldering multiple myeloma: impact on early progression. Leukemia 2018;32:1427–34.

29. Ravi P, Kumar S, Larsen JT, et al. Evolving changes in disease biomarkers and risk of early progression in smoldering multiple myeloma. Blood Cancer J 2016;6:e454.

30. Rajkumar SV, Landgren O, Mateos MV. Smoldering multiple myeloma. Blood 2015;125:3069–75.

31. Mateos MV, Hernandez MT, Giraldo P, et al. Lenalidomide plus dexamethasone versus observation in patients with high-risk smouldering multiple myeloma (QuiRedex): long-term follow-up of a randomised, controlled, phase 3 trial. Lancet Oncol 2016;17:1127–36.

32. Lonial S, Jacobus S, Fonseca R, et al. Randomized Trial of Lenalidomide Versus Observation in Smoldering Multiple Myeloma. J Clin Oncol 2020;38:1126–37.

33. Lonial S, Jacobus SJ, Weiss M, et al. E3A06: Randomized phase III trial of lenalidomide versus observation alone in patients with asymptomatic high-risk smoldering multiple myeloma. J Clin Oncol 2019;37.

34. Tsuda K, Tanimoto T, Komatsu T. Treatment for high-risk smoldering myeloma. N Engl J Med 2013;369:1763.

35. Mateos MV, San Miguel JF. Treatment for high-risk smoldering myeloma. N Engl J Med 2013;369:1764–5.

36. D'Arena G, Gobbi PG, Broglia C, et al, Gimema Gruppo Italiano Malattie Emato-logiche Dell'Adulto, Multiple Myeloma Working Party, Gisl Gruppo Italiano Studio Linfomi Cooperative Group. Pamidronate versus observation in asymptomatic myeloma: final results with long-term follow-up of a randomized study. Leuk Lymphoma 2011;52:771–5.
37. Musto P, Petrucci MT, Bringhen S, et al, GIMEMA Italian Group for Adult Hematologic Diseases/Multiple Myeloma Working Party and the Italian Myeloma Network. A multicenter, randomized clinical trial comparing zoledronic acid versus observation in patients with asymptomatic myeloma. Cancer 2008;113: 1588–95.
38. Mateos M-V, Martinez Lopez J, Rodriguez-Otero P, et al. Curative strategy for high-risk smoldering myeloma (GEM-CESAR): carfilzomib, lenalidomide and dexamethasone (KRd) as induction followed by HDT-ASCT, consolidation with KRd and maintenance with Rd. Blood 2017;130:402.

Cereblon-Targeting Ligase Degraders in Myeloma

Mechanisms of Action and Resistance

Holly Lee, MD, MSc, Paola Neri, MD, PhD, Nizar J. Bahlis, MD*

KEYWORDS

- IMiDs • CELMoDs • Thalidomide • Lenalidomide • Pomalidomide • Iberdomide
- Mezigdomide

KEY POINTS

- Cereblon ligase degraders bind the adaptor cereblon (CRBN) of the CUL4-RING E3 ubiquitin ligase (CRL4) neomorphing its substrate bindings.
- Immunomodulatory imide drugs (IMiDs) and cereblon E3 ligase modulators (CELMoDs) promote the proteasomal degradation of two plasma cells essential transcription factors Ikaros and Aiolos, decommissioning myeloma active promoters and oncogenic enhancers they regulate and their targets (*MYC, IRF4, and so forth*).
- Resistance to IMiDs and CeLMoDs is largely mediated by mutations in CRBN and CRL4 subunits as well as transcriptional plasticity at the myeloma oncogenic enhancers.

INTRODUCTION

Cereblon-targeting degraders, such as immunomodulatory imide drugs (IMiDs) lenalidomide and pomalidomide and their derivative cereblon E3 ligase modulators (CELMoDs) iberdomide and mezigdomide, have exhibited clear anti-myeloma activity. The integration of this class of drugs into various therapeutic regimens and disease stages in multiple myeloma (MM) underscores their pivotal therapeutic role. Despite their pronounced anti-MM activity, it is worth noting that ~ 5% to 10% of patients demonstrate primary refractoriness to lenalidomide and patients invariably develop resistance to this class of drugs. Consequently, an improved understanding of both the mechanisms of action and the mechanisms underlying their resistance is critical for the refining and development of novel therapeutic combinations with this class of drugs.

Arnie Charbonneau Cancer Institute, University of Calgary, Heritage Medical Research Building, 3330 Hospital Drive N.W., Calgary, Alberta T2N 4N1, Canada
* Corresponding author.
E-mail address: nbahlis@ucalgary.ca

Hematol Oncol Clin N Am 38 (2024) 305–319
https://doi.org/10.1016/j.hoc.2024.01.001
0889-8588/24/© 2024 Elsevier Inc. All rights reserved.

MECHANISMS OF ACTION
Structural Basis of Immunomodulatory Imide Drugs and Cereblon E3 Ligase Modulators

Thalidomide, α-N-phthalimido-glutarimide, consists of two moieties, phthalimide and glutarimide, and serves as the foundational structure from which IMiDs as well as CEL-MoDs are derived. Although these molecules share the glutarimide moiety which is essential for binding to the adaptor protein cereblon (CRBN), each is distinguished by their phthaloyl ring variations which define their unique pharmacokinetic and pharmacodynamic properties, as summarized in **Fig. 1** and **Table 1**.

CUL4-RING E3 Ubiquitin Ligase Complex Assembly and Immunomodulatory Imide Drug/Cereblon E3 Ligase Modulator Binding

CRBN, in conjunction with the DNA damage-binding protein 1 (DDB1), cullin 4 (CUL4), and RING-box protein 1 (Roc1) assemble to form the CUL4-RING E3 ubiquitin ligase (CRL4) complex (Cul4A^{CRBN}), as depicted in **Figs. 2** and **3**. IMiDs and CELMoDs execute their cellular functions through engagement with CRBN[1] and neomorphing substrates binding to the CRL4 E3 ligase, rendering the substrates for polyubiquitination and degradation by the 26S proteasome.

The glutarimide moiety of IMiDs and CELMoDs engages into a shallow hydrophobic pocket of CRBN formed by three tryptophan residues (Trp380, Trp386, and Trp400) located within the thalidomide binding domain (TBD) of CRBNs C terminus (exons 10–11)[2] (**Fig. 4**). Both thalidomide and pomalidomide's glutarimide rings establish two hydrogen bonds with the peptide backbone of His378 and Trp380 of CRBN.

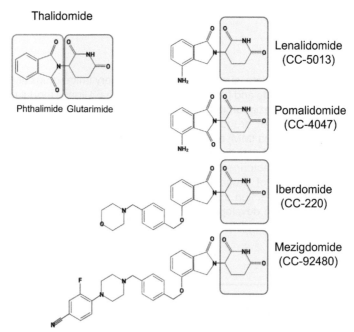

Fig. 1. Chemical structures of immunomodulatory drugs (IMiDs) and cereblon E3 ligase modulators (CELMoDs). The glutarimide ring (in *blue*) is present in all IMiDs and CELMoDs, whereas differences in the phthaloyl ring (in *yellow*) distinguish the distinctive pharmacokinetic and pharmacodynamic properties of each molecule.

Table 1
IMiD and CELMoD chemical structure and pharmacokinetics

	Lenalidomide (CC-5013)	Pomalidomide (CC-4047)	Iberdomide (CC-220)	Mezigdomide (CC-92480)
Molecular formula	$C_{13}H_{13}N_3O_3$	$C_{13}H_{11}N_3O_4$	$C_{25}H_{27}N_3O_5$	$C_{32}H_{30}FN_5O_4$
Molecular weight (g/mol)	259.3	273.2	449.5	567.6
Half-life (hours)	3–5	7.5–9.5	9–13	16–19
Renal dosing	Adjustments for CrCl <60 mL/min	Adjustments for severe renal impairment requiring dialysis	No available data	No available data
Liver metabolism	Minimal	Partially metabolized by CYP1A2, CYP3A4, substrate for p-glycoprotein CYP2C19, CYP2D6, CYP3A4	Primarily metabolized by CYP3A	Primarily liver metabolized

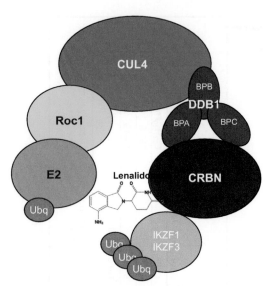

Fig. 2. CRBN E3 ligase complex (Cul4A^CRBN). The Cul4A^CRBN complex is formed by CRBN, DNA damage-binding protein 1 (DDB1), cullin 4 (CUL4), and RING-box protein 1 (Roc1). Roc1 recruits E2 ubiquitin conjugating enzyme (E2). Lenalidomide (or other IMiDs/CELMoDs) binds CRBN and induces the recruitment of substrates (such as IKZF1 or IKZF3) which undergo ubiquitination (Ubq).

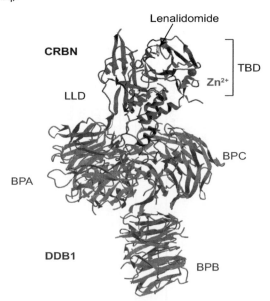

Fig. 3. Crystal structure of human Cereblon, CRBN, (in *blue*) in complex with DNA damage-binding protein 1, DDB1 (in *pink*), and lenalidomide. CRBN contains thalidomide binding domain (TBD) and LON-like domain (LLD). DDB1 consists of three domains including β-propeller A (BPA), β-propeller B (BPB), and β-propeller C (BPC). (Figure was adapted from crystal structure deposited in Protein Data Bank (PDB ID: 4TZ4) by Chamberlain et al. 2014 (Reference 12: Hansen JD, Correa M, Nagy MA, et al. Discovery of CRBN E3 Ligase Modulator CC-92480 for the Treatment of Relapsed and Refractory Multiple Myeloma. J Med Chem 2020;63(13):6648-6676).)

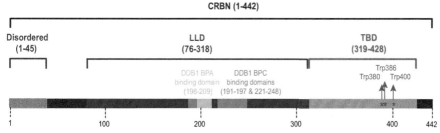

Fig. 4. Cereblon (CRBN) interaction domains. Depicted in this figure are the disordered domain, LON-like domain (LLD), and thalidomide binding domain (TBD). LLD contains DDB1 BPA and BPC binding domains. TBD domain contains three tryptophan residues (Trp 380, 386, and 400), which form the shallow hydrophobic pocket of CRBN.

Lenalidomide forms an additional third hydrogen bond with the side chain of His378 of CRBN.[2] On the docking of the glutarimide moiety to CRBN, the isoindolinone ring (of lenalidomide) or phthalimide ring (of pomalidomide) remains exposed on the surface of the CRBN complex. These structures retain the C4 amine with unquenched hydrogen molecules. This configuration contributes to defining target substrate specificity, influencing interactions with various substrates at the neomorphic interface.[2]

A cornerstone of IMIDs anti-MM activity hinges on CRBN E3 ligase dependent modulation of various transcriptional networks, effectively accomplished by the degradation of neo-substrates, including zinc finger (ZF) proteins IKZF1 (Ikaros) and IKZF3 (Aiolos), two canonical plasma cell transcription factors[3–10] with MYC and IRF4 as their downstream transcriptional targets.

Cereblon E3 Ligase Modulators Offer Enhanced Interaction, Binding Affinity, and Potency

CELMoDs, including iberdomide (CC-220) and mezigdomide (CC-92480), exhibit substantially greater potency by eliciting modulated CRBN substrate specificity compared with IMIDs. Of note, they have higher binding affinities to CRBN, as highlighted in **Table 2**, compared with those of lenalidomide and pomalidomide.[11,12]

Iberdomide, by its common glutarimide ring shared with IMIDs, interacts with CRBN. The molecule further integrates extensive modifications involving phenyl and morpholino moieties to the isoindolinone ring. These adaptations foster additional interactions with CRBN and/or substrates.[11] Indeed, iberdomide exhibits approximately 20-fold stronger affinity for CRBN compared with lenalidomide or pomalidomide, resulting in more efficient and rapid degradation of IKZF1 and IKZF3, as outlined in **Table 2**.[11] Iberdomide and mezigdomide exhibited varying degrees of IMiD resistance

Table 2				
IMiD and CELMoD half-maximal inhibitory and effective concentrations				
	Lenalidomide (CC-5013)	Pomalidomide (CC-4047)	Iberdomide (CC-220)	Mezigdomide (CC-92480)
CRBN binding (C50	1.5 μM	1.2 μM	0.06 μM	0.03 μM
CRBN closed conformation	–	20%	50%	100%
IKZF1 degradation EC50	67 nM	24 nM	1 nM	–
IKZF3 degradation EC50	87 nM	22 nM	0.5 nM	–

reversal in MM cell lines with reduced CRBN levels.[12,13] This CELMoDs improved binding affinity to CRBN stems from an extended area of contact between CRBN and the extended chemical moieties present in CELMoDs.[13] Cryo-electron microscopy-based structural analyses have characterized the allosteric modulation of CRBNs conformation, transitioning between open and closed states on IMiD or CELMoD binding.[14] This analysis revealed that mezigdomide extends its interaction to the TBD and the Lon domain of CRBN, leading to CRBNs closed conformation in 100% of the time, whereas pomalidomide primarily induces closure by binding to the TBD with only 20% of CRBN in closed confirmation. Mezigdomide and iberdomide's ability to stabilize the closed CRBN conformation without relying on the N-terminal belt contributes to their superior enhanced neosubstrate recruitment and therapeutic efficacy.[14]

Diverse Neo-Substrates Targeted by Immunomodulatory Imide Drug and Cereblon E3 Ligase Modulators

Recently, C-terminal cyclic imides, emerging from posttranslational modifications via intramolecular cyclization of glutamine or asparagine residues, were characterized to be the endogenous CRBN substrates.[15] IMiD or CELMoD-bound CRBN extends these substrates to IKZF1 and IKZF3 and differentially influences a broad spectrum of Cys_2-His_2 (C2H2) ZF proteins[16] such as ZFP91 that is uniquely targeted by pomalidomide, iberdomide, and mezigdomide, but not thalidomide or lenalidomide.[17,18] In addition to targeting shared neo-substrates, each IMiD and CELMoD confer distinct neo-substrate specificities as recently summarized in a review.[19] The spectrum of neo-substrates expands further to include substrates that lack ZF domains, such as casein kinase 1 alpha (CSNK1A1),[20,21] GSPT1,[22] and DTWD1.[18] CSNK1A1 degradation forms the basis of lenalidomide specific action in myelodysplastic syndrome with deletion of chromosome 5q.[20,21] The extent to which these substrates, beyond IKZF1 and IKZF3, contribute to IMiD and CELMoD anti-myeloma activity remains to be defined.

Altogether, the anti-MM effects of IMiDs and CelMoDs are largely linked to the integrity and expression levels of CRBN and the CRL4 E3 ligase subunits. Hence, resistance to these drugs in MM has been well documented in both primary plasma cells and cell lines that exhibit reduced or mutated CRBN.[7,23]

Additional Mechanisms of Action: Chaperon-Like Function, H_2O_2 Decomposition

Apart from its role within the E3 ligase complex, CRBN is reported to exhibit a chaperone-like function promoting the maturation and stabilization of CD147 and MCT1 proteins, which together form CD147-MCT1 transmembrane complex that supports malignant cells proliferation.[24] It has been proposed that IMiDs competitively interact with CRBN, disrupting and countering the CD147-MCT1 complex function, contributing to an additional anti-MM mechanism of IMiDs.[24] In a separate study, however, knockdown of CD147 and subsequent MCT1 downregulation did not correlate with MM cell viability or lenalidomide sensitivity.[25]

IMiDs also affect their anti-MM activity by inhibiting intracellular H_2O_2 decomposition within MM cells, with pomalidomide as the most potent agent.[26] MM cells with lower capacity for H_2O_2 decomposition were more susceptible to lenalidomide-induced cytotoxicity, regardless of CRBN protein expression levels. Lenalidomide was shown to reduce intracellular H_2O_2 decomposition, increasing intracellular oxidative stress. Elevated H_2O_2 contributed to the downregulation of IKZF1 and IKZF3 by directly attenuating their expression as well as precipitated and endoplasmic reticulum stress response with BH3 protein Bim activation and apoptotic cell death.

Immunomodulatory Effects of Immunomodulatory Imide Drugs and Cereblon E3 Ligase Modulators

IMiDs also exhibit a broad range of effects beyond their direct antitumor actions, influencing various aspects of the adaptive and innate immune system and the tumor microenvironment. IMiDs exert immunomodulatory activities by facilitating co-stimulation of CD4+ and CD8+ T cells through activation of CD28 axis, enabling them to bypass co-stimulation from antigen-presenting cell interactions. Furthermore, they enhance interleukin-2 (IL-2) and interferon gamma (IFNγ) production, while also boosting AP-1 transcriptional activity.[27–30] In T cells, IKZF1 and IKZF3 bind the promoter of IL-2 gene and repress gene transcription,[4,28,31–33] and therefore, the degradation of IKZF1 and IKZF3 by IMiDs further supports IL-2 expression.[4,34] Of note, pomalidomide and CELMoDs exhibit a more potent T-cell stimulatory effect compared with lenalidomide or thalidomide.[35]

Beyond T-cell activation, CRBN-dependent degraders contribute to the expansion and activation of NK and NK T cells, resulting in increased IFNγ production and enhanced antibody-dependent cellular cytotoxicity.[35–39] This activation of NK cells creates a positive feedback loop that promotes immune responses and the secretion of cytokines that further attract T cells and dendritic cells, ultimately enhancing local cellular immunity.[40] In addition, IMiDs have also been shown to restrain regulatory T-cell activity, further strengthening their immunomodulatory effects.[41]

Apart from the direct immunomodulation of T- and NK-cell functions, this class of drugs also modulate the bone marrow environment through reported anti-inflammatory properties[35] as well as antiangiogenic effects by inhibiting among others basic fibroblast growth factor and vascular endothelial growth factors.[42–45] In addition, IMiDs modulate the interaction between bone marrow stromal cells and plasma cells by downregulating adhesion molecules receptors and ligands reducing adhesion-mediated drug resistance. This attenuated MM cell–stromal interactions also result in reduced secretion of pro-survival cytokines, counteraction of osteoclastogenesis, and inhibition of IL-6 secretion from bone marrow stromal cells.[35,44,46–48]

MECHANISMS OF RESISTANCE TO IMMUNOMODULATORY IMIDE DRUGS AND CEREBLON E3 LIGASE MODULATORS

Resistance to CRBN-dependent degraders can be generally classified as CRBN or non-CRBN mediated. A summary of some of these reported mechanisms of resistance is depicted in **Fig. 5**.

Cereblon-Dependent Resistance Mechanisms

Cereblon, encoded by the CRBN gene on chromosome 3p26.2, is a key target of acquired resistance to IMiDs and CELMoDs in MM. Of note, genetic alterations within CRBN are detected in approximately 30% of patients on progression from IMiDs.[49] The frequency of missense or truncating mutations increases as patients progress from newly diagnosed-to lenalidomide- and pomalidomide-refractory MM with the incidence rates rising from 0.5% in newly diagnosed cases to 2.2% and 9% in lenalidomide and pomalidomide refractory patients, respectively. Furthermore, structural variations, encompassing copy number loss, inversions, or translocations, follow a similar pattern of escalation from newly diagnosed to refractory cases, with incidences of 1.5%, 7.9%, and 24%, respectively.[49] CRBN mutations often emerge as subclonal mutations and are observed more frequently with extended duration of IMiD therapy in the relapsed refractory setting.[50]

CRBN modifications can also result from alteration of CRBN transcripts through exon 10 splicing, which generates a stable protein that retains its interaction capacity

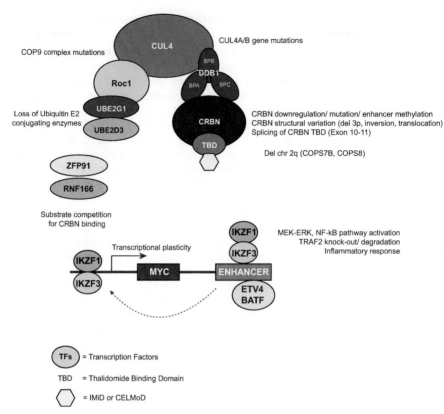

Fig. 5. Summary of mechanisms of resistance to CRBN-dependent degraders.

with DDB1 and CUL4A, but loses its ability to bind the glutarimide moiety of lenalidomide and pomalidomide.[51] The ratio between the exon 10 splice variant and the full-length transcript has been shown to correlate with the clinical response to IMiDs.[49,51] Tumors harboring CRBN exon-10 splice variants exhibit elevated TNF alpha signaling via NF-κB pathway activation, accompanied by a heightened inflammatory response characterized by elevated IL-1 and IL-10 signaling, and activation of transcriptional programs, including EZH2.[52] In this context, a potential for therapeutically leveraging molecular vulnerability arises, wherein EZH2 inhibitors could potentially address IMiD-resistant MM driven by the exon-10 splice variant of CRBN.[53]

Epigenetic regulation of CRBN was also reported.[54] DNA hypermethylation in an active intronic CRBN enhancer was observed in IMiD-refractory patients and correlated with decreased CRBN levels and in vitro DNA methyltransferase inhibitor sensitized myeloma cells to lenalidomide.

Posttranscriptional resistance mechanisms of resistance also reported competitive binding to CRBN or its substrates by other molecules hindering degradation of Ikaros and Aiolos.[55,56]

CRBN-INDEPENDENT RESISTANCE MECHANISMS
Transcriptional Plasticity

Oncogenic enhancers drive the aberrant expression of key drivers of myeloma cells survival and proliferation such as MYC and IRF4. Translocations involving the activation of potent myeloma superenhancers such as IGLL5 on chr.22 were associated with decreased response to IMiDs.[57] Chromatin immunoprecipitation sequencing studies of IKZF1 revealed the mapping of this plasma cells essential transcription factors to the promoters and oncogenic enhancers and superenhancers of transcribed myeloma genes.[58,59] Although IMiDs efficiently deplete Ikaros and Aiolos from oncogenic myeloma enhancers in both IMiDs sensitive and resistant cell lines, they only displace of the acetyltransferase (EP300) and the bromodomain acetyl mark reader (BRD4) at these enhancers in sensitive cell lines. This retention of EP300/BRD4 at these enhancers was recently revealed to result from the co-occupancy of these myeloma enhancers by other transcription factors along IKZF1 and IKZF3. Such factors included, among others, the ETS family member ETV4[58] and the bZIP family member BATF.[59] Silencing of these factors indeed sensitized IMiDs resistant myeloma cell lines to lenalidomide or pomalidomide. Therapeutically, direct targeting of the acetyl transferase EP300 with small molecule inhibitors exhibited cytotoxicity toward myeloma cell lines and synergized with IMiDs.[59,60]

Mutations in COP9 Signasolome Complex

A CRISPR-based genome wide screens have demonstrated the importance of Cul4A^{CRBN} complex regulators, including components of the COP9 signalosome, in driving IMiDs' anti-MM effectiveness.[61–64] UBE2M and COP9 signalosome complex constituents regulate Cul4A^{CRBN} complex neddylation—the covalent addition of the ubiquitin-like activator NEDD8 protein—and deneddylation of the cullin backbone. This modulation dictates the ligase's active and inactivate states.[61,65] Altered neddylation of the CUL4A complex was shown to attenuate IMiD-induced Cul4A^{CRBN} activity.[61] E2 ubiquitin-conjugating enzymes, UBE2D3, and UBE2G1 prime the neo-substrates of Cul4A^{CRBN} by monoubiquitination, with subsequent polyubiquitination formed by UBE2G1 through lysine 48-linked ubiquitin chains.[61,66] Inactivation of the cullin-RING ligase regulators by targeting of COPS5, UBE2D3, and UBE2G1 led to IMiD resistance.[45] Of note, although UBE2G1 deficiency rendered MM cells resistant to lenalidomide and pomalidomide, iberdomide retained its activity.[66]

Copy number loss in chromosome 2q37, which carries vital COP9 signalosome constituents COPS7B and COPS8, is reported to be frequently observed as patients progress from initial MM diagnosis to the more refractory stages following lenalidomide and pomalidomide treatment.[67] The incidence rates were 5.5%, 10%, and 16.5%, respectively, underscoring the potential of this alteration as a predictive marker for clinical response to IMiDs.[67]

MEK-ERK Pathway Activation

An alternative facet of IMiD resistance, distinct from the CUL4A-CRBN-IKZF1/3 axis, involves TRAF2 downregulation,[68] which leads to the activation of the noncanonical NF-kB and ERK pathways, and culminates in the elevation of phosphorylated mitogen-activated protein kinase 1 or 2 (ERK1-2) levels and upstream mitogen-activated protein kinase kinase 1 (MEK1) activity. Of note, engagement of the ERK pathway is evident in nearly all (97%) cases of relapse post-lenalidomide maintenance.[68] TNF alpha, secreted by bone marrow stromal cells, lowers TRAF2 levels and attenuates the efficacy of IMiD-induced anti-MM cytotoxicity. TNF alpha mediates this effect, independent of CRBN expression, by the activation of both the ERK and noncanonical NF-kB pathways. Importantly, the bone marrow microenvironment contributes to IMiD resistance by secreting TNF alpha and IL-6, which directly fuels ERK signaling.[68] Collectively, this demonstrates that the presence of soluble factors, by orchestrating MEK-ERK activation, shields MM cells from IMiD effect within the bone marrow.[68]

Resistance within this context was overcome by MEK inhibitor, AZD6244, suggesting the potential use of MEK/ERK inhibitors for restoration of IMiD sensitivity.[68,69]

Other Reported CRBN-Independent Mechanisms of Resistance

In a genome wide screening using short hairpin RNA (shRNA) libraries, KPNB1 was identified as a critical factor for nuclear import of CRBN, and its deficiency led to resistance to pomalidomide by inhibiting nuclear import of CRBN and reducing pomalidomide-dependent degradation of IKZF3.[63] Disturbance in the subcellular localization of CRBN had significant impact on the effectiveness of CRBN modulators, underscoring the significance of "spatial overlap" between CRBN and its targets to ensure effective ubiquitination.[63]

Epigenetically an increase in genome-wide DNA methylation and reduction in chromatin accessibility were observed in MM cells lines derived to acquire resistance to lenalidomide and pomalidomide with SMAD3 downregulation. In these cells, simultaneous inhibition of DNA methyl transferases and EZH2 restored myeloma cells to sensitivity to IMiDs in a CRBN-independent mechanism.[70]

IL6 and STAT3 activation has also been implicated in IMiD resistance both in in vitro generated lenalidomide-resistant cell lines and validated in a comprehensive genomic data set of newly diagnosed MM patients, revealing a notable correlation between heightened IL6 and STAT3 expression and shorter treatment response.[25]

SUMMARY

CRBN-dependent degraders represent a remarkable class of drugs with a pleotropic mechanisms of action with direct anti-MM as well as immunomodulatory effects. Defining the mechanisms of action and resistance to these molecules allowed the development of next-generation CRBN-dependent degraders (iberdomide, mezigdomide, CFT7455) with enhanced activity and potency compared with first-generation IMiDs. Ongoing explorations of these molecules and the combination of CRBN-dependent degraders with other novel anti-myeloma therapeutics with further unravel the pandora box effects of this class of drugs.

CLINICS CARE POINTS

- Cereblon-targeting ligase degraders neomorphe the CRL4 E3 ubiquitin ligase substrates binding and degradation with two myeloma essential transcription factors IKZF1 and IKZF3. In addition, these molecules are potent inducers of T- and NK-cell activation and expansion.

- Mutations in *CRBN*, CRL4 E3 ligase, or the COP9 signalosome subunits as well as transcriptional plasticity are the major mediators of resistance to cereblon-targeting ligase degraders

- Therapeutically, among cereblon-targeting ligase degraders, novel molecules with enhanced binding affinity for CRBN and ability to retain it in a close confirmation, exhibit more potent anti-myeloma activity and in some instances overcome resistance to earlier generation of CRBN binders. Furthermore, epigenetic modifiers such as the acetyltransferase EP300 or BRD4 inhibitors display potent preclinical synergy with cereblon-targeting ligase degraders.

- Cereblon-degraders are potent activators of innate and adaptive immunity and hence represent ideal partners to T cells redirecting antibodies and chimeric antigen receptor engineered T cells in multiple myeloma.

DISCLOSURE

N.J. Bahlis has received research funding from: Pfizer, and is a consultant/ advisory board member for Abbvie, BMS, Janssen, and Pfizer. P. Neri is a consultant/ advisory board member for BMS, Janssen, and Sanofi.

REFERENCES

1. Ito T, Ando H, Suzuki T, et al. Identification of a primary target of thalidomide teratogenicity. Science (New York, NY) 2010;327(5971):1345-50.
2. Chamberlain PP, Lopez-Girona A, Miller K, et al. Structure of the human Cereblon-DDB1-lenalidomide complex reveals basis for responsiveness to thalidomide analogs. Nat Struct Mol Biol 2014;21(9):803-9.
3. Lu G, Middleton RE, Sun H, et al. The myeloma drug lenalidomide promotes the cereblon-dependent destruction of Ikaros proteins. Science (New York, NY) 2014; 343(6168):305 9.
4. Krönke J, Udeshi ND, Narla A, et al. Lenalidomide causes selective degradation of IKZF1 and IKZF3 in multiple myeloma cells. Science (New York, NY) 2014; 343(6168):301-5.
5. Georgopoulos K, Bigby M, Wang JH, et al. The Ikaros gene is required for the development of all lymphoid lineages. Cell 1994;79(1):143-56.
6. Cortes M, Wong E, Koipally J, et al. Control of lymphocyte development by the Ikaros gene family. Curr Opin Immunol 1999;11(2):167-71.
7. Zhu YX, Braggio E, Shi CX, et al. Cereblon expression is required for the antimyeloma activity of lenalidomide and pomalidomide. Blood 2011;118(18):4771-9.
8. Nückel H, Frey UH, Sellmann L, et al. The IKZF3 (Aiolos) transcription factor is highly upregulated and inversely correlated with clinical progression in chronic lymphocytic leukaemia. Br J Haematol 2009;144(2):268-70.
9. Morgan B, Sun L, Avitahl N, et al. Aiolos, a lymphoid restricted transcription factor that interacts with Ikaros to regulate lymphocyte differentiation. Embo j 1997; 16(8):2004-13.
10. Cortés M, Georgopoulos K. Aiolos is required for the generation of high affinity bone marrow plasma cells responsible for long-term immunity. J Exp Med 2004;199(2): 209-19.
11. Matyskiela ME, Zhang W, Man HW, et al. A Cereblon Modulator (CC-220) with Improved Degradation of Ikaros and Aiolos. J Med Chem 2018;61(2):535-42.
12. Hansen JD, Correa M, Nagy MA, et al. Discovery of CRBN E3 Ligase Modulator CC-92480 for the Treatment of Relapsed and Refractory Multiple Myeloma. J Med Chem 2020;63(13):6648-76.
13. Bjorklund CC, Kang J, Amatangelo M, et al. Iberdomide (CC-220) is a potent cereblon E3 ligase modulator with antitumor and immunostimulatory activities in lenalidomide- and pomalidomide-resistant multiple myeloma cells with dysregulated CRBN. Leukemia 2020;34(4):1197-201.
14. Watson ER, Novick S, Matyskiela ME, et al. Molecular glue CELMoD compounds are regulators of cereblon conformation. Science (New York, NY) 2022;378(6619): 549-53.
15. Ichikawa S, Flaxman HA, Xu W, et al. The E3 ligase adapter cereblon targets the C-terminal cyclic imide degron. Nature 2022;610(7933):775-82.
16. Sievers QL, Petzold G, Bunker RD, et al. Defining the human C2H2 zinc finger degrome targeted by thalidomide analogs through CRBN. Science (New York, NY) 2018;362(6414).

17. An J, Ponthier CM, Sack R, et al. pSILAC mass spectrometry reveals ZFP91 as IMiD-dependent substrate of the CRL4(CRBN) ubiquitin ligase. Nat Commun 2017;8:15398.

18. Donovan KA, An J, Nowak RP, et al. Thalidomide promotes degradation of SALL4, a transcription factor implicated in Duane Radial Ray syndrome. Elife 2018;7:e38430.

19. Bird S, Pawlyn C. IMiD resistance in multiple myeloma: current understanding of the underpinning biology and clinical impact. Blood 2023;142(2):131–40.

20. Krönke J, Fink EC, Hollenbach PW, et al. Lenalidomide induces ubiquitination and degradation of CK1α in del(5q) MDS. Nature 2015;523(7559):183–8.

21. Petzold G, Fischer ES, Thomä NH. Structural basis of lenalidomide-induced CK1α degradation by the CRL4(CRBN) ubiquitin ligase. Nature 2016; 532(7597):127–30.

22. Matyskiela ME, Lu G, Ito T, et al. A novel cereblon modulator recruits GSPT1 to the CRL4(CRBN) ubiquitin ligase. Nature 2016;535(7611):252–7.

23. Lopez-Girona A, Mendy D, Ito T, et al. Cereblon is a direct protein target for immunomodulatory and antiproliferative activities of lenalidomide and pomalidomide. Leukemia 2012;26(11):2326–35.

24. Eichner R, Heider M, Fernández-Sáiz V, et al. Immunomodulatory drugs disrupt the cereblon-CD147-MCT1 axis to exert antitumor activity and teratogenicity. Nat Med 2016;22(7):735–43.

25. Zhu YX, Shi C-X, Bruins LA, et al. Identification of lenalidomide resistance pathways in myeloma and targeted resensitization using cereblon replacement, inhibition of STAT3 or targeting of IRF4. Blood Cancer J 2019;9(2):19.

26. Sebastian S, Zhu YX, Braggio E, et al. Multiple myeloma cells' capacity to decompose H(2)O(2) determines lenalidomide sensitivity. Blood 2017;129(8): 991–1007.

27. LeBlanc R, Hideshima T, Catley LP, et al. Immunomodulatory drug costimulates T cells via the B7-CD28 pathway. Blood 2004;103(5):1787–90.

28. Haslett PA, Corral LG, Albert M, et al. Thalidomide costimulates primary human T lymphocytes, preferentially inducing proliferation, cytokine production, and cytotoxic responses in the CD8+ subset. J Exp Med 1998;187(11):1885–92.

29. Schafer PH, Gandhi AK, Loveland MA, et al. Enhancement of cytokine production and AP-1 transcriptional activity in T cells by thalidomide-related immunomodulatory drugs. J Pharmacol Exp Therapeut 2003;305(3):1222–32.

30. Payvandi F, Wu L, Naziruddin SD, et al. Immunomodulatory drugs (IMiDs) increase the production of IL-2 from stimulated T cells by increasing PKC-theta activation and enhancing the DNA-binding activity of AP-1 but not NF-kappaB, OCT-1, or NF-AT. J Interferon Cytokine Res 2005;25(10):604–16.

31. Thompson EC, Cobb BS, Sabbattini P, et al. Ikaros DNA-binding proteins as integral components of B cell developmental-stage-specific regulatory circuits. Immunity 2007;26(3):335–44.

32. Avitahl N, Winandy S, Friedrich C, et al. Ikaros sets thresholds for T cell activation and regulates chromosome propagation. Immunity 1999;10(3):333–43.

33. Quintana FJ, Jin H, Burns EJ, et al. Aiolos promotes TH17 differentiation by directly silencing Il2 expression. Nat Immunol 2012;13(8):770–7.

34. Gandhi AK, Kang J, Havens CG, et al. Immunomodulatory agents lenalidomide and pomalidomide co-stimulate T cells by inducing degradation of T cell repressors Ikaros and Aiolos via modulation of the E3 ubiquitin ligase complex CRL4(CRBN.). Br J Haematol 2014;164(6):811–21.

35. Quach H, Ritchie D, Stewart AK, et al. Mechanism of action of immunomodulatory drugs (IMiDS) in multiple myeloma. Leukemia 2010;24(1):22–32.
36. Davies FE, Raje N, Hideshima T, et al. Thalidomide and immunomodulatory derivatives augment natural killer cell cytotoxicity in multiple myeloma. Blood 2001; 98(1):210–6.
37. Hayashi T, Hideshima T, Akiyama M, et al. Molecular mechanisms whereby immunomodulatory drugs activate natural killer cells: clinical application. Br J Haematol 2005;128(2):192–203.
38. Chang DH, Liu N, Klimek V, et al. Enhancement of ligand-dependent activation of human natural killer T cells by lenalidomide: therapeutic implications. Blood 2006; 108(2):618–21.
39. Zhu D, Corral LG, Fleming YW, et al. Immunomodulatory drugs Revlimid (lenalidomide) and CC-4047 induce apoptosis of both hematological and solid tumor cells through NK cell activation. Cancer immunology, immunotherapy CII 2008; 57(12):1849–59.
40. Roda JM, Parihar R, Magro C, et al. Natural killer cells produce T cell-recruiting chemokines in response to antibody-coated tumor cells. Cancer Res 2006; 66(1):517–26.
41. Galustian C, Meyer B, Labarthe MC, et al. The anti-cancer agents lenalidomide and pomalidomide inhibit the proliferation and function of T regulatory cells. Cancer immunology, immunotherapy CII 2009;58(7):1033–45.
42. Dredge K, Marriott JB, Macdonald CD, et al. Novel thalidomide analogues display anti-angiogenic activity independently of immunomodulatory effects. Br J Cancer 2002;87(10):1166–72.
43. Dredge K, Horsfall R, Robinson SP, et al. Orally administered lenalidomide (CC-5013) is anti-angiogenic in vivo and inhibits endothelial cell migration and Akt phosphorylation in vitro. Microvasc Res 2005;69(1–2):56–63.
44. Gupta D, Treon SP, Shima Y, et al. Adherence of multiple myeloma cells to bone marrow stromal cells upregulates vascular endothelial growth factor secretion: therapeutic applications. Leukemia 2001;15(12):1950–61.
45. D'Amato RJ, Loughnan MS, Flynn E, et al. Thalidomide is an inhibitor of angiogenesis. Proc Natl Acad Sci USA 1994;91(9):4082–5.
46. Geitz H, Handt S, Zwingenberger K. Thalidomide selectively modulates the density of cell surface molecules involved in the adhesion cascade. Immunopharmacology 1996;31(2–3):213–21.
47. Breitkreutz I, Raab MS, Vallet S, et al. Lenalidomide inhibits osteoclastogenesis, survival factors and bone-remodeling markers in multiple myeloma. Leukemia 2008;22(10):1925–32.
48. Bolzoni M, Storti P, Bonomini S, et al. Immunomodulatory drugs lenalidomide and pomalidomide inhibit multiple myeloma-induced osteoclast formation and the RANKL/OPG ratio in the myeloma microenvironment targeting the expression of adhesion molecules. Exp Hematol 2013;41(4):387–97.e381.
49. Gooding S, Ansari-Pour N, Towfic F, et al. Multiple cereblon genetic changes are associated with acquired resistance to lenalidomide or pomalidomide in multiple myeloma. Blood 2021;137(2):232–7.
50. Kortüm KM, Mai EK, Hanafiah NH, et al. Targeted sequencing of refractory myeloma reveals a high incidence of mutations in CRBN and Ras pathway genes. Blood 2016;128(9):1226–33.
51. Neri P, Maity R, Keats JJ, et al. Cereblon Splicing of Exon 10 Mediates IMiDs Resistance in Multiple Myeloma: Clinical Validation in the CoMMpass Trial. Blood 2016;128(22):120.

52. Gupta VA, Barwick BG, Matulis SM, et al. Venetoclax sensitivity in multiple myeloma is associated with B-cell gene expression. Blood 2021;137(26): 3604–15.

53. Karagoz K, Stokes M, Ortiz-Estévez M, et al. Multiple Myeloma Patient Tumors With High Levels of Cereblon Exon-10 Deletion Splice Variant Upregulate Clinically Targetable Pro-Inflammatory Cytokine Pathways. Front Genet 2022;13: 831779.

54. Haertle L, Barrio S, Munawar U, et al. Cereblon enhancer methylation and IMiD resistance in multiple myeloma. Blood 2021;138(18):1721–6.

55. Zhou N, Gutierrez-Uzquiza A, Zheng XY, et al. RUNX proteins desensitize multiple myeloma to lenalidomide via protecting IKZFs from degradation. Leukemia 2019; 33(8):2006–21.

56. Sperling AS, Burgess M, Keshishian H, et al. Patterns of substrate affinity, competition, and degradation kinetics underlie biological activity of thalidomide analogs. Blood 2019;134(2):160–70.

57. Barwick BG, Neri P, Bahlis NJ, et al. Multiple myeloma immunoglobulin lambda translocations portend poor prognosis. Nat Commun 2019;10(1):1911.

58. Neri P, Barwick BG, Jung D, et al. ETV4-Dependent Transcriptional Plasticity Maintains MYC Expression and Results in IMiD Resistance in Multiple Myeloma. Blood Cancer Discov 2024;5(1):56–73.

59. Welsh SJ, Barwick BG, Meermeier EW, et al. Transcriptional Heterogeneity Overcomes Super-Enhancer Disrupting Drug Combinations in Multiple Myeloma. Blood Cancer Discov 2024;5(1):34–55.

60. Nicosia L, Spencer GJ, Brooks N, et al. Therapeutic targeting of EP300/CBP by bromodomain inhibition in hematologic malignancies. Cancer Cell 2023;41(12): 2136–53.e2113.

61. Sievers QL, Gasser JA, Cowley GS, et al. Genome-wide screen identifies cullin-RING ligase machinery required for lenalidomide-dependent CRL4CRBN activity. Blood 2018;132(12):1293–303.

62. Liu J, Song T, Zhou W, et al. A genome-scale CRISPR-Cas9 screening in myeloma cells identifies regulators of immunomodulatory drug sensitivity. Leukemia 2019;33(1):171–80.

63. Tateno S, Iida M, Fujii S, et al. Genome-wide screening reveals a role for subcellular localization of CRBN in the anti-myeloma activity of pomalidomide. Sci Rep 2020;10(1):4012.

64. Costacurta M, Vervoort SJ, Hogg SJ, et al. Whole genome CRISPR screening identifies TOP2B as a potential target for IMiD sensitization in multiple myeloma. Haematologica 2021;106(7):2013–7.

65. Cavadini S, Fischer ES, Bunker RD, et al. Cullin–RING ubiquitin E3 ligase regulation by the COP9 signalosome. Nature 2016;531(7596):598–603.

66. Lu G, Weng S, Matyskiela M, et al. UBE2G1 governs the destruction of cereblon neomorphic substrates. Elife 2018;7.

67. Gooding S, Ansari-Pour N, Kazeroun M, et al. Loss of COP9 signalosome genes at 2q37 is associated with IMiD resistance in multiple myeloma. Blood 2022; 140(16):1816–21.

68. Liu J, Hideshima T, Xing L, et al. ERK signaling mediates resistance to immunomodulatory drugs in the bone marrow microenvironment. Sci Adv 2021;7(23).

69. Ocio EM, Fernández-Lázaro D, San-Segundo L, et al. In vivo murine model of acquired resistance in myeloma reveals differential mechanisms for lenalidomide

and pomalidomide in combination with dexamethasone. Leukemia 2015;29(3): 705–14.

70. Dimopoulos K, Søgaard Helbo A, Fibiger Munch-Petersen H, et al. Dual inhibition of DNMTs and EZH2 can overcome both intrinsic and acquired resistance of myeloma cells to IMiDs in a cereblon-independent manner. Mol Oncol 2018; 12(2):180–95.

Proteasome Inhibitors in Multiple Myeloma

Biological Insights on Mechanisms of Action or Resistance Informed by Functional Genomics

Constantine S. Mitsiades, MD, PhD[a,b,c,d],*

KEYWORDS

- Proteasome inhibitors • Multiple myeloma • Functional genomics
- Nuclear Factor-kappa B (NF-κB) • Endoplasmic reticulum-associated degradation
- CRISPR

KEY POINTS

- *Proteasome Inhibitors in Multiple Myeloma (MM)*: Essential for MM therapy, proteasome inhibitors have been pivotal in the last 2 decades.
- *Evolution of MM Research*: This review tracks the evolving mechanistic understanding of proteasome inhibitors' activity in MM.
- *Limited Applications Beyond MM*: Despite success in MM, proteasome inhibitors have limited clinical use outside plasma cell dyscrasias.
- *Nuclear Factor-Kappa B (NF-κB) Pathway and Endoplasmic Reticulum (ER)-Associated Degradation*: Recent functional genomics studies highlight the NF-κB pathway and ER-associated degradation as key in the clinical activity of proteasome inhibitors against MM.
- *Molecular Determinants in MM*: The review identifies NF-κB and ER-associated degradation as crucial molecular factors driving proteasome inhibitors' clinical activity in MM.

INTRODUCTION

During the last 20 years, the clinical management of multiple myeloma (MM), the second most commonly diagnosed hematologic malignancy in the western world, has been radically transformed by the introduction into the therapeutic armamentarium of a series of pharmacologic agents, monoclonal antibodies, and cell-based immunotherapies. One of the earliest events in this transformation was the documentation of the anti-MM clinical activity of thalidomide,[1] but soon thereafter proteasome inhibitors

[a] Department of Medical Oncology, Dana-Farber Cancer Institute, Boston, MA, USA; [b] Harvard Medical School, Boston, MA, USA; [c] Broad Institute of Massachusetts Institute of Technology (MIT) and Harvard, Cambridge, MA, USA; [d] Ludwig Center at Harvard, Boston, MA, USA
* Department of Medical Oncology, Dana-Farber Cancer Institute, Boston, MA.
E-mail address: constantine_mitsiades@dfci.harvard.edu

Hematol Oncol Clin N Am 38 (2024) 321–336
https://doi.org/10.1016/j.hoc.2023.12.016
0889-8588/24/© 2024 Elsevier Inc. All rights reserved.

(PIs) were introduced into the therapeutic management of MM[2–4] and have remained, as a pharmacologic class, a therapeutic cornerstone for this disease.

It is understandable that given the central role of this pharmacologic class in the therapeutic management of MM, a large body of literature has focused on PIs. This has included original articles and also even many comprehensive reviews on several different aspects of this drug class. These original or review studies include, but are not limited to detailed recaps of the preclinical literature on the anti-MM activity of PIs in different preclinical systems (eg, Refs[5–13]); the proposed mechanisms contributing to the action of PIs against MM cells (eg, Refs[5,10,14]); characterization of therapeutic agents that modify the sensitivity of MM cells to PIs (eg, Refs[10,15–25]); and genomic and other molecular profiling efforts to characterize the features of PI-resistant MM cells (eg, Refs[15,26–28]). In addition, large numbers of studies have summarized the results of clinical trials of PIs and their different combinations with established or investigational agents for the therapeutic management of MM (eg, Refs[3,4,29–34]). The current report does not intend to provide a "review of reviews" but rather revisit certain aspects of the existing knowledge on the mechanism of action of PIs in MM under the light of some more recent developments regarding our understanding on the biology of MM. Specifically, the current review seeks to explain how recently published functional genomic data on the molecular vulnerabilities of MM cells[35] shed new light into our knowledge of the molecular mechanisms that are responsible for the activity of PIs in MM. Moreover, these functional genomics data explain why PIs have limited, if any, therapeutic implications in diseases beyond the context of plasma cell dyscrasias.[36] Based on these more recent data, the current review seeks to explain gaps that still remain in our understanding of the molecular mechanisms of resistance to PI-based therapies and how recently developed technologies for functional genomic assessment may be able to provide such insights in the near future.

THE PROTEASOME COMPLEX AND ITS INHIBITORS

The 26S proteasome is a large macromolecular complex located in the cytoplasm and nucleus.[37–39] Its main role is to degrade intracellular proteins which are "decorated" with covalently attached ubiquitin (Ub) chains. These Ub chains are typically attached to proteins which should be destined for degradation because they have been misfolded, aged, oxidized, or otherwise damaged or because the expression and function of these proteins is not required by a given cell at that particular moment. Indeed, an important aspect of the proteasome function is to help regulate the intracellular levels and also intracellular localization and function of different types of regulatory proteins. The biochemistry, structural biology, and functional connections between the components of the proteasome complex and its upstream regulators have been extensively reviewed, for example, in Refs.[40–47] Briefly, the 26S proteasome includes two 19S regulatory complexes which are positioned on the opposite ends of a hollow core particle (called 20S proteasome). In order for target proteins to be marked for proteasomal degradation, a complex enzymatic system operates upstream of the 26S proteasome. This system contains Ub-activating enzymes (E1s) which use energy derived from adenosine triphosphate (ATP) hydrolysis to catalyze the transfer of Ub residues to one of 30+ Ub-conjugating enzymes (E2s), which in turn engage one of several hundred E3 ligases (E3s), as previously reviewed, for example, in Refs.[40–44] The E3 ligases covalently attach Ub chains to specific lysine residues in different groups of substrates.[44] The 19S proteasome particles engage these ubiquitinated substrates, remove their Ub chains, promote unfolding of the target protein substrates, and transfer them to the interior of the 20S proteasome chamber, through which the disassembled Ub chains are then recycled.[45] The chamber of the 20S proteasome complex contains three types of proteolytic subunits, β5, β2, and β1[45]: each of these subunits causes protein degradation at positions within the substrate proteins, which are preferentially situated after large hydrophobic, basic, or acidic residues (chymotrypsin-like, trypsin-like, and caspase-like activities, respectively).[46] In most tissues, the main and constitutively expressed form of the proteasome is the canonical 20S proteasome. In cells of the immune system, the so-called immunoproteasome can also be present, as previously reviewed in several studies, for example,[47] especially after exposure to certain proinflammatory cytokines. The immunoproteasome contains different catalytic subunits (β1i, β2i, and β5i) and often engages distinct 11S regulatory complexes; these distinguishing features of the immunoproteasome (compared with the canonical 20S proteasome) are considered to optimize its ability to generate antigenic peptides that can then be presented through major histocompatibility complex molecules to facilitate immune responses. The pharmacologic PIs, bortezomib, carfilzomib, and ixazomib, inhibit the chymotrypsin-like activity of the β5 subunit. The pharmacologic properties of these inhibitors have been extensively reviewed elsewhere (eg, Refs[48–58]).

THE EVOLVING CONCEPTUAL FRAMEWORK ON MOLECULAR MECHANISMS MEDIATING ANTI-MULTIPLE MYELOMA EFFECTS OF PROTEASOME INHIBITION

In the first few years after the initial preclinical development and early clinical studies of PIs, the prevailing views on the mechanism(s) of action of this drug class in MM centered around the inhibition of nuclear factor-kappa B (NF-κB) transcription factors and specifically the notion that the suppression of the proteasomal degradation of IκB (nuclear factor of kappa light polypeptide gene enhancer in B-cells inhibitor), an inhibitor of the nuclear translocation of NF-κB, would decrease the transcriptional activity of these key molecules. This mechanistic explanation resonated with the MM field for multiple reasons, including the known significance of NF-κB in many biological systems and the particular role of these transcription factors on regulation of key genes for B-cell differentiation and plasma cell biology.

However, a set of papers published in mid- to late-2000s highlighted an alternative notion that the mechanism of anti-MM action of PIs involved a strong component of perturbation of endoplasmic reticulum (ER) stress and specifically a disruption of the balance between the so called "proteasome load" versus "proteasome capacity." For instance, in 2006, Obeng and colleagues reported[59] that because MM cells constitutively produce very high levels of immunoglobulins and are subject to higher levels of endoplasmic reticulum (ER) stress at their own baseline (in the absence of any treatment), proteasome inhibition further increases their ER stress to such an extent that the functional reserves available for MM cells to tolerate such increases are already constrained,[59] thus allowing PIs to kill MM cells at concentrations that can be tolerated by other types of cells which do not exhibit a similar role as "professional secretory" cells.

Obeng and colleagues also reported that although bortezomib-induced proteasome inhibition is associated with suppression of the transcriptional activity of NF-κB, the exposure of MM cells to other pharmacologic agents that can inhibit NF-κB activity, such as an inhibitor of IκB phosphorylation (BAY 11–7082), does not phenocopy the effects of in vitro exposure to PIs.[59] Similar experiments were reported with the selective IκB kinase inhibitor PS-1145 by Hideshima and colleagues.[60] A common observation in these experiments was that small molecular weight inhibitors of IκB kinase (IKK) function required, compared with bortezomib or other PIs, much higher concentrations (often in high micromolar levels) and longer durations of exposure to achieve major anti-MM effects. In fact, some MM cell lines did not appear to respond even to the highest IKK inhibitor concentrations tested. At that time, these highly heterogeneous responses of MM cells to IKK inhibitor treatment in vitro, and their contrast to the more homogeneous responses of MM cells to PIs, were collectively interpreted to suggest that inhibition of NF-κB could not be considered the sole or primary explanation for the anti-MM effect of PIs. These considerations further strengthened the interest and emphasis of MM research on the "professional secretory" function of MM cells and their associated ER stress as the mechanistic basis for PIs.

This interest was consolidated a few years after the Obeng and colleagues study, when additional observations by Bianchi and colleagues[61] confirmed and extended the notion that the response of MM cells to proteasome inhibition can be linked to the relationship between the "proteasomal load" versus "proteasome capacity."[61] These two studies[59,61] and additional ones[62–65] conducted in MM or in other experimental systems (eg, models of terminal differentiation of normal B cells to plasma cells),[62–65] concordantly highlighted the significance of the ER stress/unfolded protein response as an important determinant of the extent of MM/plasma cell response to proteasome inhibition. It is notable that the studies of Obeng and colleagues or Bianchi and colleagues[59,61] did not specifically advocate that the role of NF-κB on the mechanism of action of PIs should be completed excluded, yet the ER-oriented views highlighted by these studies became during the last 15 years accepted as the central, if not the sole, mechanistic explanation for the preferential biological and clinical effects of proteasome inhibition in MM.

A factor that further solidified these views is the astute observation by Boise and colleagues, in a review article from 2014,[36] that all pharmacologic and antibody-based therapies which had demonstrated clinical activity in MM since the late 1990s/early 2000s and until the time of that review publication (for example, PIs, thalidomide derivatives, and antibodies targeting CD38) do not target the malignant plasma cells of MM because they are malignant but because of their biology as plasma cells.[36] Boise and colleagues also pointed out that these treatments target plasma cells, malignant or not, and not the genomic lesions that are responsible for malignant transformation of plasma cells. This can explain why the responsiveness of MM cells to these therapies does not seem to be predicated on specific genomic features of the MM cells. More broadly, this review article presented the notion of the "Tao of myeloma," that is, the biology of MM cells is shaped by both the "cancer-related" biology of the cells (as determined by the genomic lesions causing their malignant transformation) and the "lineage-related" biology of MM cells as plasma cells.[36] With ER stress as a built-in feature of plasma cell biology for both nonmalignant cells and in MM cells, the distinct ability of proteasome inhibition to target this pathway became widely accepted, especially because additional novel anti-MM therapies that were developed after 2014 (eg, therapies targeting B-cell maturation antigen [BCMA][66–75] or G-protein coupled receptor family C group 5 member D [GPRC5D][76–78]) were again consistent with the premise of the "Tao of myeloma."

Moreover, in the 2010s, reports emerged that MM cells derived from patients with advanced MM/refractoriness to combination therapies based on PIs often exhibited variable degrees of "dedifferentiation," manifested through decreased expression (but not necessarily elimination) of plasma cell-specific markers (often associated with decreased production of intact immunoglobulin or with light chain escape),[79] which suggested that the broader attenuation of the "plasma cell" state of these MM cells could contribute to less pronounced dependence on ER stress that is contributing to the decreased responsiveness to PIs or combinations thereof. Another aspect that further solidified the notion of PIs as preferential perturbagens for ER-stressed plasma cells was the emergence of clinical data highlighting the activity of bortezomib in autoimmune conditions, such as systemic lupus erythematosus, in which suppression of nonmalignant plasma cells was observed and considered to correlate with clinical activity.[80–83]

Collectively, the evidence about the contribution of the ER stress to the molecular sequelae of proteasome inhibition combined with the emerging understanding of the "plasma cell state" of MM cells as a molecular vulnerability in its own right led to a broader acceptance of the notion that the PIs target MM cells via disruption of the ER-associated protein degradation.

However, a key set of questions related to NF-κB and its contribution to the mechanism of action of PIs remained in the background. For instance, in the late 2000s, genomic data from MM cell lines and patient samples documented that a substantial proportion of MM exhibits loss-of-function mutations or DNA copy number losses for negative regulators of NF-κB (eg, TRAF3 and CYLD) or in some cases overexpression of positive upstream regulators of NF-κB activity.[84,85] In fact, data from these studies indicated that MM patients whose tumor cells are harboring some forms of constitutive activation of NF-κB may exhibit, when receiving PI-based therapy, higher rates of response, and longer progression-free survival compared with patients whose tumor cells lack those molecular features.[84] Still, the contribution of NF-κB inhibition to the mechanism of action of PIs remained underappreciated for an extensive period of time.

However, in retrospect, some notable nuances were worth considering. For instance, the transcriptional activity of NF-κB is shaped by the aggregate function of different members of this family and involves both a constitutive level of activity of these factors, conceivably determined by the genomic features of an individual tumor cell, and also an "inducible" component of NF-κB activity which is determined by upstream signaling mechanisms that can be triggered by external stimuli (eg, cytokines, growth factors, and interaction with stromal substrates). IKK function represents one of these upstream regulatory mechanisms of NF-κB function. Therefore, perhaps it should not have been expected that pharmacologic inhibitors of IKK, which suppress the inducible but may not completely suppress the constitutive component of NF-κB activity, must phenocopy all effects of proteasome inhibition.

Moreover, the original studies comparing the phenotypic effects of pharmacologic inhibitors of IKK versus PIs (eg, Refs[59,60]) had typically involved continuous in vitro treatment of MM cells, for example, 24 hours. However, more recent studies indicated that the in vitro assessment of response to continuous in vitro treatment with a PI for 24 hours may not be translationally relevant.[86–89] Instead, it was recommended that shorter durations of exposure and drug washout have to precede the formal evaluation of MM cell responsiveness to PIs. With these modified protocols of in vitro exposure to PIs, the MM responses were overall less pronounced and more heterogeneous.[86–89] These latter studies did not formally compare the patterns of responses of MM cells to these more translationally relevant PI exposures with those of IKK inhibitors. Therefore, it remains to be determined whether pharmacologic inhibitors upstream of NF-κB factors themselves can phenocopy the effect of brief pulses of PI treatment. More broadly, however, it is now clearer that inferring a connection (or its absence) between NF-κB transcription factors and the mechanism(s) of action of PIs simply based on the patterns of phenotypic results with extended in vitro exposures may have to be approached with caution.

The shift in MM research from an NF-κB-oriented view of the mechanism of action of PIs to an ER-stress/"proteasome load versus proteasome capacity" concept was largely stimulated by the concern that the NF-κB-oriented view could not provide a clear correlation between the baseline level of NF-κB activity and the quantitative heterogeneity of responsiveness to PI treatment in vitro or in clinical samples. It can be argued however that a similar conceptual gap may also apply, at least in part, for the "proteasome load versus capacity" concept, in the sense that there are limited, if any, clinically applicable tests that can specifically ascertain this relationship and correlate it with clinical outcomes in molecularly annotated series of patient samples. In preclinical and translational studies, extensive efforts by many groups (eg, evaluation of data sets from the Cancer Cell Line Encyclopedia effort[90]) have attempted to correlate many different types of transcriptional, proteomic, genomic, and other molecular features of cell lines in MM and beyond with the extent of in vitro responsiveness to PIs; despite extensive attempts for univariate and multivariate analyses, no definitive biomarkers, individually or in clusters, emerged to explain the variability of responses to PIs across MM cell lines. Similarly, despite extensive transcriptional profiling of purified MM tumor cells from patients participating in early clinical trials (eg, the SUMMIT and APEX studies) of the PI bortezomib in advanced MM, no definitive biomarkers correlating with response or resistance emerged.[27]

In the years that followed the initial clinical development of bortezomib, the opportunities to study patient-derived samples for potential biomarkers of response versus resistance (including biomarkers for the relative roles of ER stress or NF-κB pathway) became more limited. This was largely due to the early realization, initially pre-clinically and then in clinical studies[91,92] that PIs can be readily combined with other, established or investigational, anti-MM agents, yielding increased rates, depth and durability of clinical responses without causing unmanageable increases in the extent and severity of adverse events. Consequently, the early window of opportunity to understand the patterns of responses of MM cells based on samples from patients receiving bortezomib monotherapy (or its combination with dexamethasone) closed. This was an unavoidable collateral consequence of the pronounced therapeutic benefit associated with PI-based combinations, especially the backbone combining PIs with thalidomide derivatives.

INSIGHTS FROM FUNCTIONAL GENOMICS OF MULTIPLE MYELOMA ON THE MEDIATORS OF PROTEASOME INHIBITOR ACTIVITY

As the MM field shifted toward combined use of PIs with other pharmacologic agents (eg, glucocorticoids and thalidomide derivatives) and more recently antibody-based therapies (eg, anti-CD38 monoclonal antibodies), it can be argued that at least until recently, there was limited interest or opportunity to revisit the question of the mechanistic basis for PIs. However, new information recently emerged from CRISPR (Clustered Regularly Interspaced Short Palindromic Repeats)-based functional genomic studies to shed light into this question.

The "Tao of myeloma" review by Boise and colleagues[36] clearly vocalized the plasma cell-selective nature of the clinically successful therapies developed for MM over the last 20 years and thereby stimulated the hypothesis that a more systematic functional characterization of the molecular vulnerabilities of MM cells could not only identify essential drivers of cell-autonomous survival and proliferation of MM cells but could also determine which of these vulnerabilities are comparatively more important in MM versus other, non-plasma cell-related, hematologic malignancies or solid tumors. This motivated our laboratory and collaborators to apply CRISPR-based genome-scale gene-editing screens to identify which dependencies exhibit a pronounced and recurrent role in MM cells but are largely redundant for non-MM cells across other hematologic malignancies and in solid tumors.[35]

The results of this recently reported effort[35] led to identification of 116 MM-preferential dependencies. It was reassuring that several of those molecular vulnerabilities have established roles in the biology and therapeutic targeting of MM, including plasma cell lineage-defining transcription factors (IRF4, PRDM1, XBP1); transcription factors or kinases activated by translocations preferentially detected in MM (eg, MAF, FGFR3); and, importantly, the targets/mediators of the anti-MM activity of certain established therapies, (eg, IKZF1, IKZF3, and ARID2 as neosubstrates for thalidomide derivatives). The identification of these molecules as MM-preferential dependencies served as "positive controls" that enhanced the confidence in the biological relevance of other genes identified in this study.[35]

The identification of these MM preferential dependencies, beyond their broader biological and therapeutic implications, yielded results with direct relevance to the mechanistic basis for the anti-MM activity of PIs. Specifically, these CRISPR-based studies identified that transcription factors of the NF-κB pathway (eg, *NFKB1, RELB*), as well as the kinases *IKBKB* (IKK-β) and *CHUK* (IKK-α), which serve as upstream activators of NF-κB transcription factors, emerged as MM-preferential dependencies.[35] Notably, genes encoding other transcription factors of the NF-κB pathway, such as *RELA* and *NFKB2*, also emerged as recurrent dependencies for MM cells, even though they did not meet all formal criteria of this study for significantly more pronounced and recurrent essentiality in MM compared with non-MM tumor cells.[35]

In addition, in a manner compatible with the highly secretory nature of plasma cells, a large number of the identified MM-preferential dependencies are genes implicated in ER function. Some of these genes are coding for members of ER membrane protein complexes that mediate dislocation of misfolded proteins from the luminal side of the ER to the cytosol (eg, HERPUD1 and SEL1L). Other MM-preferential dependencies serve as ER-specific E2 Ub conjugating enzymes (eg, UBE2J1, UBE2G2); perform E3 ligase functions (SYVN1); are involved in the surveillance of quality control for luminal ER glycoproteins (eg, DPM1, ALG3, or MPDU1); participate in the chaperoning of misfolded ER proteins (eg, DNAJB11; and operate as ER stress-sensor (for instace, *ERN1*, also referred to as IRE1a [inositol-requiring enzyme 1α]) or are a target (*XBP1*) of the RNA processing activity of IRE1a. A large collection of other molecules involved in ER stress sensing or in transport of proteins from the ER to the Golgi network were also determined to be preferentially essential for MM cells. In this study, additional functional experiments with CRISPR-based approaches confirmed the biological signifi cance in vitro or in vivo for multiple genes that were previously understudied or underappreciated in MM pathophysiology but were now identified based on CRISPR studies to function as ER-associated degradation (ERAD)-associated MM preferential dependencies.[35] When the patterns of essentiality of all ER-associated genes were examined in MM versus other cancers, it was notable that a minority of these genes are "core essential" genes (functioning as dependencies for >80%–90% of cell lines across all human neoplasias) and a large proportion were essential for few, if any, cancer cell lines.[35] Several other ER-associated genes did not meet all criteria for formal classification as MM-preferential dependencies, are not broadly essential across all cancers, but are recurrently essential for many MM cell lines: this latter category included AUP1, AMFR, and RNF139 (which are involved in dislocation of misfolded ER proteins to the cytosol) and additional molecules participating in N-glycan-dependent quality control for luminal ER glycoproteins.[35]

Collectively, these observations highlighted that members of both NF-κB and ERAD pathways are prominently enriched among the genes identified as MM preferential dependencies, whereas additional members of these pathway are also identified as recurrent dependencies in MM, often with more pronounced or more recurrent essentiality in MM compared with other neoplasias.[35] It is also notable that although other neoplasias may exhibit recurrent essentiality for some members of the NF-κB pathway (eg, some forms of lymphomas) or for ERAD (eg, in some forms of solid tumors), MM was the only disease for which both NF-κB and ERAD genes emerged as prominent preferential dependencies.[35]

We interpret these results as direct functional evidence in support of the notion that the pronounced activity of PIs against plasma cell neoplasias (versus limited activity against most other tumor types) cannot be attributed to only the role of NF-κB or only the ERAD for unfolded proteins. Instead, both pathways represent important biological vulnerabilities for MM cells, given the central role of the NF-κB pathway for the survival and proliferation of the plasma cell lineage and the ERAD to protect plasma cells, malignant or not, from the proteotoxic stress associated with immunoglobulin production. Of note, these CRISPR-based studies identified ERAD-related molecules with previously underappreciated roles in MM (eg, UBE2J1, SYVN1; SEL1IL, and HER-PUD1); these molecules and their respective complexes may represent therapeutic targets in MM.

These functional genomics observations should not be interpreted to suggest that the molecular sequelae of proteasome inhibition in MM cells are related only to suppression of NF-κB activity and disruption of ERAD/induction of proteotoxic stress. The accumulation of diverse types of ubiquitinated/undegraded proteins is expected to lead to extensive molecular changes involving multiple levels of many different molecular pathways. However, the functional genomic studies of MM cells indicate that, among all possible molecular pathways that may be modulated as a result of the exposure of MM cells to PIs, the combined effect on NF-κB and ERAD function represents the most plausible explanation for why this class of pharmacologic agents has pronounced activity against MM but limited clinical applications outside the context of plasma cell dyscrasias.

CURRENT STATE AND FUTURE PERSPECTIVES ON MECHANISMS OF RESISTANCE TO PROTEASOME INHIBITORS

After 2 decades of research on pharmacologic inhibition of the proteasome, a multitude of potential mechanisms of resistance have been proposed (eg, Refs[16,93–113]), with many articles (eg, Refs[99,114–117]) summarizing this literature, yet arguably this topic remains unresolved. Several key challenges have prevented this research area from reaching definitive conclusions. For instance, it is possible that several proposed mechanisms of resistance identified through in vitro studies may not be pertinent in vivo. One such example is the identification of "gatekeeper" mutations of the PSMB5 gene, which have been reproducibly identified by several groups during the development of bortezomib-resistant MM cell lines in vitro,[104,118–122] but have not been identified in substantial numbers of patients with resistance to PI-based regimens. Increased activity of alternative pathways for protein degradation (eg, autophagy/lysosomes PI, aggresome[24,123,124]) or a state of increased tolerance to PIs due to "dedifferentiated" B-lymphocyte-like molecular state associated with decreased immunoglobulin production and suppressed proteasome "load"[79] or due to decreased expression of regulatory subunits of the 19S proteasome have been proposed[95,96] to be associated with resistance to proteasome inhibition. However, clinical information supporting these findings is still difficult to obtain, in part because clinical administration of PIs almost always involves combinations with other classes of treatments, confounding the interpretation of molecular information from the respective samples.

FUTURE PERSPECTIVES ON THE BASIC AND TRANSLATIONAL STUDIES OF PROTEASOME INHIBITION

After 2 decades of extensive preclinical, translational, and clinical studies on PIs, a wealth of information still remains to be acquired and deconvoluted regarding this class of pharmacologic agents. What are the short-term versus long-term effects of PIs on MM cells and how do these effects change when PIs are applied as monotherapy versus in combination with other treatments? Which potential biomarkers may help predict the extent of response to (or early relapse from) PI-based combination regimens? Which therapeutic strategies should be used in combination or sequentially with PIs to delay, prevent, or overcome the development of resistance? What is the precise impact of PIs on responses to established or investigational immunotherapies for MM? The first 20+ years of research on PIs have provided several important lessons, including the significance of translationally relevant in vitro and in vivo models for preclinical characterization of the performance of this drug class; the importance of functional genomics tools to dissect which molecular events correlate with versus are etiologically associated with differential responsiveness or resistance; as well as the value of large series of carefully annotated and ideally serially collected samples from patients receiving the respective treatments. These lessons remain relevant now and in the foreseeable future. The advent of new technologies for molecular and functional characterization of tumor cells provides a sense of optimism that many questions on the role of PIs in MM will in fact be answered more definitively and in a translationally actionable manner in the near future.

ACKNOWLEDGMENTS

The work of the Mitsiades Lab has been supported by grants from NIH (R01CA276156 and U01CA225730); the de Gunzburg Myeloma Research Fund; Leukemia and Lymphoma Society (LLS) Translational Research Program; Cobb Family Myeloma Research Fund, Shawna Ashlee Corman Investigatorship in Multiple Myeloma Research, Chambers Family Advanced Myeloma Research Fund; International Waldenstrom's Macroglobulinemia Foundation; and International Myeloma Society. The author apologizes in advance for the inability to reference within this article all possible studies the content of which may be relevant to the topic of this review.

COMPETING INTERESTS

C.S.M. serves on the Scientific Advisory Board of Adicet Bio and discloses consultant/honoraria from Genentech, Fate Therapeutics, Ionis Pharmaceuticals, FIMECS, Secura Bio and Oncopeptides, and research funding from Merck KGaA/EMD Serono, Karyopharm, Sanofi, Nurix, BMS, H3 Biomedicine/Eisai, Springworks, Abcuro, Novartis and OPNA.

REFERENCES

1. Singhal S, Mehta J, Desikan R, et al. Antitumor activity of thalidomide in refractory multiple myeloma. N Engl J Med 1999;341:1565–71.
2. Orlowski RZ, Stinchcombe TE, Mitchell BS, et al. Phase I trial of the proteasome inhibitor PS-341 in patients with refractory hematologic malignancies. J Clin Oncol 2002;20:4420–7.
3. Richardson PG, Barlogie B, Berenson J, et al. A phase 2 study of bortezomib in relapsed, refractory myeloma. N Engl J Med 2003;348:2609–17.

4. Richardson PG, Sonneveld P, Schuster MW, et al. Assessment of Proteasome Inhibition for Extending Remissions I. Bortezomib or high-dose dexamethasone for relapsed multiple myeloma. N Engl J Med 2005;352:2487–98.
5. Hideshima T, Richardson P, Chauhan D, et al. The proteasome inhibitor PS-341 inhibits growth, induces apoptosis, and overcomes drug resistance in human multiple myeloma cells. Cancer Res 2001;61:3071–6.
6. Adams J. Proteasome inhibition: a novel approach to cancer therapy. Trends Mol Med 2002;8:S49–54.
7. Adams J. Development of the proteasome inhibitor PS-341. Oncol 2002;7:9–16.
8. Adams J, Kauffman M. Development of the proteasome inhibitor Velcade (Bortezomib). Cancer Invest 2004;22:304–11.
9. LeBlanc R, Catley LP, Hideshima T, et al. Proteasome inhibitor PS-341 inhibits human myeloma cell growth in vivo and prolongs survival in a murine model. Cancer Res 2002;62:4996–5000.
10. Mitsiades N, Mitsiades CS, Poulaki V, et al. Molecular sequelae of proteasome inhibition in human multiple myeloma cells. Proc Natl Acad Sci U S A 2002; 99:14374–9.
11. Chesi M, Robbiani DF, Sebag M, et al. AID-dependent activation of a MYC transgene induces multiple myeloma in a conditional mouse model of post-germinal center malignancies. Cancer Cell 2008;13:167–80.
12. Chesi M, Matthews GM, Garbitt VM, et al. Drug response in a genetically engineered mouse model of multiple myeloma is predictive of clinical efficacy. Blood 2012;120:376–85.
13. Larrayoz M, Garcia-Barchino MJ, Celay J, et al. Preclinical models for prediction of immunotherapy outcomes and immune evasion mechanisms in genetically heterogeneous multiple myeloma. Nat Med 2023;29:632–45.
14. Mitsiades N, Mitsiades CS, Poulaki V, et al. Apoptotic signaling induced by immunomodulatory thalidomide analogs in human multiple myeloma cells: therapeutic implications. Blood 2002;99:4525–30.
15. Hideshima T, Chauhan D, Ishitsuka K, et al. Molecular characterization of PS-341 (bortezomib) resistance: implications for overcoming resistance using lysophosphatidic acid acyltransferase (LPAAT)-beta inhibitors. Oncogene 2005;24: 3121–9.
16. Sharma A, Nair R, Achreja A, et al. Therapeutic implications of mitochondrial stress-induced proteasome inhibitor resistance in multiple myeloma. Sci Adv 2022;8:eabq5575.
17. Gu Y, Barwick BG, Shanmugam M, et al. Downregulation of PA28alpha induces proteasome remodeling and results in resistance to proteasome inhibitors in multiple myeloma. Blood Cancer J 2020;10:125.
18. Catley L, Weisberg E, Tai YT, et al. NVP-LAQ824 is a potent novel histone deacetylase inhibitor with significant activity against multiple myeloma. Blood 2003; 102:2615–22.
19. Chauhan D, Li G, Shringarpure R, et al. Blockade of Hsp27 overcomes Bortezomib/proteasome inhibitor PS-341 resistance in lymphoma cells. Cancer Res 2003;63:6174–7.
20. Hideshima T, Chauhan D, Hayashi T, et al. Proteasome inhibitor PS-341 abrogates IL-6 triggered signaling cascades via caspase-dependent downregulation of gp130 in multiple myeloma. Oncogene 2003;22:8386–93.
21. Mitsiades N, Mitsiades CS, Richardson PG, et al. The proteasome inhibitor PS-341 potentiates sensitivity of multiple myeloma cells to conventional chemotherapeutic agents: therapeutic applications. Blood 2003;101:2377–80.

22. Chauhan D, Li G, Podar K, et al. Targeting mitochondria to overcome conventional and bortezomib/proteasome inhibitor PS-341 resistance in multiple myeloma (MM) cells. Blood 2004;104:2458–66.
23. Chauhan D, Li G, Podar K, et al. The bortezomib/proteasome inhibitor PS-341 and triterpenoid CDDO-Im induce synergistic anti-multiple myeloma (MM) activity and overcome bortezomib resistance. Blood 2004;103:3158–66.
24. Catley L, Weisberg E, Kiziltepe T, et al. Aggresome induction by proteasome inhibitor bortezomib and alpha-tubulin hyperacetylation by tubulin deacetylase (TDAC) inhibitor LBH589 are synergistic in myeloma cells. Blood 2006;108: 3441–9.
25. Garcia-Gomez A, Quwaider D, Canavese M, et al. Preclinical activity of the oral proteasome inhibitor MLN9708 in Myeloma bone disease. Clin Cancer Res 2014;20:1542–54.
26. Mulligan G, Lichter DI, Di Bacco A, et al. Mutation of NRAS but not KRAS significantly reduces myeloma sensitivity to single-agent bortezomib therapy. Blood 2014;123:632–9.
27. Mulligan G, Mitsiades C, Bryant B, et al. Gene expression profiling and correlation with outcome in clinical trials of the proteasome inhibitor bortezomib. Blood 2007;109:3177–88.
28. Chng WJ, Kumar S, Vanwier S, et al. Molecular dissection of hyperdiploid multiple myeloma by gene expression profiling. Cancer Res 2007;67:2982–9.
29. Jakubowiak A, Usmani SZ, Krishnan A, et al. Daratumumab Plus Carfilzomib, Lenalidomide, and Dexamethasone in Patients With Newly Diagnosed Multiple Myeloma. Clin Lymphoma Myeloma Leuk 2021;21:701–10.
30. Jakubowiak AJ, Dytfeld D, Griffith KA, et al. A phase 1/2 study of carfilzomib in combination with lenalidomide and low-dose dexamethasone as a frontline treatment for multiple myeloma. Blood 2012;120:1801–9.
31. Jakubowiak AJ, Jasielec JK, Rosenbaum CA, et al. Phase 1 study of selinexor plus carfilzomib and dexamethasone for the treatment of relapsed/refractory multiple myeloma. Br J Haematol 2019;186:549–60.
32. Jakubowiak AJ, Siegel DS, Martin T, et al. Treatment outcomes in patients with relapsed and refractory multiple myeloma and high-risk cytogenetics receiving single-agent carfilzomib in the PX-171-003-A1 study. Leukemia 2013;27: 2351–6.
33. Costa LJ, Davies FE, Monohan GP, et al. Phase 2 study of venetoclax plus carfilzomib and dexamethasone in patients with relapsed/refractory multiple myeloma. Blood Adv 2021;5:3748–59.
34. Derman BA, Zonder J, Reece D, et al. Phase 1/2 study of carfilzomib, pomalidomide, and dexamethasone with and without daratumumab in relapsed multiple myeloma. Blood Adv 2023;7:5703–12.
35. de Matos Simoes R, Shirasaki R, Downey-Kopyscinski SL, et al. Genome-scale functional genomics identify genes preferentially essential for multiple myeloma cells compared to other neoplasias. Nat Cancer 2023;4:754–73.
36. Boise LH, Kaufman JL, Bahlis NJ, et al. The Tao of myeloma. Blood 2014;124: 1873–9.
37. Finley D. Recognition and processing of ubiquitin-protein conjugates by the proteasome. Annu Rev Biochem 2009;78:477–513.
38. Goldberg AL. Protein degradation and protection against misfolded or damaged proteins. Nature 2003;426:895–9.
39. Goldberg AL, Dice JF. Intracellular protein degradation in mammalian and bacterial cells. Annu Rev Biochem 1974;43:835–69.

40. Pohl C, Dikic I. Cellular quality control by the ubiquitin-proteasome system and autophagy. Science 2019;366:818–22.
41. Kannt A, Dikic I. Expanding the arsenal of E3 ubiquitin ligases for proximity-induced protein degradation. Cell Chem Biol 2021;28:1014–31.
42. Cable J, Weber-Ban E, Clausen T, et al. Targeted protein degradation: from small molecules to complex organelles-a Keystone Symposia report. Ann N Y Acad Sci 2022;1510:79–99.
43. Dikic I, Schulman BA. An expanded lexicon for the ubiquitin code. Nat Rev Mol Cell Biol 2023;24:273–87.
44. Berndsen CE, Wolberger C. New insights into ubiquitin E3 ligase mechanism. Nat Struct Mol Biol 2014;21:301–7.
45. Adams J. The proteasome: structure, function, and role in the cell. Cancer Treat Rev 2003;29(Suppl 1):3–9.
46. Dong Y, Zhang S, Wu Z, et al. Cryo-EM structures and dynamics of substrate-engaged human 26S proteasome. Nature 2019;565:49–55.
47. Murata S, Takahama Y, Kasahara M, et al. The immunoproteasome and thymo-proteasome: functions, evolution and human disease. Nat Immunol 2018;19:923–31.
48. Herndon TM, Deisseroth A, Kaminskas E, et al. Food and Drug Administration approval: carfilzomib for the treatment of multiple myeloma. Clin Cancer Res 2013;19:4559–63.
49. Landgren O, Sonneveld P, Jakubowiak A, et al. Carfilzomib with immunomodu-latory drugs for the treatment of newly diagnosed multiple myeloma. Leukemia 2019;33:2127–43.
50. Chim CS, Kumar SK, Orlowski RZ, et al. Management of relapsed and refractory multiple myeloma: novel agents, antibodies, immunotherapies and beyond. Leukemia 2018;32:252–62.
51. Wang J, Fang Y, Fan RA, et al. Proteasome Inhibitors and Their Pharmacokinetics, Pharmacodynamics, and Metabolism. Int J Mol Sci 2021;22.
52. Voorhees PM, Orlowski RZ. The proteasome and proteasome inhibitors in cancer therapy. Annu Rev Pharmacol Toxicol 2006;46:189–213.
53. Elliott PJ, Ross JS. The proteasome: a new target for novel drug therapies. Am J Clin Pathol 2001;116:637–46.
54. Kisselev AF. Site-Specific Proteasome Inhibitors. Biomolecules 2021;12.
55. Fogli S, Galimberti S, Gori V, et al. Pharmacology differences among proteasome inhibitors: Implications for their use in clinical practice. Pharmacol Res 2021;167:105537.
56. Fricker LD. Proteasome Inhibitor Drugs. Annu Rev Pharmacol Toxicol 2020;60:457–76.
57. Wang Z, Yang J, Kirk C, et al. Clinical pharmacokinetics, metabolism, and drug-drug interaction of carfilzomib. Drug Metab Dispos 2013;41:230–7.
58. Besse A, Besse L, Kraus M, et al. Proteasome Inhibition in Multiple Myeloma: Head-to-Head Comparison of Currently Available Proteasome Inhibitors. Cell Chem Biol 2019;26:340–351 e343.
59. Obeng EA, Carlson LM, Gutman DM, et al. Proteasome inhibitors induce a terminal unfolded protein response in multiple myeloma cells. Blood 2006;107:4907–16.
60. Hideshima T, Chauhan D, Richardson P, et al. NF-kappa B as a therapeutic target in multiple myeloma. J Biol Chem 2002;277:16639–47.

61. Bianchi G, Oliva L, Cascio P, et al. The proteasome load versus capacity balance determines apoptotic sensitivity of multiple myeloma cells to proteasome inhibition. Blood 2009;113:3040–9.

62. Cenci S, Mezghrani A, Cascio P, et al. Progressively impaired proteasomal capacity during terminal plasma cell differentiation. EMBO J 2006;25:1104–13.

63. Masciarelli S, Fra AM, Pengo N, et al. CHOP-independent apoptosis and pathway-selective induction of the UPR in developing plasma cells. Mol Immunol 2010;47:1356–65.

64. Cenci S. The proteasome in terminal plasma cell differentiation. Semin Hematol 2012;49:215–22.

65. Pengo N, Scolari M, Oliva L, et al. Plasma cells require autophagy for sustainable immunoglobulin production. Nat Immunol 2013;14:298–305.

66. Carpenter RO, Evbuomwan MO, Pittaluga S, et al. B-cell maturation antigen is a promising target for adoptive T-cell therapy of multiple myeloma. Clin Cancer Res 2013;19:2048–60.

67. Ali SA, Shi V, Maric I, et al. T cells expressing an anti-B-cell maturation antigen chimeric antigen receptor cause remissions of multiple myeloma. Blood 2016; 128:1688–700.

68. Brudno JN, Maric I, Hartman SD, et al. T Cells Genetically Modified to Express an Anti-B-Cell Maturation Antigen Chimeric Antigen Receptor Cause Remissions of Poor-Prognosis Relapsed Multiple Myeloma. J Clin Oncol 2018;36: 2267–80.

69. Raje N, Berdeja J, Lin Y, et al. Anti-BCMA CAR T-Cell Therapy bb2121 in Relapsed or Refractory Multiple Myeloma. N Engl J Med 2019;380:1726–37.

70. Cappell KM, Kochenderfer JN. Long-term outcomes following CAR T cell therapy: what we know so far. Nat Rev Clin Oncol 2023;20:359–71.

71. Lin Y, Raje NS, Berdeja JG, et al. Idecabtagene vicleucel for relapsed and refractory multiple myeloma: post hoc 18-month follow-up of a phase 1 trial. Nat Med 2023;29:2286–94.

72. Ramadoss NS, Schulman AD, Choi SH, et al. An anti-B cell maturation antigen bispecific antibody for multiple myeloma. J Am Chem Soc 2015;137:5288–91.

73. Usmani SZ, Garfall AL, van de Donk N, et al. Teclistamab, a B-cell maturation antigen x CD3 bispecific antibody, in patients with relapsed or refractory multiple myeloma (MajesTEC-1): a multicentre, open-label, single-arm, phase 1 study. Lancet 2021;398:665–74.

74. Bahlis NJ, Costello CL, Raje NS, et al. Elranatamab in relapsed or refractory multiple myeloma: the MagnetisMM-1 phase 1 trial. Nat Med 2023;29:2570–6.

75. Lesokhin AM, Tomasson MH, Arnulf B, et al. Elranatamab in relapsed or refractory multiple myeloma: phase 2 MagnetisMM-3 trial results. Nat Med 2023;29: 2259–67.

76. Atamaniuk J, Gleiss A, Porpaczy E, et al. Overexpression of G protein-coupled receptor 5D in the bone marrow is associated with poor prognosis in patients with multiple myeloma. Eur J Clin Invest 2012;42:953–60.

77. Kodama T, Kochi Y, Nakai W, et al. Anti-GPRC5D/CD3 Bispecific T-Cell-Redirecting Antibody for the Treatment of Multiple Myeloma. Mol Cancer Ther 2019;18: 1555–64.

78. Smith EL, Harrington K, Staehr M, et al. GPRC5D is a target for the immunotherapy of multiple myeloma with rationally designed CAR T cells. Sci Transl Med 2019;11.

79. Leung-Hagesteijn C, Erdmann N, Cheung G, et al. Xbp1s-negative tumor B cells and pre-plasmablasts mediate therapeutic proteasome inhibitor resistance in multiple myeloma. Cancer Cell 2013;24:289–304.

80. Neubert K, Meister S, Moser K, et al. The proteasome inhibitor bortezomib depletes plasma cells and protects mice with lupus-like disease from nephritis. Nat Med 2008;14:748–55.

81. Walhelm T, Gunnarsson I, Heijke R, et al. Clinical Experience of Proteasome Inhibitor Bortezomib Regarding Efficacy and Safety in Severe Systemic Lupus Erythematosus: A Nationwide Study. Front Immunol 2021;12:756941.

82. Sjowall C, Hjorth M, Eriksson P. Successful treatment of refractory systemic lupus erythematosus using proteasome inhibitor bortezomib followed by belimumab: description of two cases. Lupus 2017;26:1333–8.

83. Alexander T, Sarfert R, Klotsche J, et al. The proteasome inhibitior bortezomib depletes plasma cells and ameliorates clinical manifestations of refractory systemic lupus erythematosus. Ann Rheum Dis 2015;74:1474–8.

84. Keats JJ, Fonseca R, Chesi M, et al. Promiscuous mutations activate the noncanonical NF-kappaB pathway in multiple myeloma. Cancer Cell 2007;12:131–44.

85. Annunziata CM, Davis RE, Demchenko Y, et al. Frequent engagement of the classical and alternative NF-kappaB pathways by diverse genetic abnormalities in multiple myeloma. Cancer Cell 2007;12:115–30.

86. Shabaneh TB, Downey SL, Goddard AL, et al. Molecular basis of differential sensitivity of myeloma cells to clinically relevant bolus treatment with bortezomib. PLoS One 2013;8:e56132.

87. Downey-Kopyscinski S, Daily EW, Gautier M, et al. An inhibitor of proteasome beta2 sites sensitizes myeloma cells to immunoproteasome inhibitors. Blood Adv 2018;2:2443–51.

88. Chen T, Ho M, Briere J, et al. Multiple myeloma cells depend on the DDI2/NRF1-mediated proteasome stress response for survival. Blood Adv 2022;6:429–40.

89. Downey-Kopyscinski SL, Srinivasa S, Kisselev AF. A clinically relevant pulse treatment generates a bortezomib-resistant myeloma cell line that lacks proteasome mutations and is sensitive to Bcl-2 inhibitor venetoclax. Sci Rep 2022;12:12788.

90. Barretina J, Caponigro G, Stransky N, et al. The Cancer Cell Line Encyclopedia enables predictive modelling of anticancer drug sensitivity. Nature 2012;483:603–7.

91. Richardson PG, Weller E, Jagannath S, et al. Multicenter, phase I, dose-escalation trial of lenalidomide plus bortezomib for relapsed and relapsed/refractory multiple myeloma. J Clin Oncol 2009;27:5713–9.

92. Richardson PG, Xie W, Jagannath S, et al. A phase 2 trial of lenalidomide, bortezomib, and dexamethasone in patients with relapsed and relapsed/refractory myeloma. Blood 2014;123:1461–9.

93. Franke NE, Niewerth D, Assaraf YG, et al. Impaired bortezomib binding to mutant beta5 subunit of the proteasome is the underlying basis for bortezomib resistance in leukemia cells. Leukemia 2012;26:757–68.

94. Meng L, Carpenter K, Mollard A, et al. Inhibition of Nek2 by small molecules affects proteasome activity. BioMed Res Int 2014;2014:273180.

95. Acosta-Alvear D, Cho MY, Wild T, et al. Paradoxical resistance of multiple myeloma to proteasome inhibitors by decreased levels of 19S proteasomal subunits. Elife 2015;4:e08153.

96. Tsvetkov P, Sokol E, Jin D, et al. Suppression of 19S proteasome subunits marks emergence of an altered cell state in diverse cancers. Proc Natl Acad Sci U S A 2017;114:382–7.

97. Tsvetkov P, Detappe A, Cai K, et al. Mitochondrial metabolism promotes adaptation to proteotoxic stress. Nat Chem Biol 2019;15:681–9.

98. Wallington-Beddoe CT, Sobieraj-Teague M, Kuss BJ, et al. Resistance to proteasome inhibitors and other targeted therapies in myeloma. Br J Haematol 2018; 182:11–28.

99. Gonzalez-Santamarta M, Quinet G, Reyes-Garau D, et al. Resistance to the Proteasome Inhibitors: Lessons from Multiple Myeloma and Mantle Cell Lymphoma. Adv Exp Med Biol 2020;1233:153–74.

100. Besse L, Besse A, Mendez-Lopez M, et al. A metabolic switch in proteasome inhibitor-resistant multiple myeloma ensures higher mitochondrial metabolism, protein folding and sphingomyelin synthesis. Haematologica 2019;104:e415–9.

101. Besse A, Stolze SC, Rasche L, et al. Carfilzomib resistance due to ABCB1/ MDR1 overexpression is overcome by nelfinavir and lopinavir in multiple myeloma. Leukemia 2018;32:391–401.

102. Farrell ML, Reagan MR. Soluble and Cell-Cell-Mediated Drivers of Proteasome Inhibitor Resistance in Multiple Myeloma. Front Endocrinol 2018;9:218.

103. Meul T, Berschneider K, Schmitt S, et al. Mitochondrial Regulation of the 26S Proteasome. Cell Rep 2020;32:108059.

104. Allmeroth K, Horn M, Kroef V, et al. Bortezomib resistance mutations in PSMB5 determine response to second-generation proteasome inhibitors in multiple myeloma. Leukemia 2021;35:887–92.

105. Leonardo-Sousa C, Carvalho AN, Guedes RA, et al. Revisiting Proteasome Inhibitors: Molecular Underpinnings of Their Development, Mechanisms of Resistance and Strategies to Overcome Anti-Cancer Drug Resistance. Molecules 2022;27.

106. Ferguson ID, Lin YT, Lam C, et al. Allosteric HSP70 inhibitors perturb mitochondrial proteostasis and overcome proteasome inhibitor resistance in multiple myeloma. Cell Chem Biol 2022;29:1288–302.e7.

107. Haertle L, Buenache N, Cuesta Hernandez HN, et al. Genetic Alterations in Members of the Proteasome 26S Subunit, AAA-ATPase (PSMC) Gene Family in the Light of Proteasome Inhibitor Resistance in Multiple Myeloma. Cancers 2023;15.

108. Haertle L, Barrio S, Munawar U, et al. Single-Nucleotide Variants and Epimutations Induce Proteasome Inhibitor Resistance in Multiple Myeloma. Clin Cancer Res 2023;29:279–88.

109. Wang Q, Zhao D, Xian M, et al. MIF as a biomarker and therapeutic target for overcoming resistance to proteasome inhibitors in human myeloma. Blood 2020;136:2557–73.

110. Wang Q, Shinkre BA, Lee JG, et al. The ERAD inhibitor Eeyarestatin I is a bifunctional compound with a membrane-binding domain and a p97/VCP inhibitory group. PLoS One 2010;5:e15479.

111. Wang Q, Mora-Jensen H, Weniger MA, et al. ERAD inhibitors integrate ER stress with an epigenetic mechanism to activate BH3-only protein NOXA in cancer cells. Proc Natl Acad Sci U S A 2009;106:2200–5.

112. Darawshi O, Muz B, Naamat SG, et al. An mTORC1 to HRI signaling axis promotes cytotoxicity of proteasome inhibitors in multiple myeloma. Cell Death Dis 2022;13:969.

113. Cohen YC, Zada M, Wang SY, et al. Identification of resistance pathways and therapeutic targets in relapsed multiple myeloma patients through single-cell sequencing. Nat Med 2021;27:491–503.
114. McConkey DJ, Zhu K. Mechanisms of proteasome inhibitor action and resistance in cancer. Drug Resist Updat 2008;11:164–79.
115. Niewerth D, Jansen G, Assaraf YG, et al. Molecular basis of resistance to proteasome inhibitors in hematological malignancies. Drug Resist Updat 2015;18: 18–35.
116. Bo Kim K. Proteasomal adaptations to FDA-approved proteasome inhibitors: a potential mechanism for drug resistance? Cancer Drug Resist 2021;4:634–45.
117. Patino-Escobar B, Talbot A, Wiita AP. Overcoming proteasome inhibitor resistance in the immunotherapy era. Trends Pharmacol Sci 2023;44:507–18.
118. Barrio S, Stuhmer T, Da-Via M, et al. Spectrum and functional validation of PSMB5 mutations in multiple myeloma. Leukemia 2019;33:447–56.
119. Cloos J, Roeten MS, Franke NE, et al. (Immuno)proteasomes as therapeutic target in acute leukemia. Cancer Metastasis Rev 2017;36:599–615.
120. Verbrugge SE, Assaraf YG, Dijkmans BA, et al. Inactivating PSMB5 mutations and P-glycoprotein (multidrug resistance-associated protein/ATP-binding cassette B1) mediate resistance to proteasome inhibitors: ex vivo efficacy of (immuno)proteasome inhibitors in mononuclear blood cells from patients with rheumatoid arthritis. J Pharmacol Exp Ther 2012;341:174–82.
121. Ri M, Iida S, Nakashima T, et al. Bortezomib-resistant myeloma cell lines: a role for mutated PSMB5 in preventing the accumulation of unfolded proteins and fatal ER stress. Leukemia 2010;24:1506–12.
122. Oerlemans R, Franke NE, Assaraf YG, et al. Molecular basis of bortezomib resistance: proteasome subunit beta5 (PSMB5) gene mutation and overexpression of PSMB5 protein. Blood 2008;112:2489–99.
123. Hideshima T, Bradner JE, Wong J, et al. Small-molecule inhibition of proteasome and aggresome function induces synergistic antitumor activity in multiple myeloma. Proc Natl Acad Sci U S A 2005;102:8567–72.
124. Nawrocki ST, Carew JS, Pino MS, et al. Aggresome disruption: a novel strategy to enhance bortezomib-induced apoptosis in pancreatic cancer cells. Cancer Res 2006;66:3773–81.

Monoclonal Antibodies in the Treatment of Multiple Myeloma

Niels W.C.J. van de Donk, MD, PhD[a,b,*],
Sonja Zweegman, MD, PhD[a,b]

KEYWORDS

- Monoclonal antibody • Myeloma • CD38 • SLAMF7 • BCMA • Daratumumab
- Isatuximab • Elotuzumab

KEY POINTS

- The incorporation of naked antibodies into myeloma treatment has improved the survival of patients with this disease.
- Elotuzumab has no single-agent activity, but the combination of elotuzumab plus immunomodulatory drugs (IMiD)/dexamethasone is superior to IMiD/dexamethasone alone.
- CD38-targeting antibodies (daratumumab/isatuximab) have single-agent activity.
- Addition of a CD38-targeting antibody to a backbone regimen improves response rate and progression-free survival, and in some studies with longer follow-up also overall survival, both in newly diagnosed patients and in patients with relapsed/refractory disease.

INTRODUCTION

The incorporation of immunomodulatory drugs (IMiDs; lenalidomide and pomalidomide) and proteasome inhibitors (bortezomib, ixazomib, and carfilzomib) in the treatment of multiple myeloma (MM) has significantly improved the survival of patients with both newly diagnosed and relapsed/refractory MM.[1] In addition, during the last decade, naked monoclonal antibodies significantly changed the treatment landscape of MM(2). The naked CD38-targeting antibody daratumumab was initially approved as a monotherapy for patients with heavily pretreated disease, but soon thereafter large studies showed that CD38-targeting antibodies (daratumumab and isatuximab) are good partner drugs with a favorable safety profile. Although the SLAMF7-targeting antibody elotuzumab has no single-agent activity, it markedly enhances the activity of IMiD-based regimens in patients with relapsed/refractory MM. Combination therapies

[a] Department of Hematology, Amsterdam UMC, Vrije Universiteit Amsterdam, De Boelelaan 1117, Amsterdam 1081 HV, the Netherlands; [b] Cancer Center Amsterdam, Cancer Biology and Immunology, Amsterdam, the Netherlands
* Corresponding author.
E-mail address: n.vandedonk@amsterdamumc.nl

Hematol Oncol Clin N Am 38 (2024) 337–360
https://doi.org/10.1016/j.hoc.2023.12.002
0889-8588/24/© 2023 Elsevier Inc. All rights reserved.

hemonc.theclinics.com

were initially evaluated in patients with relapsed/refractory disease, but soon thereafter also in the newly diagnosed setting with promising results of CD38-targeting antibody-based regimens in transplant-eligible (TE) patients as well as in elderly patients. Here, the authors will provide an overview of the activity, safety profile, and management of monoclonal antibodies for the treatment of MM.

CD38-TARGETING ANTIBODIES
Mode of Action

CD38 is highly expressed on normal and malignant plasma cells, but also on subsets of other immune cells. Next to expression in the hematopoietic system, it is also expressed at low levels in other tissues of non-hematopoietic origin including prostatic epithelial cells, pancreatic islet cells, as well as in the perikaryon and dendrites of some neurons. Other CD38-positive cells include airway-striated muscle cells, renal tubules, retinal gangliar cells, and corneal cells.[2] CD38 functions as a receptor for CD31 and also has ectoenzymatic activities (NADase).[3] CD38-targeting antibodies have direct on-tumor activities including complement-dependent cytotoxity (CDC), antibody-dependent cell-mediated cytotoxicity (ADCC), antibody-dependent cellular phagocytosis (ADCP), apoptosis induction upon Fcγ receptor cross-linking, and direct induction of apoptosis (**Fig. 1**).[2–7] Next to these Fc-dependent immune effector mechanisms, CD38-targeting antibodies also have immunomodulatory effects including elimination of CD38-positive regulatory T-cells, regulatory B-cells, and myeloid-derived suppressor cells, which is followed by an increase in T-cells with enhanced killing capacity (see **Fig. 1**).[8–10] CD38-targeting antibodies also modulate the enzymatic function of the CD38 molecule (see **Fig. 1**).[11]

There are currently 2 CD38-targeting antibodies approved for the treatment of MM: the fully human IgG1-kappa antibody daratumumab and the humanized IgG1-kappa isatuximab.

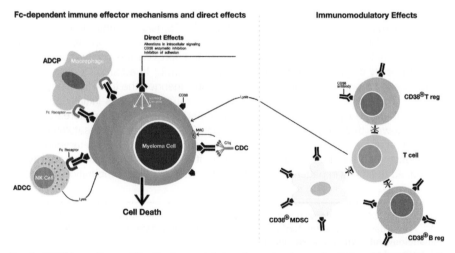

Fig. 1. CD38-targeting antibodies have pleiotropic mechanisms of action, which can be subdivided into Fc-dependent immune effector mechanisms, direct effects, and immunomodulatory effects. (*From* van de Donk N, Richardson PG, Malavasi F. CD38 antibodies in multiple myeloma: back to the future. Blood. 2018;131(1):13-29; with permission (Figure 2A in original).[2])

Daratumumab induces superior CDC, compared to isatuximab, while isatuximab has more potent direct anti-MM activity.[2–7] Extent of ADCC, ADCP, and cell death in the presence of Fc receptor cross-linking is similar when comparing daratumumab and isatuximab in *in vitro* assays.[12]

Because IMiDs have potent immune-stimulating properties including enhancement of natural killer (NK) cell function,[13,14] these drugs are potent partner drugs for CD38-targeting antibodies. Indeed, in preclinical experiments, IMiDs synergistically enhanced daratumumab-mediated MM lysis through activation of NK cells.[15] This formed the rationale for several clinical studies that evaluated the combination of a CD38-targeting antibody in combination with lenalidomide or pomalidomide (see below). Preclinical studies also showed that the efficacy of CD38-targeting antibodies can be enhanced by proteasome inhibitors.[15–17]

Resistance to CD38-Targeting Antibodies

Resistance to CD38-targeting antibodies is multifactorial and includes the upregulation of complement inhibitory proteins on the tumor cell surface, NK cell depletion, NK cell exhaustion, and downregulation of the target protein.[18–21] Bone marrow stromal cells also confer resistance to CD38-targeting antibodies.[22] Although poor risk conferred by high-risk cytogenetic abnormalities is not completely abrogated by adding a CD38-targeting antibody to the backbone regimen, patients with high-risk cytogenetic abnormalities also benefit from CD38-targeting antibodies.[23–27] However, the survival of patients with 2 or more high-risk cytogenetic abnormalities (double-hit MM) remains very poor also with CD38-targeting antibody-based therapy.[28–30]

Single-Agent Activity

In 2008, the first MM patient was treated with a very low-dose of daratumumab in the first-in-human phase 1 GEN501 study. This study, together with the SIRIUS trial, showed that daratumumab has single-agent activity with an overall response rate of 30% in heavily pretreated patients (87% double-refractory).[31–33] Isatuximab also has single-agent activity in patients with a median of 4 prior therapy lines (overall response rate: 23.9%). Addition of dexamethasone to isatuximab increased the response rate to 43.6%.[34]

Importantly, the subcutaneous formulation of daratumumab is equally effective, compared to the intravenous formulation, but the frequency of infusion-related reactions is markedly lower (13% with subcutaneous administration vs 34% with intravenous daratumumab).[35] An additional benefit of the subcutaneous formulation is that the administration duration is significantly shorter, which is important for patients as well as the organization of the outpatient clinic.[35] The randomized phase 3 IRAKLIA study is evaluating whether subcutaneous isatuximab has a comparable activity and safety profile as intravenous isatuximab, both being combined with pomalidomide-dexamethasone.

Specific Management Issues with CD38-Targeting Antibodies

Infusion-related reactions
Intravenous administration of CD38-targeting antibodies is frequently associated with the occurrence of infusion-related reactions, typically during the first infusion (**Fig. 2**). Symptoms include nasal congestion, cough, chills, and nausea.[31] Premedication with steroids, anti-histamine, and acetaminophen mitigates the severity of infusion-related reactions. Also montelukast, a leukotriene receptor antagonist, probably reduces the frequency and severity of infusion-related reactions. In case an infusion-related reaction develops, management consists of extra anti-histamines or corticosteroids (and

Management Aspect	Applicable to	Management and Developments
Administration -Duration of infusion -Infusion-related reactions	All antibodies	Appropriate pre- and post-infusion medication; subcutaneous administration of daratumumab
Interference of therapeutic antibody with SPEP/IFE assays	All antibodies but dependent on plasma concentrations	Shift assays; mass spectrometry
Auto-immune adverse events	PD-1/PD-L1 neutralizing antibodies (not observed with CD38 antibodies)	Institution of appropriate treatment (including prompt treatment with prednisone)
Interference with blood transfusion tests	CD38-targeting antibodies (and CD44-targeting antibodies)	DTT, anti-idiotype, serotyping/genotyping before start therapy; provide patients with blood transfusion card
Infections	Dependent on antibody type and other drugs in combination regiments	Herpes zoster prophylaxis is recommended for CD38 antibodies

Fig. 2. Practical aspects of management of monoclonal antibody-based therapy in MM. (*From* van de Donk N, Richardson PG, Malavasi F. CD38 antibodies in multiple myeloma: back to the future. Blood. 2018;131(1):13-29; with permission (Figure 3 in original).[2])

interruption of the intravenous infusion).[2] However, maybe most important is the observation that with subcutaneous administration of daratumumab the frequency of infusion-related reactions is markedly reduced.[35,36]

Interference with laboratory-based blood group compatibility tests
Red blood cells also express low levels of CD38, and this explains why patients treated with CD38-targeting antibodies have pan-reactive indirect antiglobulin tests on antibody screens (see **Fig. 2**).[2,37] The interference of CD38-targeting antibodies with routine methods for compatibility testing for blood transfusions may cause delays in the delivery of compatible blood products, as underlying allo-antibodies cannot be detected. Mitigation methods that can be used by blood banks to safely and timely provide blood products include red blood cell phenotyping or genotyping in patients who will be treated with a CD38-targeting antibody. In case of a blood transfusion, phenotypically or genotypically matched red blood cell units should be given to the patient. Other less frequently used strategies include the application of dithiothreitol which denatures CD38 on test red blood cells, or the neutralization of the CD38-targeting antibody in serum obtained from the patient.[2]

Interference with response evaluation assays (serum protein electrophoresis /immune fixation electrophoresis)
Therapeutic antibodies can interfere with response assessment (serum protein electrophoresis [SPEP]/serum immune fixation electrophoresis [IFE]) because these drugs can be detected in these assays as a monoclonal band (see **Fig. 2**).[38] This mainly causes confusion when the M-protein has the same heavy-chain and light-chain isotype as the therapeutic antibody (daratumumab, isatuximab, and elotuzumab are all IgG-kappa antibodies), and also migrates into the same region.[2] In this situation,

the 2 bands cannot be discriminated from each other, without the use of additional techniques, such as the commercially available daratumumab shift assay (daratumumab-specific IFE reflex assay; DIRA).[2] In clinical studies with isatuximab or elotuzumab, this issue may lead to underestimation of complete response rates because of limited availability for novel assays that adjust for isatuximab or elotuzumab interference in M-protein measurement by standard immunofixation assays.[39–41]

Combination Therapy with a CD38-Targeting Antibody

Daratumumab is mostly used in combination with other agents because several studies have clearly shown that this strategy results in improved clinical outcomes including response, PFS and, in some studies with longer follow-up, also OS(2). The rate of minimal residual disease (MRD)-negativity was also higher with CD38-targeting antibody combination regimens compared to those without.[39,42] Achieving MRD-negative status is relevant because this translates into improved PFS, compared to patients who remain MRD-positive.[39,42] Based on these results, various daratumumab and isatuximab-based combinations are currently approved for the treatment of patients with newly diagnosed or relapsed/refractory MM.

CD38-Targeting Antibodies in Newly Diagnosed Multiple Myeloma

Both in non-transplant eligible (NTE) and transplant eligible (TE) newly diagnosed MM, daratumumab-based triplet and quadruplets are highly effective, FDA and EMA-approved, treatment regimens, with significantly improved response rate and PFS, compared to regimens without daratumumab.[24–27,43–45] In the studies with longer follow-up also, OS benefit was observed with daratumumab-containing regimens.[24,43]

Non-transplant eligible newly diagnosed multiple myeloma

In NTE newly diagnosed MM patients, it was shown that treatment with daratumumab in combination with bortezomib-melphalan-prednisone (VMP) resulted in a superior PFS as compared to VMP (median PFS: 36.4 vs 19.3 months).[24,25] Pre-specified subgroup analysis showed that superiority was irrespective of age, International Staging System (ISS) disease stage, and renal impairment. With longer follow-up, OS was also superior with daratumumab-VMP (OS at 36-months: 78.0% vs 67.9% with VMP), with the caveat that at the time of publication only 8% of patients who relapsed following VMP received daratumumab-based therapy.[24] The incidence of severe grade 3 and 4 side effects was comparable, with the exception of infections which occurred more frequent in patients treated with daratumumab-VMP, compared to VMP (23.1% vs 14.7%, with pneumonia in 11.3% vs 4.0%).[25]

The MAIA trial showed that daratumumab in combination with lenalidomide-dexamethasone resulted in a superior PFS, when compared to lenalidomide-dexamethasone in patients with NTE newly diagnosed MM (median PFS: not reached [52.2% of patients alive and free of progression at 60 months] vs 34.4 months).[26,43] All subgroups experienced benefit from adding daratumumab to the lenalidomide-dexamethasone backbone. At a median follow-up of 56.2 months, the median OS has not been reached in both arms, however, OS was superior with daratumumab-lenalidomide-dexamethasone, compared to lenalidomide-dexamethasone (60-month OS: 66.3% vs 53.1%). Prespecified subgroup analysis showed that superiority in OS with daratumumab-lenalidomide-dexamethasone was consistent across subgroups and irrespective of age, ISS disease stage, and renal impairment.[43]

With daratumumab-lenalidomide-dexamethasone, there was a higher incidence of neutropenia (50% vs 35.3%), infections (32.1% vs 23.3%), pneumonia (13.7% vs 7.9%), and fatigue (8% vs 3.8%) as compared to lenalidomide-dexamethasone.[26]

In both studies, the impact of the level of frailty on clinical outcomes has been investigated.[46,47] This is of importance as the median age of MM patients is 70 years and approximately half of the patients are defined frail according to the International Myeloma Frailty Index (IMWG-FI). This index classifies patients as fit, intermediate fit, and frail based on age, comorbidities, and activities of daily living.[48] Although in both studies the PFS was inferior in frail versus non-frail patients, it was found that also frail patients experienced benefit from the addition of daratumumab to VMP or lenalidomide-dexamethasone.[46,47] In the ALCYONE trial, the median PFS in non-frail patients was 45.7 months with daratumumab-VMP versus 19.1 months with VMP. Accordingly, in frail patients, a longer PFS was achieved with daratumumab-VMP versus VMP alone (median PFS: 32.9 vs 19.5 months).[46] In the MAIA trial, the median PFS in non-frail patients was significantly longer with daratumumab-lenalidomide-dexamethasone; not reached versus 41.7 months with lenalidomide-dexamethasone.[47] Likewise, in the frail patients, the addition of daratumumab prolonged PFS, compared to lenalidomide-dexamethasone alone (median PFS: not reached vs 30.4 months).[47] Also with respect to OS, the added value of daratumumab was found to be independent of frailty level. It is important to realize that these frailty subanalyses were performed retrospectively and that information on the activities of daily living were lacking. Therefore, the simplified frailty index was used to identify the frailty level, replacing patient-reported activities of daily living with physician-reported WHO performance status. This probably overestimates the level of fitness,[49] which might explain the unprecedented outcomes in frail patients. It also questions whether daratumumab is feasible in patients defined frail using the IMWG-FI. However, a Dutch trial, specifically designed for frail patients, showed that daratumumab-based therapy was feasible.[50] Therefore, daratumumab should not be withheld in first-line treatment of NTE newly diagnosed MM patients, even if frail. However, in this frail population, extra attention should be payed to prevention and early treatment of adverse events, such as infections, as the incidence of severe adverse events is higher in frail patients.

The ALCYONE and MAIA trials led to the registration of daratumumab-based regimens in NTE newly diagnosed MM patients.[51] Although daratumamab-VMP and daratumumab-lenalidomide-dexamethasone are not head-to-head compared, the median PFS of more than 60 months with the latter and consistency of efficacy across subgroups supports the use of daratumumab-lenalidomide-dexamethasone, irrespective of age, renal function, and cytogenetic risk status.

Currently, several ongoing phase 3 trials are exploring novel CD38-targeting antibody-based regimens to further improve the results obtained with daratumumab-lenalidomide-dexamethasone. In 2 randomized phase 3 trials, the value of adding daratumumab (CEPHEUS) or isatuximab (IMROZ) to bortezomib-lenalidomide-dexamethasone (VRd) is investigated. In addition, in the EQUATE trial, it will be investigated whether intensification of therapy, by consolidation with daratumumab-VRd, improves outcome in patients who are MRD-positive following standard induction therapy with daratumumab-lenalidomide-dexamethasone. In non-frail patients, a phase 3 trial comparing isatuximab-lenalidomide-dexamethasone versus isatuximab-VRd will be initiated in NTE newly diagnosed MM patients aged ≥65 and ≤ 80 years.

Transplant eligible newly diagnosed multiple myeloma

Two pivotal trials showed benefit of the addition of daratumumab to both induction and consolidation therapy in newly diagnosed MM patients who underwent an autologous stem cell transplantation (auto-SCT).[27,44,45] In part 1 of the phase 3 CASSIOPEIA trial, patients were randomized to pre-transplant induction (4 cycles) and post-transplant consolidation (2 cycles) with bortezomib-thalidomide-dexamethasone (VTd) with or without daratumumab.[27] Part 1 of the trial showed that addition of daratumumab to VTd resulted in a superior stringent complete response rate at day 100 after transplantation (29% vs 20%), a higher frequency of MRD-negativity, and improved PFS (median PFS not reached in either group; 18-month PFS rate: 93% in the daratumumab-VTd group and 85% in the VTd group).[27] In part 2 of the CASSIOPEIA study, patients were randomized to daratumumab maintenance therapy for 2 years following consolidation therapy or observation only.[44] Daratumumab maintenance resulted in a superior PFS, compared to observation only (median PFS: not reached vs 46.7 months).[44] Importantly, a pre-specified analysis showed that PFS was comparable between patients who received daratumumab-VTd plus daratumumab maintenance versus daratumumab-VTd plus observation only, suggesting that with the current follow-up daratumumab maintenance therapy is not of added value in case daratumumab is used during induction and consolidation.[44]

In the randomized phase 2 GRIFFIN trial there was a comparable design, except for the fact that daratumumab was added to VRd instead of VTd and patients in the daratumumab group received maintenance therapy with daratumumab-lenalidomide versus lenalidomide alone in the non-daratumumab group, the latter being standard of care when the study was designed.[45] Similar to the results from the CASSIOPEIA trial, the stringent complete response rate was higher in the daratumumab arm (42.4% vs 32%).[45] Moreover, the MRD-negativity rate and PFS were superior when daratumumab was added to standard-of-care induction/consolidation, and maintenance.[45] These trials led to the registration of daratumumab for the treatment of TE newly diagnosed MM patients.

Ongoing trials are evaluating the value of daratumumab plus lenalidomide maintenance after auto-SCT (eg, DRAMMATIC trial).[52] In addition, the combination of daratumumab with carfilzomib-lenalidomide-dexamethasone (KRd) in conjunction with auto-SCT has been investigated in the phase 2 MASTER trial.[30] Consolidation therapy with daratumumab-KRd was started and continued based on MRD status. It was found to be safe to discontinue Dara-KRd in patients with 2 consecutive MRD-negative assessments, provided there were less than 2 high-risk cytogenetic features.[30]

Isatuximab is also being evaluated in TE newly diagnosed MM patients. In part 1 of the phase 3 GMMG-HD7 trial, patients were randomized between three 42-day induction cycles with either isatuximab-VRd or VRd.[53] Addition of isatuximab resulted in a superior MRD-negativity rate after induction therapy (50% vs 36%).[53] Data on PFS are lacking because of short follow-up.[53] Part 2 is ongoing and is focused on the value of addition of isatuximab to lenalidomide maintenance after auto-SCT.[53] The phase 3 IsKia study will provide information on the added value of isatuximab to KRd as pre-transplant induction and post-transplant consolidation therapy. Early results from the ongoing phase 2 GMMG-CONCEPT trial have already shown that front-line treatment with isatuximab-KRd is promising with induction of rapid and deep remissions in patients with high-risk MM.[54] In the phase 2 RADAR trial, several maintenance approaches are being investigated based on MRD-status, including the strategy of adding isatuximab to lenalidomide or lenalidomide-bortezomib.[55]

CD38-Targeting Antibodies in Relapsed/Refractory Multiple Myeloma

Various daratumumab and isatuximab-based combination regimens are approved for the treatment of relapsed/refractory MM. These regimens are IMiD-based (**Table 1**) or proteasome inhibitor-based (**Table 2**).

Table 1
Randomized clinical studies evaluating antibody/IMiD-based triplets in relapsed/refractory MM

Study (Number of Patients)	Regimen	Patient Population	Median Follow-Up	≥PR	(s)CR	Median PFS	Median OS	Important Toxicity
POLLUX[58–60] (569)	dara-Rd vs Rd	• At least 1 prior line of therapy; len-refractory patients were excluded • Creatinine clearance ≥ 30 mL/min	79.7 months	92.9% vs 76.4%	51.2% vs 21.0%	45.0 vs 17.5 months	67.6 vs 51.8 months	• IRR in 47.7% vs not applicable • Grade 3/4 neutropenia: 57.6% vs 41.6% • Grade 3/4 infections: 44.5 vs 28.1%
APOLLO[62] (304)	dara-Pd vs Pd	• At least 1 prior line of therapy, including lenalidomide and PI (if only 1 prior therapy patients had to be len-refractory) • Creatinine clearance ≥ 30 mL/min	16.9 months	69% vs 46%	25% vs 4%	12.4 vs 6.9 months	OS data immature	• IRR in 5% vs not applicable • Grade 3/4 neutropenia: 68% vs 51% • Grade 3/4 infections: 28% vs 23%
IKARIA[40,63] (307)	isa-Pd vs Pd	• At least 2 prior lines of therapy • Creatinine clearance ≥ 30 mL/min	35.3 months	63% vs 33%	10% vs 3%	11.1 vs 5.9 months	24.6 vs 17.7 months	• IRR in 38% vs not applicable • Grade 3/4 neutropenia: 50% vs 35% • Grade 3/4 infections: 58% vs 39%

Trial	Comparison	Key inclusion criteria	Median follow-up	ORR	(s)CR	PFS	OS	Safety
ELOQUENT-2[41,87,88] (646)	elo-Rd vs Rd	• 1–3 prior lines of therapy; len-refractory patients were excluded • Creatinine clearance ≥ 30 mL/min	70.6 months	79% vs 66%	5% vs 9%	19.4 vs 14.9 months	48.3 vs 39.6 months	• IRR in 11% vs not applicable • Grade 3/4 lymphocytopenia in 8% vs 4%
ELOQUENT-3[89,90,117]	elo-Pd vs Pd	• ≥2 prior lines of therapy and previous treatment with len and PI • Creatinine clearance ≥ 45 mL/min	45 months	53% vs 26%	8% vs 2%	10.3 vs 4.7 months	29.8 vs 17.4 months	• IRR in 3% vs not applicable • Grade 3/4 lymphopenia in 8.3% vs 1.8%

Abbreviations: (s)CR, (stringent) complete response; dara-Pd, daratumumab-pomalidomide-dexamethasone; dara-Rd, daratumumab-lenalidomide-dexamethasone; elo-Pd, elotuzumab-pomalidomide-dexamethasone; elo-Rd, elotuzumab-lenalidomide-dexamethasone; IRR, infusion-related reaction; isa-Pd, isatuximab-pomalidomide-dexamethasone; len, lenalidomide; OS, overall survival; Pd, pomalidomide-dexamethasone; PFS, progression-free survival; PI, proteasome inhibitor; PR, partial response; Rd, lenalidomide-dexamethasone.

Table 2
Randomized clinical studies evaluating antibody/proteasome inhibitor-based triplets in relapsed/refractory MM

Study (Number of Patients)	Regimen	Patient Population	Median Follow-Up	≥PR	(s)CR	Median PFS	Median OS	Important Toxicity
CASTOR[64,65,116] (498)	dara-Vd vs Vd	• At least 1 prior line of therapy; bort-refractory patients were excluded • Creatinine clearance ≥ 20 mL/min	72.6 months	83.8% vs 63.2%	28.8% vs 9.8%	16.7 vs 7.1 months	49.6 vs 38.5 months	• IRR in 45.3% vs not applicable • All-grade peripheral neuropathy: 49.8% vs 38.0% • Grade 3/4 thrombocytopenia: 46% vs 33%
NCT01478048[92] (152)	elo-Vd vs Vd	• 1–3 prior lines of therapy; PI-refractory patients were excluded • Creatinine clearance ≥ 30 mL/min	15.9 months in the elo-Vd group, and 11.7 months in the Vd group	66% vs 63%	4% vs 4%	9.7 vs 6.9 months	Median OS not yet reported; 1-year OS: 85% vs 74%	• IRR in 5% vs not applicable • All-grade peripheral neuropathy: 36% vs 36%
CANDOR[66-68] (466)	dara-Kd vs Kd	• 1–3 prior lines of therapy • Creatinine clearance ≥ 20 mL/min	50.6 months in the dara-Kd arm and 50.1 months in the Kd arm	84% vs 73%	33% vs 13%	28.4 vs 15.2 months	50.8 vs 43.6 months	• ≥ Grade 3 peripheral neuropathy: 2% vs 0% • ≥ Grade 3 hypertension: 21% vs 15% • ≥ Grade 3 cardiac failure: 4% vs 8% • ≥ Grade 3 acute renal failure: 3% vs 7%

| IKEMA[39,117] (302) | isa-Kd vs Kd | • 1–3 prior lines of therapy • Creatinine clearance ≥ 15 mL/min | 44 months | 86.6% vs 83.7% | 44.1% vs 28.5% | 35.7 vs 19.2 months | Median OS: not yet reported; OS at 3 years: 68.7% vs 62.9% | • ≥ Grade 3 hypertension: 22.6% vs 23.0% • ≥ Grade 3 cardiac failure: 4.5% vs 4.1% |

Abbreviations: (s)CR, (stringent) complete response; t.ort, bortezomib; dara-Vd, daratumumab-bortezomib-dexamethasone; elo-Vd, elotuzumab-bortezomib-dexamethasone; IRR, infusion-related reaction; isa-Kd, isatuximab-carfilzomib-dexamethasone; Kd, carfilzomib-dexamethasone; OS, overall survival; PFS, progression-free survival; PI, proteasome inhibitor; PR, partial response; Vd, bortezomib-dexamethasone.

Combination Therapies Containing a CD38-Targeting Antibody and immunomodulatory drug

CD38-targeting antibody plus lenalidomide

Phase 1 studies showed that isatuximab and daratumumab could be effectively and safely combined with lenalidomide-dexamethasone.[56,57] Results from these trials formed the basis for the large randomized phase 3 POLLUX study, which evaluated daratumumab plus lenalidomide-dexamethasone versus lenalidomide-dexamethasone alone in patients with at least 1 prior therapy.[58–60] Superior response rates and markedly enhanced PFS was observed when daratumumab was added to lenalidomide-dexamethasone, and with longer follow-up also an OS advantage occurred in the triplet arm.[58–60] Daratumumab-lenalidomide-dexamethasone treatment was associated with a higher rate of neutropenia and infections (especially respiratory tract infections).[58–60]

CD38-targeting antibody plus pomalidomide

A phase 1b study showed that the triplet of daratumumab plus pomalidomide-dexamethasone was well tolerated in patients with heavily pretreated MM (≥2 prior lines of therapy) with at least partial response (PR) in 60% of patients.[61] These promising results led to the initiation of the phase 3 APOLLO study which evaluated daratumumab plus pomalidomide-dexamethasone versus pomalidomide-dexamethasone alone in 304 patients with relapsed/refractory MM who had received at least 1 previous line of therapy, including lenalidomide and a proteasome inhibitor. The addition of daratumumab to pomalidomide-dexamethasone increased the response rate (≥PR: 69% vs 46%) and improved PFS (median PFS: 12.4 vs 6.9 months) compared to pomalidomide-dexamethasone alone.[62] There was a higher rate of grade 3 or 4 neutropenia in the daratumumab-pomalidomide-dexamethasone group than in the pomalidomide-dexamethasone group. Also any grade infections were more common in the triplet arm than in the pomalidomide-dexamethasone arm (70% vs 55%; mostly respiratory tract infections).

Comparable improvements in clinical outcomes were observed in the IKARIA study, which randomized patients, who had received at least 2 prior therapies, to treatment with isatuximab-pomalidomide-dexamethasone or pomalidomide-dexamethasone (≥PR: 63% vs 33%; median PFS: 11.1 vs 5.9 months).[40,63]

Combination Therapies Containing a CD38-Targeting Antibody plus Proteasome Inhibitor

The phase 3 CASTOR study showed that addition of daratumumab to the bortezomib-dexamethasone backbone was superior to bortezomib-dexamethasone alone with significantly improved response rates, PFS, and OS.[64,65.] OS benefit was most pronounced in patients with 1 prior line of therapy, supporting early use of CD38-targeting antibodies.[64] Grade 3/4 infections were more common in the daratumumab arm.[64] In this study, bortezomib was given for a fixed treatment duration because development of neuropathy precludes continuous treatment with bortezomib.[64,65]

Three-drug regimens containing a CD38-targeting antibody plus the second generation proteasome inhibitor carfilzomib, and dexamethasone, are increasingly used to treat patients who experience first relapse and who are not refractory to CD38-targeting antibodies. This is based on 2 randomized phase 3 studies which showed that addition of isatuximab (IKEMA) or daratumumab (CANDOR) to carfilzomib-dexamethasone resulted in a substantial deepening of response and superior PFS compared to carfilzomib-dexamethasone alone.[66–68] There was also a trend toward enhanced OS with daratumumab-carfilzomib-dexamethasone versus carfilzomib-dexamethasone.[66–68] Such improvements were consistent across subgroups including patients with lenalidomide-refractory disease. Monitoring and management of cardiovascular risk factors, such as blood pressure and volume status, may prevent cardiac toxicities associated with carfilzomib.[69] The PFS obtained with daratumumab or isatuximab plus carfilzomib-dexamethasone is superior to that obtained with daratumumab-bortezomib-dexamethasone. Although cross-trial comparisons should be done with caution, these differences may be related to higher activity of carfilzomib compared to bortezomib, but also trial design (fixed duration bortezomib vs continuous treatment with carfilzomib).[70,71]

Retreatment with CD38-Targeting Antibodies

Retrospective studies suggest clinical efficacy of retreatment with a CD38-targeting antibody after developing CD38-targeting antibody-refractory disease, with switching of the partner drug.[72–74] However, prospective studies should be performed to better understand efficacy of this approach and to investigate whether a treatment-free interval is required in order to allow for NK cell recovery and to restore CD38 expression to baseline levels. The randomized phase 2 LYNX study, which evaluated the efficacy and safety of daratumumab retreatment, was recently stopped for futility (recommendation of the data review committee).[75]

SLAMF7-Targeting Antibodies

Elotuzumab, a humanized IgG1-kappa monoclonal antibody, is currently the only approved SLAMF7-targeting antibody in MM. SLAMF7 is highly expressed on the MM cell surface and on subsets of normal immune cells (such as NK cells and T-cells).[76] This antibody eliminates MM cell death via induction of ADCC and ADCP, but is also capable of direct NK cell stimulation.[77–79] The SLAMF7-targeting antibody elotuzumab mediates its anti-MM activity in part via NK cells.[76] Decreased NK cell numbers induced by CD38 antibodies may impair the efficacy of elotuzumab after daratumumab treatment. Indeed, in 2 retrospective studies, prior therapy with daratumumab had a negative impact on response to elotuzumab in subsequent lines of therapy.[80,81]

Infusion-related reactions are relatively infrequent with elotuzumab with preinfusion prophylaxis with dexamethasone, anti-histamines, and acetaminophen (see **Fig. 2**) (7%–10%, mostly during the first infusion).[3] As already discussed earlier, elotuzumab can be detected in SPEP and IFE assays, and therefore may interfere with the assessment of complete response (see **Fig. 2**).[3]

Elotuzumab in Newly Diagnosed Multiple Myeloma

In the ELOQUENT-1 trial, elotuzumab-lenalidomide-dexamethasone was compared with lenalidomide-dexamethasone in patients with newly diagnosed MM who were ineligible for auto-SCT(82). Although safe without increase in non-hematologic side effects, no improvement in PFS was observed by adding elotuzumab to the lenalidomide-dexamethasone backbone (median PFS: 31.4 months for elotuzumab-lenalidomide-dexamethasone vs 29.5 months for lenalidomide-dexamethasone).[82] In addition, the randomized phase 3 GMMG-HD6 study showed that addition of elotuzumab to VRd induction/consolidation therapy and lenalidomide maintenance did not result in improved PFS or OS in TE newly diagnosed MM patients.[83] The randomized phase 2 SWOG-1211 trial also showed no benefit of adding elotuzumab to VRd in patients with untreated, high-risk MM (median PFS: 33.6 for VRd and 31.5 months for elotuzumab-VRd).[84]

In conclusion, all these studies in newly diagnosed MM showed no benefit of integrating elotuzumab with VRd or lenalidomide-dexamethasone, and therefore there is currently no role for elotuzumab in newly diagnosed MM. However, a randomized phase 3 study which compared KRd with elotuzumab-KRd for induction/consolidation in conjunction with auto-SCT (DSMM XVII) recently demonstrated an increased proportion of patients with $\geq$very good partial response and MRD-negativity with elotuzumab-KRd versus KRd (49.8% vs 35.4%).[85] Follow-up is ongoing to assess whether this difference in depth of response will translate into improved PFS and OS(85).

Elotuzumab in Relapsed/Refractory Multiple Myeloma

Although elotuzumab has no single-agent activity in relapsed/refractory MM, the ELOQUENT-2 and ELOQUENT-3 studies showed that anti-MM activity of the combination of elotuzumab plus an IMiD is superior to the IMiD backbone alone (see **Table 1**).[86]

The randomized phase 3 ELOQUENT-2 study enrolled patients with 1 to 3 prior lines of therapy and randomized these patients to treatment with elotuzumab-lenalidomide-dexamethasone or lenalidomide-dexamethasone alone.[41,87,88] Patients who were treated with the elotuzumab-containing triplet regimen had a superior overall response rate, PFS, and OS with an acceptable long-term safety and tolerability profile.[41,87,88] The randomized phase 2 ELOQUENT-3 study showed that patients with at least 2 prior regimens and exposure to lenalidomide and proteasome inhibitor experienced benefit from elotuzumab plus pomalidomide-dexamethasone, compared to pomalidomide-dexamethasone, with improved response rate and PFS, and with longer follow-up also an OS advantage.[89,90] The addition of elotuzumab to pomalidomide-dexamethasone generally did not lead to an increase in the incidence of grade 3/4 adverse events compared to pomalidomide-dexamethasone alone.[89,90]

Preclinical studies showed that elotuzumab in combination with bortezomib exhibited markedly enhanced anti-MM activity.[91] This formed the preclinical rationale for a randomized phase 2 study evaluating elotuzumab-bortezomib-dexamethasone versus bortezomib-dexamethasone alone. This study showed that addition of elotuzumab to bortezomib-dexamethasone resulted in improved PFS in patients with 1 to 3 prior therapies (see **Table 2**).[92]

BCMA-Targeting Monoclonal Antibodies

B-cell maturation antigen (BCMA)-targeting chimeric antigen receptor (CAR) T-cell therapies, antibody drug conjugates, and bispecific antibodies (BsAbs) are highly effective anti-MM agents.[93–98] In addition, naked BCMA-targeting antibodies are also in clinical development. Naked BCMA-targeting antibodies induce MM cell death in preclinical experiments via ADCC, ADCP, and through inhibition of BCMA-mediated pro-survival signaling.[99] SEA-BCMA is a humanized, nonfucosylated immunoglobulin (Ig)G1 monoclonal anti-BCMA antibody.[100] Preliminary results from the phase 1 dose-escalation study showed a favorable safety profile and anti-tumor activity in heavily pretreated patients. Three (14%) of 22 patients who received 1600 mg SEA-BCMA every 2 weeks as monotherapy achieved a PR or better.[100,101] The response rate appears to increase (at least PR: 27%) with a more intensive administration schedule (weekly during 2 cycles, and then every 2 weeks).[100,101] Combination therapy with SEA-BCMA is also being investigated in patients with relapsed/refractory MM.

Ongoing Developments

Several studies are currently evaluating CD38-or SLAMF7-targeting monoclonal antibodies with novel anti-MM agents. Newer cereblon E3 ligase modulators (eg, iberdomide and mezigdomide[102,103]) are interesting combination partners for naked antibodies because these drugs have enhanced tumoricidal and immune-stimulatory effects compared with lenalidomide and pomalidomide.[104] Early results of the combination of iberdomide-daratumumab-dexamethasone show a promising activity and safety profile.[105] The phase 3 EXCALIBER-RRMM study is currently evaluating iberdomide-daratumumab-dexamethasone versus daratumumab-bortezomib-dexamethasone in patients with relapsed/refractory MM. An ongoing study is evaluating iberdomide combined with elotuzumab-dexamethasone.

The combination of a CD38-targeting antibody plus a T-cell redirecting BsAb is also explored. The rationale for this combination therapy is the observation that resistance to T-cell redirecting BsAbs is in part mediated by immunosuppressive regulatory T-cells, which can be eliminated by CD38-targeting antibodies.[8,106] Preclinical experiments showed that daratumumab enhanced the activity of teclistamab and talquetamab by improving T-cell function.[107,108] These studies formed the rationale for the TRIMM study, which evaluates novel combinations with teclistamab or talquetamab. Preliminary data from the combination of talquetamab plus daratumumab showed a promising efficacy profile with toxicity in line with what is observed with both agents alone.[109,110]

Another strategy to improve response is to combine CD38-targeting antibody-based therapy with adoptive NK cell therapy. Preclinical studies have already shown that addition of NK cells enhances response to CD38-targeting antibodies.[20,111] NK cells with CD38 deletion to eliminate daratumumab-induced fratricide may be most effective in the setting of NK cell therapy.[111] The DARA/ATRA study showed that addition of all-trans retinoic acid at the time of resistance to daratumumab, resulted in a temporary increase in CD38 expression on the tumor cell surface, but there was only limited clinical activity of this combination.[112]

Next to improving combination therapy, another strategy to improve clinical outcomes is to modify the molecular format of the naked antibody. SAR442085 is a next-generation Fc-engineered IgG1 backbone anti-CD38 monoclonal antibody with enhanced affinity for activating Fcγ receptors, compared to the affinity of daratumumab and isatuximab.[113] This translated into superior NK cell activation and degranulation against MM cells (enhanced ADCC activity) with SAR442085.[113] A phase 1 study with SAR442085 is ongoing. Another example of a next-generation CD38-targeting antibody is Hexabody-CD38.[114] This antibody has an E430 mutation in its Fc domain which facilitates the natural process of antibody hexamer formation upon binding to the tumor cell surface, resulting in enhanced binding of the complement molecule C1q and potentiated CDC, compared to daratumumab.[114] Hexabody-CD38 also induces tumor cell killing via ADCC and ADCP.[114] The safety and efficacy of Hexabody-CD38 are currently evaluated in a first-in-human study in heavily pretreated MM. Preliminary results from this study show that Hexabody-CD38 has a tolerable safety profile and clinical activity in patients with relapsed/refractory MM, including those with prior anti-CD38 antibody exposure.[115]

SUMMARY

The incorporation of CD38-targeting antibodies in the treatment of patients with newly diagnosed or relapsed/refractory MM has significantly improved survival. SLAMF7-targeting antibody elotuzumab can also be effectively and safely combined with IMiD-based backbone regimens in the setting of relapsed/refractory MM. The authors expect that novel forms of immunotherapy, such as Fc- engineered naked antibodies, T-cell redirecting bispecific antibodies, and CAR T-cell therapies, will further contribute to improved clinical outcomes of MM patients.[96,98]

CLINICS CARE POINTS

- Transplant-eligible newly diagnosed MM patients benefit from addition of daratumumab to VTd or VRd as induction and consolidation therapy in conjunction with auto-SCT.

- Daratumumab-lenalidomide-dexamethasone should be considered as first-line treatment option for newly diagnosed MM patients who are not eligible for auto-SCT.
- Therapeutic antibodies may interfere with assessment of complete response, and CD38-targeting antibodies interfere with routine methods for compatibility testing for blood transfusions.
- Elotuzumab combined with lenalidomide-dexamethasone or pomalidomide-dexamethasone is an effective regimen to treat patients with relapsed/refractory MM.

DISCLOSURE

N.W.C.J. van.de.Donk has received research support from Janssen Pharmaceuticals, United States, Amgen, United States, Celgene, United States, Novartis, Switzerland, Cellectis and BMS, and serves in advisory boards for Janssen Pharmaceuticals, AMGEN, Celgene, BMS, Takeda, Roche, Abbvie, Novartis, Bayer, Adaptive, and Servier, all paid to institution; S. Zweegman. has received research funding from Celgene, Takeda, Janssen, United States, and serves in advisory boards for Janssen, Takeda, BMS, Oncopeptides and Sanofi, all paid to institution; no funding received for this article.

REFERENCES

1. Brink M, Visser O, Zweegman S, et al. First-line treatment and survival of newly diagnosed primary plasma cell leukemia patients in the Netherlands: a population-based study, 1989-2018. Blood Cancer J 2021;11(2):22.
2. van de Donk N, Richardson PG, Malavasi F. CD38 antibodies in multiple myeloma: back to the future. Blood 2018;131(1):13–29.
3. van de Donk NW, Moreau P, Plesner T, et al. Clinical efficacy and management of monoclonal antibodies targeting CD38 and SLAMF7 in multiple myeloma. Blood 2016;127(6):681–95.
4. Zhu C, Song Z, Wang A, et al. Isatuximab Acts Through Fc-Dependent, Independent, and Direct Pathways to Kill Multiple Myeloma Cells. Front Immunol 2020;11:1771.
5. Deckert J, Wetzel MC, Bartle LM, et al. SAR650984, a novel humanized CD38-targeting antibody, demonstrates potent antitumor activity in models of multiple myeloma and other CD38+ hematologic malignancies. Clin Cancer Res 2014; 20(17):4574–83.
6. Jiang H, Acharya C, An G, et al. SAR650984 directly induces multiple myeloma cell death via lysosomal-associated and apoptotic pathways, which is further enhanced by pomalidomide. Leukemia 2016;30(2):399–408.
7. de WM, Tai YT, van d V, et al. Daratumumab, a novel therapeutic human CD38 monoclonal antibody, induces killing of multiple myeloma and other hematological tumors. J Immunol 2011;186(3):1840–8.
8. Krejcik J, Casneuf T, Nijhof IS, et al. Daratumumab depletes CD38+ immune regulatory cells, promotes T-cell expansion, and skews T-cell repertoire in multiple myeloma. Blood 2016;128(3):384–94.
9. Adams HC 3rd, Stevenaert F, Krejcik J, et al. High-Parameter Mass Cytometry Evaluation of Relapsed/Refractory Multiple Myeloma Patients Treated with Daratumumab Demonstrates Immune Modulation as a Novel Mechanism of Action. Cytometry Part A : The Journal of the International Society for Analytical Cytology 2019;95(3):279–89.

10. Feng X, Zhang L, Acharya C, et al. Targeting CD38 Suppresses Induction and Function of T Regulatory Cells to Mitigate Immunosuppression in Multiple Myeloma. Clin Cancer Res 2017;23(15):4290–300.
11. Lammerts van Bueren J, Jakobs D, Kaldenhoven N, et al. Direct *in Vitro* Comparison of Daratumumab with Surrogate Analogs of CD38 Antibodies MOR03087, SAR650984 and Ab79. Blood 2014;124(21):3474.
12. Kinder M, Bahlis NJ, Malavasi F, et al. Comparison of CD38 antibodies in vitro and ex vivo mechanisms of action in multiple myeloma. Haematologica 2021; 106(7):2004–8.
13. Quach H, Ritchie D, Stewart AK, et al. Mechanism of action of immunomodulatory drugs (IMiDS) in multiple myeloma. Leukemia 2010;24(1):22–32.
14. van de Donk NW, Görgün G, Groen RW, et al. Lenalidomide for the treatment of relapsed and refractory multiple myeloma. Cancer Manag Res 2012;4:253–68.
15. Nijhof IS, Groen RW, Noort WA, et al. Preclinical Evidence for the Therapeutic Potential of CD38-Targeted Immuno-Chemotherapy in Multiple Myeloma Patients Refractory to Lenalidomide and Bortezomib. Clin Cancer Res 2015;21(12): 2802–10.
16. van der Veer MS, de WM, van KB, et al. The therapeutic human CD38 antibody daratumumab improves the anti-myeloma effect of newly emerging multi-drug therapies. Blood Cancer J 2011;1(10):e41.
17. Cai T, Wetzel M, Nicolazzi C, et al. Preclinical chracterization of SAR650984, a humanized anti-CD38 antibody for the treatment of multiple myeloma. Clin Lymphoma Myeloma Leuk 2013;288.
18. Krejcik J, Frerichs KA, Nijhof IS, et al. Monocytes and Granulocytes Reduce CD38 Expression Levels on Myeloma Cells in Patients Treated with Daratumumab. Clin Cancer Res 2017;23(24):7498–511.
19. Nijhof IS, Casneuf T, van VJ, et al. CD38 expression and complement inhibitors affect response and resistance to daratumumab therapy in myeloma. Blood 2016;128(7):959–70.
20. Verkleij CPM, Frerichs KA, Broekmans MEC, et al. NK Cell Phenotype Is Associated With Response and Resistance to Daratumumab in Relapsed/Refractory Multiple Myeloma. Hemasphere 2023;7(5):e881.
21. Casneuf T, Xu XS, Adams HC 3rd, et al. Effects of daratumumab on natural killer cells and impact on clinical outcomes in relapsed or refractory multiple myeloma. Blood advances 2017;1(23):2105–14.
22. de Haart SJ, Holthof L, Noort WA, et al. Sepantronium bromide (YM155) improves daratumumab-mediated cellular lysis of multiple myeloma cells by abrogation of bone marrow stromal cell-induced resistance. Haematologica 2016; 101(8):e339–42.
23. Giri S, Grimshaw A, Bal S, et al. Evaluation of Daratumumab for the Treatment of Multiple Myeloma in Patients With High-risk Cytogenetic Factors: A Systematic Review and Meta-analysis. JAMA Oncol 2020;6(11):1759–65.
24. Mateos MV, Cavo M, Blade J, et al. Overall survival with daratumumab, bortezomib, melphalan, and prednisone in newly diagnosed multiple myeloma (ALCYONE): a randomised, open-label, phase 3 trial. Lancet 2020;395(10218):132–41.
25. Mateos MV, Dimopoulos MA, Cavo M, et al, ALCYONE Trial Investigators. Daratumumab plus Bortezomib, Melphalan, and Prednisone for Untreated Myeloma. N Engl J Med 2018;378(6):518–28.
26. Facon T, Kumar S, Plesner T, et al, MAIA Trial Investigators. Daratumumab plus Lenalidomide and Dexamethasone for Untreated Myeloma. N Engl J Med 2019; 380(22):2104–15.

27. Moreau P, Attal M, Hulin C, et al. Bortezomib, thalidomide, and dexamethasone with or without daratumumab before and after autologous stem-cell transplantation for newly diagnosed multiple myeloma (CASSIOPEIA): a randomised, open-label, phase 3 study. Lancet 2019;394(10192):29–38.

28. Chari A, Kaufman JL, Laubach JP, et al. Daratumumab Plus Lenalidomide, Bortezomib, and Dexamethasone (D-RVd) in Transplant-Eligible Newly Diagnosed Multiple Myeloma (NDMM) Patients (Pts): Final Analysis of Griffin Among Clinically Relevant Subgroups. Blood 2022;140(Supplement 1):7278–81.

29. Moreau P, Facon T, Usmani S, et al. Daratumumab Plus Lenalidomide and Dexamethasone (D-Rd) Versus Lenalidomide and Dexamethasone (Rd) in Transplant-Ineligible Patients (Pts) with Newly Diagnosed Multiple Myeloma (NDMM): Clinical Assessment of Key Subgroups of the Phase 3 Maia Study. Blood 2022; 140(Supplement 1):7297–300.

30. Costa LJ, Chhabra S, Medvedova E, et al. Daratumumab, Carfilzomib, Lenalidomide, and Dexamethasone With Minimal Residual Disease Response-Adapted Therapy in Newly Diagnosed Multiple Myeloma. J Clin Oncol 2022;40(25):2901–12.

31. Usmani SZ, Nahi H, Plesner T, et al. Daratumumab monotherapy in patients with heavily pretreated relapsed or refractory multiple myeloma: final results from the phase 2 GEN501 and SIRIUS trials. Lancet Haematol 2020;7(6):e447–55.

32. Lokhorst HM, Plesner T, Laubach JP, et al. Targeting CD38 with Daratumumab Monotherapy in Multiple Myeloma. N Engl J Med 2015;373(13):1207–19.

33. Lonial S, Weiss BM, Usmani SZ, et al. Daratumumab monotherapy in patients with treatment-refractory multiple myeloma (SIRIUS): an open-label, randomised, phase 2 trial. Lancet 2016;387(10027):1551–60.

34. Dimopoulos M, Bringhen S, Anttila P, et al. Isatuximab as monotherapy and combined with dexamethasone in patients with relapsed/refractory multiple myeloma. Blood 2021;137(9):1154–65.

35. Mateos MV, Nahi H, Legiec W, et al. Subcutaneous versus intravenous daratumumab in patients with relapsed or refractory multiple myeloma (COLUMBA): a multicentre, open-label, non-inferiority, randomised, phase 3 trial. Lancet Haematol 2020;7(5):e370–80.

36. Usmani SZ, Nahi H, Mateos MV, et al. Subcutaneous delivery of daratumumab in relapsed or refractory multiple myeloma. Blood 2019;134(8):668–77.

37. Oostendorp M, Lammerts van Bueren JJ, Doshi P, et al. When blood transfusion medicine becomes complicated due to interference by monoclonal antibody therapy. Transfusion 2015;55(6 Pt 2):1555–62.

38. van de Donk NW, Otten HG, El Haddad O, et al. Interference of daratumumab in monitoring multiple myeloma patients using serum immunofixation electrophoresis can be abrogated using the daratumumab IFE reflex assay (DIRA). Clin Chem Lab Med 2016;54(6):1105–9.

39. Martin T, Dimopoulos MA, Mikhael J, et al. Isatuximab, carfilzomib, and dexamethasone in patients with relapsed multiple myeloma: updated results from IKEMA, a randomized Phase 3 study. Blood Cancer J 2023;13(1):72.

40. Attal M, Richardson PG, Rajkumar SV, et al, ICARIA-MM study group. Isatuximab plus pomalidomide and low-dose dexamethasone versus pomalidomide and low-dose dexamethasone in patients with relapsed and refractory multiple myeloma (ICARIA-MM): a randomised, multicentre, open-label, phase 3 study. Lancet 2019;394(10214):2096–107.

41. Lonial S, Dimopoulos M, Palumbo A, et al, ELOQUENT-2 Investigators. Elotuzumab Therapy for Relapsed or Refractory Multiple Myeloma. N Engl J Med 2015; 373(7):621–31.

42. Cavo M, San-Miguel J, Usmani SZ, et al. Prognostic value of minimal residual disease negativity in myeloma: combined analysis of POLLUX, CASTOR, ALCYONE, and MAIA. Blood 2022;139(6):835–44.

43. Facon T, Kumar SK, Plesner T, et al. Daratumumab, lenalidomide, and dexamethasone versus lenalidomide and dexamethasone alone in newly diagnosed multiple myeloma (MAIA): overall survival results from a randomised, open-label, phase 3 trial. Lancet Oncol 2021;22(11):1582–96.

44. Moreau P, Hulin C, Perrot A, et al. Maintenance with daratumumab or observation following treatment with bortezomib, thalidomide, and dexamethasone with or without daratumumab and autologous stem-cell transplant in patients with newly diagnosed multiple myeloma (CASSIOPEIA): an open-label, randomised, phase 3 trial. Lancet Oncol 2021;22(10):1378–90.

45. Voorhees PM, Kaufman JL, Laubach J, et al. Daratumumab, lenalidomide, bortezomib, and dexamethasone for transplant-eligible newly diagnosed multiple myeloma: the GRIFFIN trial. Blood 2020;136(8):936–45.

46. Mateos MV, Dimopoulos MA, Cavo M, et al. Daratumumab Plus Bortezomib, Melphalan, and Prednisone Versus Bortezomib, Melphalan, and Prednisone in Transplant-Ineligible Newly Diagnosed Multiple Myeloma: Frailty Subgroup Analysis of ALCYONE. Clin Lymphoma, Myeloma & Leukemia 2021;21(11):785–98.

47. Facon T, Cook G, Usmani SZ, et al. Daratumumab plus lenalidomide and dexamethasone in transplant-ineligible newly diagnosed multiple myeloma: frailty subgroup analysis of MAIA. Leukemia 2022;36(4):1066–77.

48. Palumbo A, Bringhen S, Mateos MV, et al. Geriatric assessment predicts survival and toxicities in elderly myeloma patients: an International Myeloma Working Group report. Blood 2015;125(13):2068–74.

49. Facon T, Dimopoulos MA, Meuleman N, et al. A simplified frailty scale predicts outcomes in transplant-ineligible patients with newly diagnosed multiple myeloma treated in the FIRST (MM-020) trial. Leukemia 2020;34(1):224–33.

50. Stege CAM, Nasserinejad K, van der Spek E, et al. Ixazomib, Daratumumab, and Low-Dose Dexamethasone in Frail Patients With Newly Diagnosed Multiple Myeloma: The Hovon 143 Study. J Clin Oncol 2021;39(25):2758–67.

51. Korst C, van de Donk N. Should all newly diagnosed MM patients receive CD38 antibody-based treatment? Hematology American Society of Hematology Education Program 2020;2020(1):259–63.

52. Krishnan A, Hoering A, Hari P, et al. Phase III Study of Daratumumab/rhuph20 (nsc- 810307) + Lenalidomide or Lenalidomide As Post-Autologous Stem Cell Transplant Maintenance Therapyin Patients with Multiple Myeloma (mm) Using Minimal Residual Disease Todirect Therapy Duration (DRAMMATIC study): SWOG s1803. Blood 2020;136:21–2.

53. Goldschmidt H, Mai EK, Bertsch U, et al, German-Speaking Myeloma Multicenter Group GMMG HD7 investigators. Addition of isatuximab to lenalidomide, bortezomib, and dexamethasone as induction therapy for newly diagnosed, transplantation-eligible patients with multiple myeloma (GMMG-HD7): part 1 of an open-label, multicentre, randomised, active-controlled, phase 3 trial. Lancet Haematol 2022;9(11):e810–21.

54. Leypoldt LB, Besemer B, Asemissen AM, et al. Isatuximab, carfilzomib, lenalidomide, and dexamethasone (Isa-KRd) in front-line treatment of high-risk multiple myeloma: interim analysis of the GMMG-CONCEPT trial. Leukemia 2022;36(3):885–8.

55. Royle KL, Coulson AB, Ramasamy K, et al. Risk and response adapted therapy following autologous stem cell transplant in patients with newly diagnosed

multiple myeloma (RADAR (UK-MRA Myeloma XV Trial): study protocol for a phase II/III randomised controlled trial. BMJ Open 2022;12(11):e063037.

56. Plesner T, Arkenau T, Lokhorst H, et al. Preliminary Safety and Efficacy Data Of Daratumumab In Combination With Lenalidomide and Dexamethasone In Relapsed Or Refractory Multiple Myeloma. Blood 2013;122(21):1986.

57. Martin T, Baz R, Benson DM, et al. A phase 1b study of isatuximab plus lenalidomide and dexamethasone for relapsed/refractory multiple myeloma. Blood 2017;129(25):3294–303.

58. Dimopoulos MA, Oriol A, Nahi H, et al, POLLUX Investigators. Daratumumab, Lenalidomide, and Dexamethasone for Multiple Myeloma. N Engl J Med 2016; 375(14):1319–31.

59. Dimopoulos MA, San-Miguel J, Belch A, et al. Daratumumab plus lenalidomide and dexamethasone versus lenalidomide and dexamethasone in relapsed or refractory multiple myeloma: updated analysis of POLLUX. Haematologica 2018; 103(12):2088–96.

60. Dimopoulos MA, Oriol A, Nahi H, et al. Overall Survival With Daratumumab, Lenalidomide, and Dexamethasone in Previously Treated Multiple Myeloma (POLLUX): A Randomized, Open-Label, Phase III Trial. J Clin Oncol 2023;41(8):1590–9.

61. Chari A, Suvannasankha A, Fay JW, et al. Daratumumab plus pomalidomide and dexamethasone in relapsed and/or refractory multiple myeloma. Blood 2017;130(8):974–81.

62. Dimopoulos MA, Terpos E, Boccadoro M, et al, APOLLO Trial Investigators. Daratumumab plus pomalidomide and dexamethasone versus pomalidomide and dexamethasone alone in previously treated multiple myeloma (APOLLO): an open-label, randomised, phase 3 trial. Lancet Oncol 2021;22(6):801–12.

63. Richardson PG, Perrot A, San-Miguel J, et al. Isatuximab plus pomalidomide and low-dose dexamethasone versus pomalidomide and low-dose dexamethasone in patients with relapsed and refractory multiple myeloma (ICARIA-MM): follow-up analysis of a randomised, phase 3 study. Lancet Oncol 2022;23(3): 416–27.

64. Sonneveld P, Chanan-Khan A, Weisel K, et al. Overall Survival With Daratumumab, Bortezomib, and Dexamethasone in Previously Treated Multiple Myeloma (CASTOR): A Randomized, Open-Label, Phase III Trial. J Clin Oncol 2023;41(8): 1600–9.

65. Palumbo A, Chanan-Khan A, Weisel K, et al, CASTOR Investigators. Daratumumab, Bortezomib, and Dexamethasone for Multiple Myeloma. N Engl J Med 2016;375(8):754–66.

66. Dimopoulos M, Quach H, Mateos MV, et al. Carfilzomib, dexamethasone, and daratumumab versus carfilzomib and dexamethasone for patients with relapsed or refractory multiple myeloma (CANDOR): results from a randomised, multicentre, open-label, phase 3 study. Lancet 2020;396(10245):186–97.

67. Usmani SZ, Quach H, Mateos MV, et al. Carfilzomib, dexamethasone, and daratumumab versus carfilzomib and dexamethasone for patients with relapsed or refractory multiple myeloma (CANDOR): updated outcomes from a randomised, multicentre, open-label, phase 3 study. Lancet Oncol 2022;23(1):65–76.

68. Usmani SZ, Quach H, Mateos MV, et al. Final analysis of carfilzomib, dexamethasone, and daratumumab vs carfilzomib and dexamethasone in the CANDOR study. Blood Advances 2023;7(14):3739–48.

69. Bringhen S, Milan A, Ferri C, et al, European Hematology Association, the European Myeloma Network and the Italian Society of Arterial Hypertension. Cardiovascular adverse events in modern myeloma therapy - Incidence and risks. A

review from the European Myeloma Network (EMN) and Italian Society of Arterial Hypertension (SIIA). Haematologica 2018;103(9):1422–32.

70. Dimopoulos MA, Goldschmidt H, Niesvizky R, et al. Carfilzomib or bortezomib in relapsed or refractory multiple myeloma (ENDEAVOR): an interim overall survival analysis of an open-label, randomised, phase 3 trial. Lancet Oncol 2017; 18(10):1327–37.

71. van de Donk NW. Carfilzomib versus bortezomib: no longer an ENDEAVOR. Lancet Oncol 2017;18(10):1288–90.

72. Nooka AK, Joseph NS, Kaufman JL, et al. Clinical efficacy of daratumumab, pomalidomide, and dexamethasone in patients with relapsed or refractory myeloma: Utility of re-treatment with daratumumab among refractory patients. Cancer 2019;125(17):2991–3000.

73. Hussain MJ, Robinson MM, Hamadeh I, et al. Daratumumab, pomalidomide and dexamethasone combination therapy in daratumumab and/or pomalidomide refractory multiple myeloma. Br J Haematol 2019;186(1):140–4.

74. Alici E, Chrobok M, Lund J, et al. Re-challenging with anti-CD38 monotherapy in triple-refractory multiple myeloma patients is a feasible and safe approach. Br J Haematol 2016;174(3):473–7.

75. Bahlis NJ, Zonder JA, Wroblewski S, et al. Subcutaneous daratumumab in patients with multiple myeloma who have been previously treated with intravenous daratumumab: A multicenter, randomized, phase II study (LYNX). J Clin Oncol 2020;38(15_suppl):TPS8553.

76. Hsi ED, Steinle R, Balasa B, et al. CS1, a potential new therapeutic antibody target for the treatment of multiple myeloma. Clin Cancer Res 2008;14(9):2775–84.

77. Kurdi AT, Glavey SV, Bezman NA, et al. Antibody-Dependent Cellular Phagocytosis by Macrophages is a Novel Mechanism of Action of Elotuzumab. Mol Cancer Therapeut 2018;17(7):1454–63.

78. Tai YT, Dillon M, Song W, et al. Anti-CS1 humanized monoclonal antibody Hu-Luc63 inhibits myeloma cell adhesion and induces antibody-dependent cellular cytotoxicity in the bone marrow milieu. Blood 2008;112(4):1329–37.

79. Collins SM, Bakan CE, Swartzel GD, et al. Elotuzumab directly enhances NK cell cytotoxicity against myeloma via CS1 ligation: evidence for augmented NK cell function complementing ADCC. Cancer Immunol Immunother 2013;62(12): 1841–9.

80. Hoylman E, Brown A, Perissinotti AJ, et al. Optimal sequence of daratumumab and elotuzumab in relapsed and refractory multiple myeloma. Leuk Lymphoma 2020;61(3):691–8.

81. Becnel M, Rubin L, Nair R, et al. Effect of Timing of Monoclonal Antibody Therapy on the Time to Next Treatment and Response Rate in Heavily Pre-Treated Patients with Myeloma Who Separately Received Both Daratumumab and Elotuzumab-Based Regimens. Blood 2018;132:3258.

82. Dimopoulos MA, Richardson PG, Bahlis NJ, et al, ELOQUENT-1 investigators. Addition of elotuzumab to lenalidomide and dexamethasone for patients with newly diagnosed, transplantation ineligible multiple myeloma (ELOQUENT-1): an open-label, multicentre, randomised, phase 3 trial. Lancet Haematol 2022; 9(6):e403–14.

83. Goldschmidt H, Mai EK, Bertsch U, et al. Elotuzumab in Combination with Lenalidomide, Bortezomib, Dexamethasone and Autologous Transplantation for Newly-Diagnosed Multiple Myeloma: Results from the Randomized Phase III GMMG-HD6 Trial. Blood 2021;138:486.

84. Usmani SZ, Hoering A, Ailawadhi S, et al, SWOG1211 Trial Investigators. Borte-zomib, lenalidomide, and dexamethasone with or without elotuzumab in patients with untreated, high-risk multiple myeloma (SWOG-1211): primary analysis of a randomised, phase 2 trial. Lancet Haematol 2021;8(1):e45–54.

85. Knop S, Stuebig T, Kull M, et al. Carfilzomib, lenalidomide, and dexamethasone (KRd) versus elotuzumab and KRd in transplant-eligible patients with newly diagnosed multiple myeloma: Post-induction response and MRD results from an open-label randomized phase 3 study. J Clin Oncol 2023;41(16_suppl):8000.

86. Zonder JA, Mohrbacher AF, Singhal S, et al. A phase 1, multicenter, open-label, dose escalation study of elotuzumab in patients with advanced multiple myeloma. Blood 2012;120(3):552–9 %19.

87. Dimopoulos MA, Lonial S, Betts KA, et al. Elotuzumab plus lenalidomide and dexamethasone in relapsed/refractory multiple myeloma: Extended 4-year follow-up and analysis of relative progression-free survival from the randomized ELOQUENT-2 trial. Cancer 2018;124(20):4032–43.

88. Dimopoulos MA, Lonial S, White D, et al. Elotuzumab, lenalidomide, and dexa-methasone in RRMM: final overall survival results from the phase 3 randomized ELOQUENT-2 study. Blood Cancer J 2020;10(9):91.

89. Dimopoulos MA, Dytfeld D, Grosicki S, et al. Elotuzumab plus Pomalidomide and Dexamethasone for Multiple Myeloma. N Engl J Med 2018;379(19):1811–22.

90. Dimopoulos MA, Dytfeld D, Grosicki S, et al. Elotuzumab Plus Pomalidomide and Dexamethasone for Relapsed/Refractory Multiple Myeloma: Final Overall Survival Analysis From the Randomized Phase II ELOQUENT-3 Trial. J Clin On-col 2023;41(3):568–78.

91. van RF, Szmania SM, Dillon M, et al. Combinatorial efficacy of anti-CS1 mono-clonal antibody elotuzumab (HuLuc63) and bortezomib against multiple myeloma. Mol Cancer Ther 2009;8(9):2616–24.

92. Jakubowiak A, Offidani M, Pegourie B, et al. Randomized phase 2 study: elotu-zumab plus bortezomib/dexamethasone vs bortezomib/dexamethasone for relapsed/refractory MM. Blood 2016;127(23):2833–40.

93. Moreau P, Garfall AL, van de Donk N, et al. Teclistamab in Relapsed or Refrac-tory Multiple Myeloma. N Engl J Med 2022;387(6):495–505.

94. Martin T, Usmani SZ, Berdeja JG, et al. Ciltacabtagene Autoleucel, an Anti-B-cell Maturation Antigen Chimeric Antigen Receptor T-Cell Therapy, for Relapsed/Re-fractory Multiple Myeloma: CARTITUDE-1 2-Year Follow-Up. J Clin Oncol 2023; 41(6):1265–74.

95. Lonial S, Lee HC, Badros A, et al. Belantamab mafodotin for relapsed or refrac-tory multiple myeloma (DREAMM-2): a two-arm, randomised, open-label, phase 2 study. Lancet Oncol 2020;21(2):207–21.

96. van de Donk N, Usmani SZ, Yong K. CAR T-cell therapy for multiple myeloma: state of the art and prospects. Lancet Haematol 2021;8(6):e446–61.

97. O'Neill C, van de Donk N. T-cell redirecting bispecific antibodies in multiple myeloma: Current landscape and future directions. EJHaem 2023;4(3):811–22.

98. van de Donk N, Zweegman S. T-cell-engaging bispecific antibodies in cancer. Lancet 2023;402(10396):142–58.

99. Ryan MC, Hering M, Peckham D, et al. Antibody targeting of B-cell maturation antigen on malignant plasma cells. Mol Cancer Therapeut 2007;6(11):3009–18.

100. Hoffman JE, Lipe B, Melear J, et al. SEA-BCMA, an Investigational Nonfucosy-lated Monoclonal Antibody: Ongoing Results of a Phase 1 Study in Patients with Relapsed/Refractory Multiple Myeloma (SGNBCMA-001). Blood 2021;138:2740.

101. Hoffman JE, Lipe B, Melear J, et al. Sea-BCMA Mono- and Combination Therapy in Patients with Relapsed/Refractory Multiple Myeloma: Updated Results of a Phase 1 Study (SGNBCMA-001). Blood 2022;140(Supplement 1):10160–2.

102. Lonial S, Popat R, Hulin C, et al. Iberdomide plus dexamethasone in heavily pre-treated late-line relapsed or refractory multiple myeloma (CC-220-MM-001): a multicentre, multicohort, open-label, phase 1/2 trial. Lancet Haematol 2022; 9(11):e822–32.

103. Richardson PG, Trudel S, Quach H, et al. Mezigdomide (CC-92480), a Potent, Novel Cereblon E3 Ligase Modulator (CELMoD), Combined with Dexamethasone (DEX) in Patients (pts) with Relapsed/Refractory Multiple Myeloma (RRMM): Preliminary Results from the Dose-Expansion Phase of the CC-92480-MM-001 Trial. Blood 2022;140(Supplement 1):1366–8.

104. Lonial S, Amatangelo M, Popat R, et al. Preclinical, Translational, and Clinical Evidence of a Differentiated Profile for the Novel CELMoD, Iberdomide (CC-220). Blood 2019;134:3119.

105. van de Donk NWCJ, Popat R, Larsen J, et al. First Results of Iberdomide (IBER; CC-220) in Combination with Dexamethasone (DEX) and Daratumumab (DARA) or Bortezomib (BORT) in Patients with Relapsed/Refractory Multiple Myeloma (RRMM). Blood 2020;136(Supplement 1):16–7.

106. Cortes-Selva D, Casneuf T, Vishwamitra D, et al. Teclistamab, a B-Cell Maturation Antigen (BCMA) x CD3 Bispecific Antibody, in Patients with Relapsed/Refractory Multiple Myeloma (RRMM): Correlative Analyses from MajesTEC-1. Blood 2022;140(Supplement 1):241–3.

107. Frerichs KA, Broekmans MEC, Marin Soto JA, et al. Preclinical Activity of JNJ-7957, a Novel BCMA×CD3 Bispecific Antibody for the Treatment of Multiple Myeloma, Is Potentiated by Daratumumab. Clin Cancer Res 2020;26(9):2203–15.

108. Verkleij CPM, Broekmans MEC, van Duin M, et al. Preclinical activity and determinants of response of the GPRC5DxCD3 bispecific antibody talquetamab in multiple myeloma. Blood Advances 2021;5(8):2196–215.

109. Rodríguez-Otero P, D'Souza A, Reece DE, et al. A novel, immunotherapy-based approach for the treatment of relapsed/refractory multiple myeloma (RRMM): Updated phase 1b results for daratumumab in combination with teclistamab (a BCMA x CD3 bispecific antibody). J Clin Oncol 2022;40(16_suppl):8032.

110. Dholaria B, Weisel K, Mateos M-V, et al. Talquetamab (tal) + daratumumab (dara) in patients (pts) with relapsed/refractory multiple myeloma (RRMM): Updated TRIMM-2 results. J Clin Oncol 2023;41(16_suppl):8003.

111. Naeimi Kararoudi M, Nagai Y, Elmas E, et al. CD38 deletion of human primary NK cells eliminates daratumumab-induced fratricide and boosts their effector activity. Blood 2020;136(21):2416–27.

112. Frerichs KA, Minnema MC, Levin MD, et al. Efficacy and safety of daratumumab combined with all-trans retinoic acid in relapsed/refractory multiple myeloma. Blood Advances 2021;5(23):5128–39.

113. Kassem S, Diallo BK, El-Murr N, et al. SAR442085, a novel anti-CD38 antibody with enhanced antitumor activity against multiple myeloma. Blood 2022;139(8): 1160–76.

114. Hiemstra IH, Santegoets KCM, Janmaat ML, et al. Preclinical anti-tumour activity of HexaBody-CD38, a next-generation CD38 antibody with superior complement-dependent cytotoxic activity. EBioMedicine 2023;93:104663.

115. Spencer A, Iversen KF, Dhakal B, et al. Preliminary Dose-Escalation Results from a Phase 1/2 Study of GEN3014 (HexaBody®-CD38) in Patients (pts) with Relapsed or Refractory Multiple Myeloma (RRMM). Blood 2022;140(Supplement 1):7320–1.

116. Spencer A, Lentzsch S, Weisel K, et al. Daratumumab plus bortezomib and dexamethasone versus bortezomib and dexamethasone in relapsed or refractory multiple myeloma: updated analysis of CASTOR. Haematologica 2018;103(12): 2079–87.
117. Moreau P, Dimopoulos MA, Mikhael J, et al, IKEMA study group. Isatuximab, carfilzomib, and dexamethasone in relapsed multiple myeloma (IKEMA): a multicentre, open-label, randomised phase 3 trial. Lancet 2021;397(10292):2361–71.

Bispecific Antibodies in the Treatment of Multiple Myeloma

Xiang Zhou, MD, Xianghui Xiao, MD, Klaus Martin Kortuem, MD,
Hermann Einsele, MD*

KEYWORDS

- Multiple myeloma • Immunotherapy bispecific antibody • CAR T cell

KEY POINTS

- Bispecific antibodies (T-cell engaging antibodies) provide a new mode of action for anti-myeloma therapy by redirecting autologous T cells toward myeloma cells to mediate anti-tumor efficacy.
- Most of the bispecific antibodies in clinical development in myeloma are targeting B-cell maturation antigen, and other targets are GPRC5D, FCRH5, CD38, and CD19.
- Bispecific antibodies are currently approved in relapsed/refractory multiple myeloma (teclistamab already approved, elranatamab and talquetamab expected to be approved in a few weeks) in greater than third line of therapy can mediate overall response rate in greater than 60%, CR of 30% to 40% of patients, and a progression-free survival of around 1 year.

INTRODUCTION

Multiple myeloma (MM), the second most common hematologic malignancy in adult, is a plasma cell neoplasm characterized by bone lesions, kidney injury, anemia, and hypercalcemia.[1] The prognosis of MM patients has been dramatically improved over the last few decades by the introduction of various novel anti-MM agents including proteasome inhibitors, immunomodulatory drugs (IMiDs) and monoclonal antibodies (mAbs) and high-dose therapy with autologous stem cell transplant (ASCT). Results from recent randomized clinical trials showed a median overall survival (OS) of more than 8 years and a 4-year OS rate of more than 80% in patients who received induction with modern quadruple regimens followed by ASCT.[1–4] Even in the transplant ineligible elderly patients, the median OS was about 5 years.[1,5,6] However, MM is still considered an incurable disease, as most of the patients suffer from relapse and develop drug resistance over time[7] and the management of patients with relapsed/refractory (RR) MM remains challenging. More recently, T-cell-based immunotherapies, for example,

Department of Internal Medicine II, University Hospital of Würzburg, Würzburg, Germany
* Corresponding author. Oberdürrbacher Street 6, Würzburg D-97080, Germany.
E-mail address: Einsele_H@ukw.de

Hematol Oncol Clin N Am 38 (2024) 361–381
https://doi.org/10.1016/j.hoc.2023.12.003
0889-8588/24/© 2023 Elsevier Inc. All rights reserved.
hemonc.theclinics.com

chimeric antigen receptor (CAR)-modified T-cells and bispecific antibodies (bsAbs), have been developed to fight against MM using the patient's own immune system.[8] To date, several CAR T-cell and bsAb products have been investigated within clinical trials and have shown promising efficacy in RRMM patients.[9,10] In the 2020s, the US Food and Drug Administration (FDA) approved the first B-cell maturation antigen (BCMA)-directed CAR T-cell therapies idecabtagene vicleucel (ide-cel or bb2121) and ciltacabtagene autoleucel (cilta-cel), and the first BCMAxCD3 bsAb teclistamab.[11–13] Moreover, CAR T-cell and bsAb products are being evaluated in earlier lines of treatment and/or as frontline therapy in newly diagnosed (ND) MM patients.[10,14] The development of CAR T-cell and bsAb are leading to a paradigm shift in the treatment of RRMM and will greatly further improve the outcome of MM patients. Unlike autologous CAR T-cell therapy, which requires ex vivo manufacturing process, bsAb presents an off-the-shelf product that is readily available and can be administered directly to the patients.[7,15] Ultimately, bsAbs are integrated into the standard of care of MM patients currently in late line but increasingly in clinical trials also in earlier lines of therapy. In this review, the authors provide an overview of potential drug targets, mechanisms of action, efficacy and safety data from recent clinical trials, resistance mechanisms, and future directions of bsAb therapies in MM.

POTENTIAL BISPECIFIC ANTIBODY TARGETS AND MECHANISMS OF ACTION

In brief, bsAb is a T-cell-based therapy that bridges the MM cells and the patients' T-cells in vivo.[16] Therefore, first, bsAbs recruit and activate T cells, for example, by binding to the T-cell co-receptor CD3.[17] Second, similar to mAbs, bsAbs recognize specifically an antigen target, which ideally is uniquely expressed on MM cells and absent on other tissue to avoid on-target off-tumor toxicity. In this way, an immune synapse is built between the MM cells and the patients' own T cells, leading to T-cell (mainly CD8+ T cells) activation and proliferation, which induce MM cell lysis by release of granzymes, perforins, and different cytokines such as interleukin (IL)-6, IL-2, inferon-gamma (INF-γ), IL-5, and monocyte chemoattractant protein-1 (MCP-1).[7,18–21] Currently, the most commonly used bsAbs in MM include bispecific T-cell engagers (BiTE, Amgen, Thousand Oaks, CA) and DuoBody (Genmab A/S, Copenhagen, Denmark).[18,22] BiTE is a molecule containing two single-chain variable fragments linked with each other, whereas DuoBody consists of two different antigen-binding fragments and a functional constant region fragment (Fc), which can extend the half-life time of the molecule.[23,24] So far, several MM-specific immune targets for bsAb have been investigated in preclinical and/or clinical setting, for example, BCMA, G-protein-coupled receptor family C group 5 member D (GPRC5D), Fc receptor-homolog 5 (FcRH5), CD38, CD138, CD19, and signaling lymphocytic activation molecule family-7 (SLAMF7).[25] Herein, the authors summarize the mechanisms of action and the preclinical development of bsAbs targeting the above-mentioned antigens.

BCMA, also known as CD269 or tumor necrosis factor receptor superfamily 17 (TNFRSF17), is highly expressed in malignant plasma cells with low expression level in healthy human tissues.[26] BCMA is a type III transmembrane glycoprotein, which binds to B-cell-activating factor and a proliferation-inducing ligand. In turn, BCMA can regulate B-cell proliferation and differentiation into plasma cells, and in MM cells, BCMA represents an important pro-survival factor by activating various antiapoptotic pathways including nuclear factor 'kappa-light-chain-enhancer' of activated B-cells (NF-κB), mitogen-activated protein kinase, and protein kinase B (AKT).[27–31] Therefore, the BCMA has been selected as an ideal drug target for MM therapy. In cell lines and/or animal models, the BCMAxCD3 bsAbs BI 836909 and JNJ-64007957 (teclistamab) could lead to selective lysis of BCMA+ MM cells.[32,33] Currently, BCMA is the most commonly used immune target for CAR T cells and bsAb in MM patients.

GPRC5D is a transmembrane receptor expressed in the hair follicle and in the bone marrow from MM patients. Although the function of GPRC5D has not yet been determined, it has been found that overexpression of GPRC5D is associated with poor prognosis in patients with MM.[34–38] GPRC5D is considered as a drug target for anti-MM immunotherapy.[39] JNJ-64407564 (talquetamab), a GPRC5DxCD3 bsAb, could induce cell death of GPRC5D+ MM cells in vitro, in patient samples ex vivo and in mouse models.[40] Currently, GPRC5D-targeted bsAbs are investigated in clinical trials.

FcRH5 (also known as FcRL5, IFGP5, BXMAS1, CD307, or IRTA2) is a surface molecule predominantly expressed on B cells and malignant plasma cells, with the function of FcRH5 remaining not fully understood.[41–43] Moreover, MM cells displayed higher FcRH5 expression level compared with healthy plasma cells, and especially MM cell lines with 1q21 copy number abnormalities showed increased FcRH5 expression, as the FcRH5 gene is located on the human chromosome 1 band 1q23.1.[19,41,42,44] The FcRH5xCD3 bsAb BFCR4350 A (cevostamab) showed effective T-cell activation, cytokine release, and MM cell death in vitro and in vivo.[19] At present, cevostamab is further developed within clinical trials.

CD38, a type II transmembrane glycoprotein, is involved in cell adhesion and signaling and acts as an ectoenzyme for intracellular calcium mobilization.[45] CD38 is overexpressed on plasma cells and considered a drug target for treatment of MM, and CD38-targeted mAbs daratumumab and isatuximab have been approved by the US FDA for the treatment of MM in different combinations.[46–48] In a recent study, AMG424, a CD38xCD3 bsAb, could kill CD38+ MM cells and induce T-cell proliferation, with attenuated cytokine release in vitro and in vivo,[49] but the further clinical development of the drug was terminated.

CD138 (also known as syndecan-1) is a transmembrane heparin sulfate proteoglycan highly expressed on MM cells and can support the cell adhesion and survival of MM cells.[50,51] In cell lines, CD138xCD3 bsAbs h-STL002 and m-STL002 showed cytotoxicity against CD138+ MM cells by T-cell activation, highlighting that CD138 might be a potential drug target of bsAb for the treatment of MM.[52]

CD19 is widely expressed in B-cell lineage, but only a low proportion of MM cells were CD19+ as demonstrated by studies using flow cytometry.[53,54] However, a recent study using single molecule-sensitive direct stochastic optical reconstruction microscopy showed that MM cells with ultra-low CD19 expression (<100 molecules per cell) could also be eliminated by anti-CD19 CAR T cells, suggesting that CD19 could be a potential target for MM immunotherapies.[55] Thus, blinatumomab, the approved bsAb for B-cell precursor acute lymphoblastic leukemia (B-ALL), might also be a candidate drug for the treatment of CD19+ MM.[56–59]

SLAMF7 (also known as CS1 or CD319) is a member of the SLAMF, which is highly expressed in plasma cells and almost absent in other healthy tissues.[60] SLAMF7 can support the interaction between MM cells and bone marrow stromal cells and can promote MM cell survival by activating ERK1/2, STAT3, and AKT pathways.[61–63] SLAMF7-targeted mAb elotuzumab has been approved by the US FDA for the treatment of RRMM.[64,65] A preclinical study has evaluated a bsAb targeting SLAMF7 and NKG2D, which is widely expressed on cytotoxic immune cells including NK cells, CD8+ T cells, $\gamma\delta$ T cells, and NKT cells; in MM cell lines and mouse models, this SLAMF7xNKG2D bsAb facilitated immune synapse between SLAMF7+ MM cells and NKG2D+ immune effector cells, leading to activation of the most cells and MM cell lysis.[66]

Taken together, several bsAbs targeting different antigens have been developed for the treatment of MM in preclinical studies. However, most of the above-mentioned bsAbs for MM should be further tested in the clinical routine, especially the bsAbs targeting "non-BCMA" antigens. At the time of writing, clinical data are only available for bsAbs targeting BCMA, GPRC5D, FcRH5, and CD38.

SELECTED CLINICAL DATA OF BISPECIFIC ANTIBODIES IN RELAPSED/REFRACTORY MULTIPLE MYELOMA

At present, several bsAbs have been approved for the treatment of RRMM, and as previously mentioned, BCMA represents the most commonly used bsAb target in RRMM. Here, the authors provide a brief summary of selected clinical data of bsAb in RRMM (**Table 1**).

BCMAxCD3 Bispecific Antibodies

AMG420, a BCMAxCD3 bsAb, is the first-in-class bsAbs developed for MM. In a phase 1 study (NCT02514239), a total of 42 RRMM patients received AMG420 at 0.2 to 800 μg/d as a continuous infusion due to its short half-life time. The overall response rate (ORR) was 31% and 70% in the entire cohort and at the maximum tolerated dose of 400 μg/d, respectively. Adverse events (AEs) ≥ grade 3 included infection (19%), peripheral polyneuropathy (5%), edema (2%), and cytokine release syndrome (CRS) (2%). Serious AEs were seen in 48% patients ($n = 20$), including infections ($n = 14$) and polyneuropathy ($n = 2$). There was no grade ≥ 3 neurotoxicity observed.[67] The drug was not further developed for it required application as a continuous infusion.

AMG701 is a BCMAxCD3 bsAb with an extended half-life time of 112 hours, which enables weekly dosing of this product. In a phase 1 study (NCT03287908), 75 RRMM patients were treated with AMG701 at 3 to 12 mg weekly as intravenous infusions until disease progression, showing an ORR of 36% in the entire group and 83% at the dose of 9 mg weekly. The median response duration was 3.8 months with a maximum duration of 23 months. Four patients with negative minimal residual disease (MRD) showed sustained MRD negativity at the last observations up to 20 months later. The most common hematological AEs included anemia (43%), neutropenia (23%), and thrombocytopenia (20%). The most common non-hematological AEs were CRS (61%), diarrhea (31%), fatigue (25%), and fever (25%). Serious AEs were observed in 29 (39%) patients, including infections ($n = 13$), CRS ($n = 7$), and asymptomatic pancreatic enzyme rise ($n = 2$). Reversible treatment-related neurotoxicity was seen in six patients (all grade 1–2).[68] Further clinical development of this drug was stopped by the sponsor.

Teclistamab (JNJ-64007957) is a humanized BCMAxCD3 bsAb. In the phase 1/2 MajesTEC-1 study (NCT03145181 and NCT04557098), teclistamab was given to RRMM patients with ≥ 3 prior treatment lines. A total of 165 patients received a subcutaneous injection of teclistamab weekly at a dose of 1.5 mg/kg after step-up doses of 0.06 mg/kg and 0.3 mg/kg. The ORR was 63.0%, including 65 patients (39.4%) with complete response (CR) or better, and 44 patients (26.7%) reached MRD negativity. Common AEs included infections (76.4%; ≥ grade 3: 44.8%), CRS (72.1%; ≥ grade 3: 0.6%), neutropenia (70.9%; ≥ grade 3: 64.2%), anemia (52.1%; ≥ grade 3: 37.0%), and thrombocytopenia (40.0%; ≥ grade 3: 21.2%). Neurotoxic events were seen in 24 (14.5%) patients, with 5 (3.0%) patients suffering from immune effector cell-associated neurotoxicity syndrome (ICANS) (all grade 1 or 2). After a median follow-up of 14.1 months, the median progression-free survival (PFS) was 11.3 months (95% CI, 8.8–17.1).[69] Moreover, in the phase 1b MajesTEC-2 study (NCT04722146),

Table 1
Selected clinical data of bispecific antibody therapy for relapsed/refractory multiple myeloma

ClinicalTrials.gov Identifier	Bispecific Antibody	Targets	Study Phase	Estimated Enrollment	Status as of July 2023	Response Rates	AEs ≥ Grade 3
NCT02514239	AMG420	BCMA/CD3	1	43 patients	Completed	42 patients were treated. ORR: 31% (13/42); at MTD of 400 µg/d: 70% (7/10) including 50% (5/10) MRD-negative CR	Infection 19%; PNP 5%; edema 2%; CRS 2%
NCT03836053	AMG420	BCMA/CD3	1/2	23 patients	Completed	N/A	N/A
NCT03269136 Magnetismm-1	Elranatamab (PF-06863135)	BCMA/CD3	1	101 patients	Active, not recruiting	58 patients were treated. ORR in part 1: 70% (14/20) including CR/sCR of 30% (6/20); ORR at the RP2D: 83% (5/6)	No CRS ≥ grade 3 Lymphopenia 64%; neutropenia 60%: anemia 38%; thrombocytopenia 31%
NCT04649359 MagnetisMM-3	Elranatamab (PF-06863135)	BCMA/CD3	2	187 patients	Active, not recruiting	123 patients were treated. ORR 61.0%. In patients with 2–3 prior lines of therapy (n = 26): ORR 73.1%	Most common AEs ≥ grade 3 were hematologic. Non-hematologic AEs ≥ grade 3: COVID-pneumonia (10.6%), hypokalemia (9.8%), pneumonia (7.3%), sepsis (6.5%), hypertension (6.5%), ALT increased (5.7%), and SARS-COV-2 test positive (5.7%)

(continued on next page)

Table 1
(continued)

ClinicalTrials.gov Identifier	Bispecific Antibody	Targets	Study Phase	Estimated Enrollment	Status as of July 2023	Response Rates	AEs ≥ Grade 3
NCT03145181 MajesTEC-1	Teclistamab (JNJ-64007957)	BCMA/CD3	1	282 patients	Recruiting	165 patients were treated. ORR: 63.0%, including 39.4% (n = 65) CR or better and 26.7% (n = 44) MRD-negative patients	CRS 0.6%, neutropenia 64.2%, anemia 37.0%, thrombocytopenia 21.2%, infections 44.8%
NCT04722146 MajesTEC-2	Teclistamab (JNJ-64007957)	BCMA/CD3	1b	140 patients	Active, not recruiting	32 patients received tec-dara-len. ORR was 13/13 evaluable patients at 0.72 mg/kg and 13/16 evaluable patients at 1.5 mg/kg	No CRS ≥ grade 3, neutropenia 68.8%, fatigue 6.3%, insomnia 3.1%, pyrexia 6.3%, febrile neutropenia 12.5%, infections 28.1%
NCT05243797 MajesTEC-4	Teclistamab (JNJ-64007957)	BCMA/CD3	3	1530 patients	Recruiting	N/A	N/A
NCT05552222 MajesTEC-7	Teclistamab (JNJ-64007957)	BCMA/CD3	3	1060 patients	Recruiting	N/A	N/A
NCT03933735	TNB-383B	BCMA/CD3	1	220 patients	Active, not recruiting	124 patients were treated. ORR: 57% including 29% CR or better	No CRS ≥ grade 3, neutropenia 67%, anemia 17% in 40 mg cohort; CRS 2%, neutropenia 35%, anemia 12%, and thrombocytopenia 12% in 60 mg cohort

NCT number	Drug	Target	Phase	Patients	Status	Results	Safety
NCT03486067	Alnuctamab (ALNUC, CC-93269)	BCMA/CD3	1	220 patients	Recruiting	70 patients were treated with IV ALNUC with ORR 39%; 47 patients were treated with SC ALNUC with ORR: 51% with 17% ≥ CR	No CRS ≥ grade 3, neutropenia 30%, and anemia 17%
NCT03287908	AMG701	BCMA/CD3	1	174 patients	Active, not recruiting	75 patients were treated with ORR 36% including 4 sCR stringent CRs, 1 MRD-negative CR, 6 VGPRs, and 6 PRs	CRS 7%, serious AEs 39% including four deaths
NCT03761108	REGN-5458	BCMA/CD3	1/2	309 patients	Active, not recruiting	252 patients were treated. ORR at 200 mg dose levels was 64%; at doses 50 mg was 50%	At 200 mg: CRS 37%, fatigue 32%, and anemia 28% At 50 mg: CRS 53%, fatigue 33%, and anemia 40% ICANS ≥ grade 3: 2% (n = 2) at 200 mg and 1% (n = 1) at 50 mg
NCT04083534	REGN-5459	BCMA/CD3	1/2	43 patients	Active, not recruiting	N/A	N/A
NCT04108195 TRIMM-2	Teclistamab (JNJ-64007957)	BCMA/CD3	1b	294 patients	Active, not recruiting	33 patients were treated with tec + dara. Partial response or better: in cohort dara + tec 1500 µg/kg (n = 13/17); in cohort dara + tec 3000 µg/kg (n = 4/4); in cohort dara + tec 300 µg/kg (n = 1/2)	66.7% of patients had grade 3/4 AEs. Neutropenia 36.4%; thrombocytopenia 33.3%, anemia 24.2%, diarrhea 3.0%
	Talquetamab (JNJ-64407564)	GPRC5D/CD3	1b	294 patients	Active, not recruiting	N/A	N/A

(continued on next page)

Table 1
(continued)

ClinicalTrials.gov Identifier	Bispecific Antibody	Targets	Study Phase	Estimated Enrollment	Status as of July 2023	Response Rates	AEs ≥ Grade 3
NCT03399799 MonumenTAL-1	Talquetamab (JNJ-64407564)	GPRC5D/CD3	1	320 patients	Recruiting	95 patients were treated with SC talquetamab. ORR was 70% at 405 µg/kg weekly dose and the ORR was 71% at 800 µg/kg biweekly dose	At the 405 µg/kg weekly dose: CRS ≥ grade 3 (n = 1), neutropenia 60%, skin-related AEs 13%, infections ≥ grade 3 (n = 1); at the 800 µg/kg biweekly dose no CRS ≥ grade 3, neutropenia 35%, skin-related AEs: 13%; infections ≥ grade 3 (n = 1)
NCT04557150	RG6234 (RO7425781, forimtamig)	GPRC5D/CD3	1	480 patients	Recruiting	ORR: 68%, including 50% ≥VGPR	CRS: 85.4% (grade 3: 2.4%) Neurologic toxicity (headache and confusion): 7.3% Skin-related AEs: 66% Dysgeusia: 36.6%
NCT03309111	ISB1342	CD38/CD3	1	245 patients	Recruiting	24 patients received ISB1342. ORR N/A	Infusion-related reactions 17%, delirium (n = 1)
NCT03445663	AMG424	CD38/CD3	1	27 patients	Terminated	N/A	N/A
NCT03275103	Cevostamab (BFCR4350 A)	FcRH5/CD3	1	420 patients	Recruiting	160 patients had been enrolled. ORR was 54.5% at 160 mg dose level; ORR was 36.7% at 90 mg dose level	CRS 1.3%, ICANS 1.4%, infections 18.8%, neurologic/psychiatric 3.8%, anemia 21.9%, and diarrhea 0.6%
NCT03173430	Blinatumomab	CD19/CD3	1	6 patients	Terminated	N/A	N/A

Abbreviations: AE, adverse event; ALT, alanine transaminase; BCMA, B-cell maturation antigen; CR, complete remission; CRS, cytokine release syndrome; CD3, CD3 (cluster of differentiation 3) is a protein complex and T cell co-receptor; ICANS, immune effector cell-associated neurotoxicity syndrome; MRD, minimal residual disease; N/A, not available; ORR, overall response rate; RP2D, recommended phase 2 dose; sCR, stringent complete remission; VGPR, very good partial remission.

teclistamab was given in combination with other anti-MM agents such as daratumumab and lenalidomide. In this study, 32 patients received weekly teclistamab with step-up dosing of 0.72 or 1.5 mg/kg together with daratumumab 1800 mg and lenalidomide 25 mg (tec-dara-len). The most common AE was CRS (81.3%, all grade 1/2), and no ICANS was reported. The ORR was 100% (13/13) at 0.72 mg/kg and 81% (13/16) at 1.5 mg/kg in evaluable patients. Infections were reported in 24 (75.0%) patients, including upper respiratory infection (21.9%, $n = 7$), COVID-19 (21.9%, $n = 7$), and pneumonia (21.9%, $n = 7$).[70] In the phase 1b TRIMM-2 trial (NCT04108195), 33 RRMM patients with a median of five prior lines therapies were treated with teclistamab in combination with daratumumab (tec + dara). Mechanistically, it was observed that daratumumab could reduce CD38+ immunosuppressive regulatory T and B cells, increasing the T-cell clonality and functional response.[71,72] Of note, the ORR was 78% (18/23) in evaluable patients in the TRIMM-2 trial. The most common AE was CRS (54.5%, all grade 1/2) and no ICANS was reported. Other frequent AEs included neutropenia (36.4%; all grade 3/4), thrombocytopenia (36.4%; $\geq$ grade 3: 33.3%), anemia (36.4%; $\geq$ grade 3: 24.2%), diarrhea (36.4%; $\geq$ grade 3: 3.0%), nausea (30.3%; all grade 1/2), pyrexia (30.3%; all grade 1/2), and infections (51.5%; $\geq$ grade 3: 24.2%). Median duration of response (DOR) was not reached, and a data update is being excepted with a longer follow-up.[73] Currently, teclistamab is being investigated in the first line in ND MM. For instance, the phase 3 MajesTEC-4 study (NCT05243797) will compare the combination "tec-len" (teclistamab, lenalidomide) versus lenalidomide alone as maintenance therapy after ASCT in NDMM. Results from this trial will provide new insights into maintenance regimens that could improve response and prolong survival duration for NDMM.[74] In addition, the phase 3 MajesTEC-7 study (NCT05552222) will investigate the combination of "Tec-DR" (teclistamab, daratumumab, lenalidomide) versus DRd (daratumumab, lenalidomide, and dexamethasone) in NDMM which is not eligible or intended for ASCT. This trial may provide insights into a possible new first-line treatment with improved efficacy in transplant ineligible NDMM.[75] In 2022, teclistamab was approved by the European Medicines Agency for adult RRMM patients, who have received $\geq$ 3 prior lines of therapy, and in the United States, teclistamab received the FDA approval for the treatment of RRMM with $\geq$ 4 prior lines of therapy.[13] Currently, the phase 2 DSMM-XX trial (NCT05695508) is evaluating teclistamab in combination with DRd with or without bortezomib as induction therapy followed by ASCT and teclistamab in combination with daratumumab and lenalidomide as posttransplant maintenance in NDMM.

Elranatamab (PF-06863135) is another BCMAxCD3 bsAb evaluated in the phase 1 MagnetisMM-1 trial (NCT03269136). A total of 58 RRMM patients received subcutaneous elranatamab as monotherapy ($n = 50$) or in combination with lenalidomide ($n = 4$) or pomalidomide ($n = 4$). CRS were reported in 48 (83%) patients (all $\leq$ grade 2). Hematological AEs included lymphopenia ($n = 37$, 64%; 12% grade 3, 52% grade 4), neutropenia ($n = 37$, 64%; 31% grade 3, 29% Grade 4), anemia ($n = 32$, 55%; 38% grade 3), injection site reaction ($n = 31$, 53%; all $\leq$ grade 2), and thrombocytopenia ($n = 30$, 52%; 14% grade 3, 17% grade 4). Among the 20 patients who received efficacious dosing (215–1000 μg/kg), the ORR was 70% (14/20) with $\geq$ CR rate of 30% (6/20). At the recommended phase 2 dose of 1000 μg/kg, the ORR was 83%.[76] In the phase 2 study MagnetisMM-3 (NCT04649359), elranatamab was administered as single agent in patients with RRMM.[77] A total of 123 patients were included, and the ORR was 61.0%. In patients who received two to three prior lines of therapy ($n = 26$), the ORR was 73.1%, including 19.2% sCR, 26.9% CR, and 23.1% very good partial remission (VGPR). The most common $\geq$ grade 3 AEs were hematologic, and COVID-pneumonia showed the most common non-hematologic AE.[78]

Alnuctamab (also referred to as BMS-986349 or CC-93269), a humanized immuno-globulin G (IgG1) BCMAxCD3 bsAb with an asymmetric 2-arm, is characterized by biva-lent binding to BCMA and monovalently binding to CD3ε in a 2 + 1 format.[79] In the most recent update of the first-in-human phase 1 study CC-93269-MM-001 (NCT03486067), 70 patients received alnuctamab intravenously and 39% of them achieved an objective response. The median DOR was 146.1 weeks in patients who reached a response with intravenous alnuctamab therapy. In addition, 47 patients were treated with CC-93269 subcutaneously in dose escalation (10 mg: $n = 6$; 15 mg: $n = 4$; 30 mg: $n = 6$; and 60 mg: $n = 3$) as well as in dose expansion (10 mg: $n = 19$; 30 mg: $n = 9$). The most common AE was CRS (53%) and all CRS events were $\leq$ grade 2. Grade 1 ICANS was reported in one patient. Subcutaneous CC-93269 exhibited an improved safety profile compared with intravenous application. This study is currently ongoing.[80]

REGN5458 (linvoseltamab) is a BCMAxCD3 bsAb been investigated in RRMM within the phase 1/2 LINKER-MM1 trial (NCT03761108). A total of 252 RRMM patients were enrolled and treated with linvoseltamab at 50 or 200 mg dose. The ORR was 64% in the 200-mg dose cohort ($n = 58$) and 50% at 50 mg ($n = 104$). The most common AEs at 200 mg were CRS 37%, fatigue 32%, and anemia 28% and at 50 mg were CRS 53%, fatigue 33%, and anemia 40%. ICANS $\geq$ grade 3 occurred in 2% patients ($n = 2$) in the 200-mg cohort and in 1% patients ($n = 1$) at 50 mg.[81]

TNB-383B (ABBV-383), a BCMAxCD3 bsAb with two BCMA binding domains, was evaluated in a phase 1 study (NCT03933735). In this study, 124 RRMM patients ($\geq$3 prior lines of therapy) received ABBV-383 intravenously in a dose escalation cohort (0.025–120 mg, $n = 73$) and a dose expansion cohort (60 mg, $n = 51$). The ORR was 57% of all evaluable patients ($n = 122$) including 29% of patients with CR or bet-ter. At the dose $\geq$ 40 mg, the ORR was 68%. The most common hematological AEs $\geq$ grade 3 were neutropenia (34%) and anemia (16%). The most common non-hematological AEs included CRS (57%) and fatigue (30%), and $\geq$ grade 3 CRS was observed in three (2%) patients.[82]

GPRC5DxCD3 Bispecific Antibodies

Talquetamab (JNJ-64407564) is the first bsAb-targeting GPRC5DxCD3 bsAb in MM.[83] In the phase 1 MonumenTAL-1 trial (NCT03399799), 232 patients with RRMM received subcutaneous talquetamab. Of note, patients previously treated with BCMA-directed therapies were eligible in this study. Overall, 30 and 44 patients received the recommen-ded phase 2 doses of 405 μg/kg weekly and 800 μg/kg biweekly, respectively, and the ORR was similar in both patient cohorts (405 μg/kg weekly: 70%; 800 μg/kg biweekly: 64%). Likewise, the CRS rates were comparable in the both groups with 77% at 405 μg/kg weekly and 80% at 800 μg/kg biweekly. Of note, skin-related AEs (all grade 1/2) were found in a significant proportion of patients (405 μg/kg weekly: 67% including 57% nail disorders; 800 μg/kg biweekly: 70% including 27% nail disorders). Moreover, dysgeu-sia represented a frequent and relevant AE that might lead to weight loss in this study (405 μg/kg weekly: 63%; 800 μg/kg biweekly: 57%).[84,85] Currently, based on these results, a biologics license application has been submitted to the FDA for talquetamab for the treatment of RRMM. Further studies investigating talquetamab either as mono-therapy (NCT04634552) or in combination with other anti-MM agents [eg, RedirecTT-1 (NCT04586426), MonumenTAL-2 (NCT05050097), MonumenTAL-3 (NCT05455320), TRIMM-2 (NCT04108195), and TRIMM-3 (NCT05338775)] are underway. Most recently, Cohen and Morillo[86] reported the first results from the RedirecTT-1 study (NCT04586426) with the combination teclistamab and talquetamab in RRMM. A total of 63 patients with RRMM pretreated with a median of five (range 1–11) therapy lines were enrolled in this trial, with the majority of the patients being penta-refractory

(40/63, 63%). Extramedullary disease (EMD) was observed in 43% (27/63) of the patients. The most common treatment-emergent AEs included CRS (81%; grade 3: 3%), neutropenia (76%; grade 3/4: 75%), and anemia (60%; grade 3/4: 43%), and one patient presented with ICANS. The ORR was 84% (52/62) and 73% (19/26) in the entire group and in patients with EMD, respectively. At the recommended phase 2 dose, the ORR was 92% (12/13) among all evaluable patients.[87]

RG6234 (also referred to as RO7425781 or forimtamig) is another GPRC5DxCD3 bsAb characterized by increased half-life with a silent Fc-region. In a phase 1 trial (NCT04557150), 41 RRMM patients received RG6234 at a dosing level of 0.006 to 10 mg. CRS occurred in 85.4% (grade 3: 2.4%, all others grade 1/2) of the patients and CNS toxicity (headache and confusion) was observed in 3 (7.3%) patients. Skin-related AEs and dysgeusia were observed in 66% and 36.6% of patients, respectively. The ORR was 68% among the 34 patients with evaluable response data, including 50% with VGPR or better.[88]

Importantly, compared with BCMAxCD3 bsAbs, GPRC5D-targeting bsAbs induces a much lower B-cell depletion and, subsequently, lower grade of hypogammaglobu-linemia and infectious complications.[89,90]

FcRH5xCD3 Bispecific Antibodies

Cevostamab (BFCR4350 A) is an FcRH5xCD3 bsAb.[19] In the updated analysis of the phase 1 GO39775 trial (NCT03275103), 160 RRMM patients received intravenous cevostamab Q3W. Cevostamab was administered for a fixed duration of 17 cycles or until progression/unacceptable toxicity. CRS occurred in 128 (80.0%) patients (grade 3: 1.3%, all others grade 1/2), and CRS-associated ICANS was reported in 21 (13.1%) patients. Anemia and neutropenia were found in 51 (31.9%; $\geq$ grade 3: 21.9%) and 24 (15.0%%; $\geq$ grade 3: 13.8%) patients, respectively. In the 158 patients with evaluable efficacy data, response was observed at the 20- to 198-mg target dose levels, and higher target dose was associated with increased efficacy. The ORR was 54.5% and 36.7% at the 160 and 90 mg target dosing, respectively. Among the 16 patients who completed the 17 cycles, 8 of them showed a sustained response of $\geq$ 6 months after completion of therapy.[91–93]

CD38xCD3 Bispecific Antibodies

ISB1342 is the first humanized CD38xCD3 bsAb for MM. A phase 1 trial of ISB1342 in RRMM patients is still ongoing (NCT03309111). In the initial analysis, ISB1342 was given in 24 RRMM patients as infusion once weekly in 6 dose-escalation groups (range: 0.2/0.3–1.0/4.0 mg/kg). The most common AEs were infusion-related reactions (42%; grade 3: 16.7%), anemia (21%; grade 3: 4.2%), CRS (17%), thrombocytopenia (17%), diarrhea (13%), and lymphopenia (8.4%, all $\geq$ grade 3). Efficacy analysis is still pending.[94]

CD19xCD3 Bispecific Antibody

Blinatumomab is a humanized CD19xCD3 bsAb mainly used in the treatment of non-Hodgkin's lymphoma and ALL.[95] Blinatumomab was investigated in a pilot study (NCT03173430) in combination with salvage ASCT in RRMM. This study was terminated in 2020 due to slow accrual.

POTENTIAL RESISTANCE MECHANISMS

Although the results of recent clinical trials have demonstrated promising efficacy of bsAbs in RRMM, there are still patients who do not respond to the therapy or suffer from relapse in the course of the disease. However, the resistance mechanism of bsAbs in RRMM is poorly understood and has yet to be further explored. So far, the following factors have been reported to be associated with bsAb resistance in RRMM: loss of antigen, T-cell exhaustion, lack of recruitment or priming of T-cells, and immunosuppressive bone marrow microenvironment.[96]

The stable presence of the target antigens is a prerequisite for a successful bsAb therapy.[26] To date, the loss of antigen has already been reported to be a tumor intrinsic resistance mechanism in CAR T-cell and bsAb therapy for different hematologic malignancies. Homozygous BCMA loss was reported as a tumor intrinsic resistance mechanism in MM patients treated with BCMA-directed CAR T-cell therapy.[97,98] In bsAbs, CD20 negative relapse was found in B-cell non-Hodgkin lymphoma patients treated with CD20xCD3 bsAb REGN1979.[99,100] In MM patients treated with BCMAxCD3 and GPRC5DxCD3 bsAbs, the underlying mechanism of antigen loss has been further elucidated using genomic diagnostics such as whole genome sequencing and single-cell RNA sequencing. The expression level of target antigen was an important determinant of response in GPRC5DxCD3 bsAb therapy JNJ-7564, and bone marrow samples with higher GPRC5D expression showed superior MM cell lysis compared with those with lower GPRC5D expression.[101] More recently, Truger and colleagues[102] found biallelic BCMA gene deletion in a patient who received BCMAxCD3 bsAb AMG420, and this patient did not respond to anti-BCMA antibody drug conjugate belantamab mafodotin. Similarly, Lee and colleagues[103] reported a patient with biallelic BCMA gene deletion at the time point of disease progression after BCMAxCD3 bsAb therapy, and clonal biallelic GPRC5D loss following GPRC5DxCD3 bsAb was detected in another patient with preexisting monoallelic GPRC5D loss in 79.2% of the cells before bsAb therapy. Moreover, monoallelic BCMA loss coupled with de novo BCMA extracellular domain point mutation c.81 G greater than C [p.(R27P)] was identified as resistance mechanism in a patient progressing after BCMAxCD3 bsAb.[104] These findings suggested that irreversible complete antigen (eg, BCMA and GPRC5D) loss caused by deletion and/or mutation of the gene encoding for the target antigen may appear after bsAb therapy in MM patients, possibly due to the high selection pressure by bsAb that may lead to expansion of a preexisting small subclone without target antigen expression before bsAb treatment.[26] Importantly, in the study of Truger and colleagues, monoallelic BCMA and GPRC5D deletions were detected in 8% and 15% of MM patients being T-cell immunotherapy naïve, respectively, and these patients may have an increased risk to develop biallelic BCMA and GPRC5D loss after T-cell-based immunotherapies such as CAR T-cells or bsAb. However, gain of FcRH5 and SLAMF7 genes (both located in chromosome 1q) were significantly enriched in RRMM compared with NDMM, suggesting a low risk of FcRH5 and SLAMF7 loss in the course of the disease.[26,102] Taken together, irreversible complete antigen loss resulted by deletion and/or mutation represents a potential resistance mechanism to bsAb therapy in MM, and the selection of a drug targeting the "most suitable" antigen by genetic/genomic analysis is a crucial step for a successful treatment.

In bsAb therapies, the patients' own T cells are activated after establishing an immune synapse between MM and T cells, leading to cytokine release and tumor elimination. Therefore, the functionality of the patient's T cells may be an important factor that correlates with the therapy outcome. Leblay and colleagues[105] reported that MM patients responding to CAR T cells or bsAb therapy displayed a higher CD4/CD8 ratio and higher proportions of memory like T cells (T memory stem cells [Tscm] and central memory T cells) in comparison to patients resistant to T-cell-based immunotherapies. Moreover, these resistant patients likewise showed increased numbers/percentages of terminally exhausted T cells and senescent cells with upregulated expression of certain T-cell checkpoint molecules such as LAG3, TIGIT, and PD1. In addition, decreased anti-MM effect of JNJ-7564, a GPRC5DxCD3 bsAb, was found in elderly patients (>67 years) with low T-cell counts and thus low effector/target ratios (E:T), and in patients with high frequency of PD1+ T cells, MHC class II cell surface receptor (HLA-DR)+ activated T cells or immunosuppressive regulatory T cells as well as bone marrow stromal cells.[101] Recently, Neri and colleagues reported that CD8+ T cells were preferentially expanded by bsAb, and CD8+ naïve and memory T cells were enriched in responders to BCMAxCD3 bsAb therapy, while increased numbers/percentages of exhausted T cells, for example, granzyme K (GZMK)+ CD8+ T cells were found in resistant patients. In general, the current application schedule of bsAbs, mainly weekly or biweekly until progression, is probably not the ideal mode of application, leading to T-cell exhaustion with reduced antitumor efficacy and a considerable risk of severe infections. In RR B-ALL patients, 28-day continuous blinatumomab infusion resulted in reduced T-cell function. In an in vitro model with the CD19xCD3 bsAb AMG562, treatment-free intervals led to strong functional reinvigoration of T cells and transcriptional reprogramming. Importantly, treatment-free intervals improved T-cell expansion and tumor control in vivo.[106] In RRMM treated with teclistamab, patients showed sustained response after the switch from weekly to a less frequent biweekly dosing schedule, with a median DOR of 20.5 (range 1–23) months since switch.[107] Altogether, a fixed duration of administration of bsAbs and treatment-free intervals may significantly reduce infectious complications without interfering with antitumor efficacy.

Furthermore, the expression of major histocompatibility complex (MHC) class I on MM cells could support the cell–cell interaction between CD8+ T cells and MM cells, leading to amplified T-cell response and may be epitope spreading and thus priming/induction of a neo-antigen-specific T-cell response. On the other hand, the loss of MHC receptor molecules was described as a bsAb-induced adaption, which might result in immune escape and resistance to bsAbs.[108,109]

Combination therapy is a strategy to enhance the efficacy of bsAbs in RRMM by modulating the immune microenvironment. For instance, IMiD and BCMAxCD3 bsAb AMG701 acted synergistically and could overcome the immunosuppressive microenvironment associated with the presence of bone marrow stromal cells and osteoclasts that contribute to MM cell proliferation and drug resistance. Moreover, IMiD enhanced AMG701 efficacy by inducing T-cell differentiation to memory phenotypes, reducing immunosuppressive regulatory T cells and increasing CD8/CD4 ratios and percentages of Tscm.[110] Similarly, in vivo, BCMAxCD3 bsAb demonstrated only limited anti-MM effect in mice with high tumor burden, and concurrent administration of pomalidomide could increase T-cell response even in IMiD resistant cases, but induced T-cell exhaustion and, in turn, resulted in rapid progression thereafter. In contrast, by the addition of cyclophosphamide, T-cell exhaustion could be lessened, and durable remission was induced by reducing tumor burden as well as depleting regulatory T cells in vivo.[111] On the other hand, the triple combination with anti-PD1 checkpoint inhibitor in addition to bsAb and IMiD showed sustained activation and expansion of non-exhausted effector T cell at tumor sites probably by IL-2 production.[112]

SUMMARY AND OUTLOOK

The treatment of MM is evolving dramatically. Novel immunotherapies, that is, CAR T cells and bsAb, are leading to a paradigm shift of the MM treatment. When compared with CAR T-cell therapies, bsAb tends to show lower grade toxicity, which is limited to the first few weeks of administration. Thus, bsAb can be administrated in outpatient setting after the first doses with hospitalization. On the other hand, the ORR, CR rates, and PFS of bsAb therapies are lower and shorter when compared with most of the CAR T-cell products.[113] In brief, although bsAb therapies have shown promising efficacy and acceptable safety profile, these novel agents are still in their "infancy" with multiple unaddressed issues. For instance, the mechanisms of toxicities, including CRS, ICANS, and prolonged cytopenia following bsAb therapies, remain poorly understood. Moreover, most of the MM patients treated with bsAbs suffer from relapse in the course of the disease, and the multiple resistance mechanisms have to be addressed to further improve their efficacy. BsAb containing combination regimens have been described in in vitro and in vivo models and are currently entering clinical trials.

CLINICS CARE POINTS

- Severe cytokine release syndrome and neurotoxicity are observed only in a minority of patients receiving bispecific antibodies, but cytopenias and especially severe infections (up to 40% of treated patients) are frequently observed.
- Modifications of the current treatment schedules, for example, combination regimens and fixed therapy duration or longer treatment-free intervals, are currently tested in clinical trials to improve efficacy and reduce infectious complications
- Bispecific antibodies are increasingly used in earlier lines of therapy (as induction or consolidation or maintenance) as well as in combination regimens to further increase the anti-myeloma efficacy

REFERENCES

1. Rajkumar SV. Multiple myeloma: 2022 update on diagnosis, risk stratification, and management. Am J Hematol 2022;97(8):1086–107.
2. Attal M, Lauwers-Cances V, Hulin C, et al. Lenalidomide, Bortezomib, and Dexamethasone with Transplantation for Myeloma. N Engl J Med 2017;376(14):1311–20.
3. Goldschmidt H, Lokhorst HM, Mai EK, et al. Bortezomib before and after high-dose therapy in myeloma: long-term results from the phase III HOVON-65/GMMG-HD4 trial. Leukemia 2018;32(2):383–90.
4. Chetter I, Arundel C, Bell K, et al. The epidemiology, management and impact of surgical wounds healing by secondary intention: a research programme including the SWHSI feasibility RCT. Southampton (UK): Programme Grants for Applied Research; 2020.
5. Durie BGM, Hoering A, Abidi MH, et al. Bortezomib with lenalidomide and dexamethasone versus lenalidomide and dexamethasone alone in patients with newly diagnosed myeloma without intent for immediate autologous stem-cell transplant (SWOG S0777): a randomised, open-label, phase 3 trial. Lancet 2017;389(10068):519–27.
6. Facon T, Kumar SK, Plesner T, et al. Daratumumab, lenalidomide, and dexamethasone versus lenalidomide and dexamethasone alone in newly diagnosed multiple myeloma (MAIA): overall survival results from a randomised, open-label, phase 3 trial. Lancet Oncol 2021;22(11):1582–96.
7. Zhou X, Einsele H, Danhof S. Bispecific Antibodies: A New Era of Treatment for Multiple Myeloma. J Clin Med 2020;9(7):2166.

8. Ho WY, Blattman JN, Dossett ML, et al. Adoptive immunotherapy: engineering T cell responses as biologic weapons for tumor mass destruction. Cancer Cell 2003;3(5):431–7.

9. Yang Q, Li X, Zhang F, et al. Efficacy and Safety of CAR-T Therapy for Relapse or Refractory Multiple Myeloma: A systematic review and meta-analysis. Int J Med Sci 2021;18(8):1786–97.

10. Cipkar C, Chen C, Trudel S. Antibodies and bispecifics for multiple myeloma: effective effector therapy. Hematology Am Soc Hematol Educ Program 2022; 2022(1):163–72.

11. Mullard A. FDA approves first BCMA-targeted CAR-T cell therapy. Nat Rev Drug Discov 2021;20(5):332.

12. Mullard A. FDA approves second BCMA-targeted CAR-T cell therapy. Nat Rev Drug Discov 2022;21(4):249.

13. Kang C. Teclistamab: First Approval. Drugs 2022;82(16):1613–9.

14. Rendo MJ, Joseph JJ, Phan LM, et al. CAR T-Cell Therapy for Patients with Multiple Myeloma: Current Evidence and Challenges. Blood Lymphat Cancer 2022; 12:119–36.

15. Kazandjian D, Kowalski A, Landgren O. T cell redirecting bispecific antibodies for multiple myeloma: emerging therapeutic strategies in a changing treatment landscape. Leuk Lymphoma 2022;63(13):3032–43.

16. Granger K, Gaffney KJ, Davis JA. Newly approved and forthcoming T-cell-redirecting bispecific antibodies for the treatment of relapsed/refractory multiple myeloma. J Oncol Pharm Pract 2023;29(3):722–6.

17. Link BK, Kostelny SA, Cole MS, et al. Anti-CD3-based bispecific antibody designed for therapy of human B-cell malignancy can induce T-cell activation by antigen-dependent and antigen-independent mechanisms. Int J Cancer 1998; 77(2):251–6.

18. Shah N, Chari A, Scott E, et al. B-cell maturation antigen (BCMA) in multiple myeloma: rationale for targeting and current therapeutic approaches. Leukemia 2020;34(4):985–1005.

19. Li J, Stagg NJ, Johnston J, et al. Membrane-Proximal Epitope Facilitates Efficient T Cell Synapse Formation by Anti-FcRH5/CD3 and Is a Requirement for Myeloma Cell Killing. Cancer Cell 2017;31(3):383–95.

20. Seckinger A, Delgado JA, Moser S, et al. Target Expression, Generation, Preclinical Activity, and Pharmacokinetics of the BCMA-T Cell Bispecific Antibody EM801 for Multiple Myeloma Treatment. Cancer Cell 2017;31(3):396–410.

21. Goldstein RL, Goyos A, Li CM, et al. AMG 701 induces cytotoxicity of multiple myeloma cells and depletes plasma cells in cynomolgus monkeys. Blood Adv 2020;4(17):4180–94.

22. Brinkmann U, Kontermann RE. The making of bispecific antibodies. mAbs 2017; 9(2):182–212.

23. Madduri D, Dhodapkar MV, Lonial S, et al. SOHO State of the Art Updates and Next Questions: T-Cell-Directed Immune Therapies for Multiple Myeloma: Chimeric Antigen Receptor-Modified T Cells and Bispecific T-Cell-Engaging Agents. Clin Lymphoma, Myeloma & Leukemia 2019;19(9):537–44.

24. Kontermann RE, Brinkmann U. Bispecific antibodies. Drug Discov Today 2015; 20(7):838–47.

25. Moreau P, Touzeau C. T-cell-redirecting bispecific antibodies in multiple myeloma: a revolution? Blood 2022;139(26):3681–7.

26. Zhou X, Rasche L, Kortum KM, et al. BCMA loss in the epoch of novel immunotherapy for multiple myeloma: from biology to clinical practice. Haematologica 2023;108(4):958–68.

27. Tai YT, Acharya C, An G, et al. APRIL and BCMA promote human multiple myeloma growth and immunosuppression in the bone marrow microenvironment. Blood 2016;127(25):3225–36.

28. Moreaux J, Legouffe E, Jourdan E, et al. BAFF and APRIL protect myeloma cells from apoptosis induced by interleukin 6 deprivation and dexamethasone. Blood 2004;103(8):3148–57.

29. Tai YT, Li XF, Breitkreutz I, et al. Role of B-cell-activating factor in adhesion and growth of human multiple myeloma cells in the bone marrow microenvironment. Cancer Res 2006;66(13):6675–82.

30. Cho SF, Anderson KC, Tai YT. Targeting B Cell Maturation Antigen (BCMA) in Multiple Myeloma: Potential Uses of BCMA-Based Immunotherapy. Front Immunol 2018;9:1821.

31. Demchenko YN, Glebov OK, Zingone A, et al. Classical and/or alternative NF-kappaB pathway activation in multiple myeloma. Blood 2010;115(17):3541–52.

32. Pillarisetti K, Powers G, Luistro L, et al. Teclistamab is an active T cell-redirecting bispecific antibody against B-cell maturation antigen for multiple myeloma. Blood Adv 2020;4(18):4538–49.

33. Hipp S, Tai YT, Blanset D, et al. A novel BCMA/CD3 bispecific T-cell engager for the treatment of multiple myeloma induces selective lysis in vitro and in vivo. Leukemia 2017;31(8):1743–51.

34. Gao Y, Wang X, Yan H, et al. Comparative Transcriptome Analysis of Fetal Skin Reveals Key Genes Related to Hair Follicle Morphogenesis in Cashmere Goats. PLoS One 2016;11(3):e0151118.

35. Inoue S, Nambu T, Shimomura T. The RAIG family member, GPRC5D, is associated with hard-keratinized structures. J Invest Dermatol 2004;122(3):565–73.

36. Kim YJ, Yoon B, Han K, et al. Comprehensive Transcriptome Profiling of Balding and Non-Balding Scalps in Trichorhinophalangeal Syndrome Type I Patient. Ann Dermatol 2017;29(5):597–601.

37. Atamaniuk J, Gleiss A, Porpaczy E, et al. Overexpression of G protein-coupled receptor 5D in the bone marrow is associated with poor prognosis in patients with multiple myeloma. Eur J Clin Invest 2012;42(9):953–60.

38. Cohen Y, Gutwein O, Garach-Jehoshua O, et al. GPRC5D is a promising marker for monitoring the tumor load and to target multiple myeloma cells. Hematology 2013;18(6):348–51.

39. Smith EL, Harrington K, Staehr M, et al. GPRC5D is a target for the immunotherapy of multiple myeloma with rationally designed CAR T cells. Sci Transl Med 2019;11(485):eaau7746.

40. Pillarisetti K, Edavettal S, Mendonca M, et al. A T-cell-redirecting bispecific G-protein-coupled receptor class 5 member D x CD3 antibody to treat multiple myeloma. Blood 2020;135(15):1232–43.

41. Elkins K, Zheng B, Go M, et al. FcRL5 as a target of antibody-drug conjugates for the treatment of multiple myeloma. Mol Cancer Therapeut 2012;11(10):2222–32.

42. Polson AG, Zheng B, Elkins K, et al. Expression pattern of the human FcRH/IRTA receptors in normal tissue and in B-chronic lymphocytic leukemia. Int Immunol 2006;18(9):1363–73.

43. Stewart AK, Krishnan AY, Singhal S, et al. Phase I study of the anti-FcRH5 anti-body-drug conjugate DFRF4539A in relapsed or refractory multiple myeloma. Blood Cancer J 2019;9(2):17.
44. Inoue J, Otsuki T, Hirasawa A, et al. Overexpression of PDZK1 within the 1q12-q22 amplicon is likely to be associated with drug-resistance phenotype in multiple myeloma. Am J Pathol 2004;165(1):71–81.
45. Funaro A, Malavasi F. Human CD38, a surface receptor, an enzyme, an adhesion molecule and not a simple marker. J Biol Regul Homeost Agents 1999; 13(1):54–61.
46. Lin P, Owens R, Tricot G, et al. Flow cytometric immunophenotypic analysis of 306 cases of multiple myeloma. Am J Clin Pathol 2004;121(4):482–8.
47. de Weers M, Tai YT, van der Veer MS, et al. Daratumumab, a novel therapeutic human CD38 monoclonal antibody, induces killing of multiple myeloma and other hematological tumors. J Immunol 2011;186(3):1840–8.
48. Zhu C, Song Z, Wang A, et al. Isatuximab Acts Through Fc-Dependent, Independent, and Direct Pathways to Kill Multiple Myeloma Cells. Front Immunol 2020;11:1771.
49. Zuch de Zafra CL, Fajardo F, Zhong W, et al. Targeting Multiple Myeloma with AMG 424, a Novel Anti-CD38/CD3 Bispecific T-cell-recruiting Antibody Optimized for Cytotoxicity and Cytokine Release. Clin Cancer Res 2019;25(13): 3921–33.
50. Akhmetzyanova I, McCarron MJ, Parekh S, et al. Dynamic CD138 surface expression regulates switch between myeloma growth and dissemination. Leukemia 2020;34(1):245–56.
51. Gotte M. Syndecans in inflammation. Faseb J 2003;17(6):575–91.
52. Chen D, Zou J, Zong Y, et al. Anti-human CD138 monoclonal antibodies and their bispecific formats: generation and characterization. Immunopharmacol Immunotoxicol 2016;38(3):175–83.
53. Robillard N, Wuilleme S, Moreau P, et al. Immunophenotype of normal and myelomatous plasma-cell subsets. Front Immunol 2014;5:137.
54. Tembhare PR, Yuan CM, Venzon D, et al. Flow cytometric differentiation of abnormal and normal plasma cells in the bone marrow in patients with multiple myeloma and its precursor diseases. Leuk Res 2014;38(3):371–6.
55. Nerreter T, Letschert S, Gotz R, et al. Super-resolution microscopy reveals ultra-low CD19 expression on myeloma cells that triggers elimination by CD19 CAR-T. Nat Commun 2019;10(1):3137.
56. Ali S, Moreau A, Melchiorri D, et al. Blinatumomab for Acute Lymphoblastic Leukemia: The First Bispecific T-Cell Engager Antibody to Be Approved by the EMA for Minimal Residual Disease. Oncol 2020;25(4):e709–15.
57. Bargou R, Leo E, Zugmaier G, et al. Tumor regression in cancer patients by very low doses of a T cell-engaging antibody. Science 2008;321(5891):974–7.
58. Kantarjian H, Stein A, Gokbuget N, et al. Blinatumomab versus Chemotherapy for Advanced Acute Lymphoblastic Leukemia. N Engl J Med 2017;376(9): 836–47.
59. Topp MS, Gokbuget N, Stein AS, et al. Safety and activity of blinatumomab for adult patients with relapsed or refractory B-precursor acute lymphoblastic leukaemia: a multicentre, single-arm, phase 2 study. Lancet Oncol 2015;16(1): 57–66.
60. Hsi ED, Steinle R, Balasa B, et al. CS1, a potential new therapeutic antibody target for the treatment of multiple myeloma. Clin Cancer Res 2008;14(9):2775–84.

61. Tai YT, Soydan E, Song W, et al. CS1 promotes multiple myeloma cell adhesion, clonogenic growth, and tumorigenicity via c-maf-mediated interactions with bone marrow stromal cells. Blood 2009;113(18):4309–18.

62. Tai YT, Dillon M, Song W, et al. Anti-CS1 humanized monoclonal antibody Hu-Luc63 inhibits myeloma cell adhesion and induces antibody-dependent cellular cytotoxicity in the bone marrow milieu. Blood 2008;112(4):1329–37.

63. Wang Y, Sanchez L, Siegel DS, et al. Elotuzumab for the treatment of multiple myeloma. J Hematol Oncol 2016;9(1):55.

64. Magen H, Muchtar E. Elotuzumab: the first approved monoclonal antibody for multiple myeloma treatment. Ther Adv Hematol 2016;7(4):187–95.

65. Ratner M. FDA approves three different multiple myeloma drugs in one month. Nat Biotechnol 2016;34(2):126.

66. Chan WK, Kang S, Youssef Y, et al. A CS1-NKG2D Bispecific Antibody Collectively Activates Cytolytic Immune Cells against Multiple Myeloma. Cancer Immunol Res 2018;6(7):776–87.

67. Topp MS, Duell J, Zugmaier G, et al. Anti-B-Cell Maturation Antigen BiTE Molecule AMG 420 Induces Responses in Multiple Myeloma. J Clin Oncol 2020; 38(8):775–83.

68. Harrison SJ, Minnema MC, Lee HC, et al. A Phase 1 First in Human (FIH) Study of AMG 701, an Anti-B-Cell Maturation Antigen (BCMA) Half-Life Extended (HLE) BiTE® (bispecific T-cell engager) Molecule, in Relapsed/Refractory (RR) Multiple Myeloma (MM). Blood 2020;136(Supplement 1):28–9.

69. Moreau P, Garfall AL, van de Donk N, et al. Teclistamab in Relapsed or Refractory Multiple Myeloma. N Engl J Med 2022;387(6):495–505.

70. Searle E, Quach H, Wong SW, et al. Teclistamab in Combination with Subcutaneous Daratumumab and Lenalidomide in Patients with Multiple Myeloma: Results from One Cohort of MajesTEC-2, a Phase1b, Multicohort Study. Blood 2022;140(Supplement 1):394–6.

71. Rodríguez-Otero P, D'Souza A, Reece DE, et al. A novel, immunotherapy-based approach for the treatment of relapsed/refractory multiple myeloma (RRMM): Updated phase 1b results for daratumumab in combination with teclistamab (a BCMA x CD3 bispecific antibody). J Clin Oncol 2022;40(16_suppl):8032.

72. Krejcik J, Casneuf T, Nijhof IS, et al. Daratumumab depletes CD38+ immune regulatory cells, promotes T-cell expansion, and skews T-cell repertoire in multiple myeloma. Blood 2016;128(3):384–94.

73. Rodriguez-Otero P, Dholaria B, Askari E, et al. Subcutaneous Teclistamab in Combination with Daratumumab for the Treatment of Patients with Relapsed/Refractory Multiple Myeloma: Results from a Phase 1b Multicohort Study. Blood 2021;138(Supplement 1):1647.

74. Zamagni E, Boccadoro M, Spencer A, et al. MajesTEC-4 (EMN30): A Phase 3 Trial of Teclistamab + Lenalidomide Versus Lenalidomide Alone As Maintenance Therapy Following Autologous Stem Cell Transplantation in Patients with Newly Diagnosed Multiple Myeloma. Blood 2022;140(Supplement 1): 7289–91.

75. Krishnan AY, Manier S, Terpos E, et al. MajesTEC-7: A Phase 3, Randomized Study of Teclistamab + Daratumumab + Lenalidomide (Tec-DR) Versus Daratumumab + Lenalidomide + Dexamethasone (DRd) in Patients with Newly Diagnosed Multiple Myeloma Who Are Either Ineligible or Not Intended for Autologous Stem Cell Transplant. Blood 2022;140(Supplement 1):10148–9.

76. Sebag M, Raje NS, Bahlis NJ, et al. Elranatamab (PF-06863135), a B-Cell Maturation Antigen (BCMA) Targeted CD3-Engaging Bispecific Molecule, for Patients

with Relapsed or Refractory Multiple Myeloma: Results from Magnetismm-1. Blood 2021;138(Supplement 1):895.

77. Lesokhin A, Iida S, Stevens D, et al. Magnetismm-3: An Open-Label, Multicenter, Non-Randomized Phase 2 Study of Elranatamab (PF-06863135) in Patients with Relapsed or Refractory Multiple Myeloma. Blood 2021;138(Supplement 1):1674.

78. Tomasson MH, Arnulf B, Bahlis NJ, et al. Elranatamab, a B-cell maturation antigen (BCMA)-CD3 bispecific antibody, for patients (pts) with relapsed/refractory multiple myeloma (RRMM): Extended follow up and biweekly administration from the MagnetisMM-3 study. J Clin Oncol 2023;41(16_suppl):8039.

79. Costa LJ, Wong SW, Bermúdez A, et al. First Clinical Study of the B-Cell Maturation Antigen (BCMA) 2+1 T Cell Engager (TCE) CC-93269 in Patients (Pts) with Relapsed/Refractory Multiple Myeloma (RRMM): Interim Results of a Phase 1 Multicenter Trial. Blood 2019;134(Supplement_1):143.

80. Wong SW, Bar N, Paris L, et al. Alnuctamab (ALNUC; BMS-986349; CC-93269), a B-Cell Maturation Antigen (BCMA) x CD3 T-Cell Engager (TCE), in Patients (pts) with Relapsed/Refractory Multiple Myeloma (RRMM): Results from a Phase 1 First-in-Human Clinical Study. Blood 2022;140(Supplement 1):400–2.

81. Bumma N, Richter JR, Dhodapkar MV, et al. LINKER-MM1 study: Linvoseltamab (REGN5458) in patients with relapsed/refractory multiple myeloma. J Clin Oncol 2023;41(16_suppl):8006.

82. D'Souza A, Shah N, Rodriguez C, et al. A Phase I First-in-Human Study of ABBV-383, a B-Cell Maturation Antigen x CD3 Bispecific T-Cell Redirecting Antibody, in Patients With Relapsed/Refractory Multiple Myeloma. J Clin Oncol 2022; 40(31):3576–86.

83. Verkleij CPM, Broekmans MEC, van Duin M, et al. Preclinical activity and determinants of response of the GPRC5DxCD3 bispecific antibody talquetamab in multiple myeloma. Blood Adv 2021;5(8):2196–215.

84. Chari A, Minnema MC, Berdeja JG, et al. Talquetamab, a T-Cell-Redirecting GPRC5D Bispecific Antibody for Multiple Myeloma. N Engl J Med 2022; 387(24):2232–44.

85. Krishnan AY, Minnema MC, Berdeja JG, et al. Updated Phase 1 Results from MonumenTAL-1: First-in-Human Study of Talquetamab, a G Protein-Coupled Receptor Family C Group 5 Member D x CD3 Bispecific Antibody, in Patients with Relapsed/Refractory Multiple Myeloma. Blood 2021;138(Supplement 1):158.

86. Cohn Y, Morillo D. First results from the RedirecTT-1 study with teclistamab (tec) + talquetamab (tal) simultaneously targeting BCMA and GPRC5D in patients (pts) with relapsed/refractory multiple myeloma (RRMM), *J Clin Oncol*, 41, (16_suppl), 2023, 8002.

87. Morillo D, Gatt ME, Sebag M, et al. First results from the RedirecTT-1 study with teclistamab (tec) + talquetamab (tal) simultaneously targeting BCMA and GPRC5D in patients (pts) with relapsed/refractory multiple myeloma (RRMM). J Clin Oncol 2023;41(16_suppl):8002.

88. Hasselbalch Riley C, Hutchings M, Yoon S-S, et al. S180: RG6234, A NOVEL GPRC5D T-CELL ENGAGING BISPECIFIC ANTIBODY, INDUCES RAPID RESPONSES IN PATIENTS WITH RELAPSED/REFRACTORY MULTIPLE MYELOMA: PRELIMINARY RESULTS FROM A FIRST-IN-HUMAN TRIAL. HemaSphere 2022;6:81–2.

89. Sim BZ, Longhitano A, Er J, et al. Infectious complications of bispecific antibody therapy in patients with multiple myeloma. Blood Cancer J 2023;13(1):34.

90. Mazahreh F, Mazahreh L, Schinke C, et al. Risk of infections associated with the use of bispecific antibodies in multiple myeloma: a pooled analysis. Blood Adv 2023;7(13):3069–74.
91. Cohen AD, Harrison SJ, Krishnan A, et al. Initial Clinical Activity and Safety of BFCR4350A, a FcRH5/CD3 T-Cell-Engaging Bispecific Antibody, in Relapsed/Refractory Multiple Myeloma. Blood 2020;136(Supplement 1):42–3.
92. Trudel S, Cohen AD, Krishnan AY, et al. Cevostamab Monotherapy Continues to Show Clinically Meaningful Activity and Manageable Safety in Patients with Heavily Pre-Treated Relapsed/Refractory Multiple Myeloma (RRMM): Updated Results from an Ongoing Phase I Study. Blood 2021;138(Supplement 1):157.
93. Lesokhin AM, Richter J, Trudel S, et al. Enduring Responses after 1-Year, Fixed-Duration Cevostamab Therapy in Patients with Relapsed/Refractory Multiple Myeloma: Early Experience from a Phase I Study. Blood 2022;140(Supplement 1):4415–7.
94. Mohan SR, Costa Chase C, Berdeja JG, et al. Initial Results of Dose Escalation of ISB 1342, a Novel CD3xCD38 Bispecific Antibody, in Patients with Relapsed/Refractory Multiple Myeloma (RRMM). Blood 2022;140(Supplement 1):7264–6.
95. Viardot A, Bargou R. Bispecific antibodies in haematological malignancies. Cancer Treat Rev 2018;65:87–95.
96. Ahn S, Leblay N, Neri P. Understanding the Mechanisms of Resistance to T Cell-based Immunotherapies to Develop More Favorable Strategies in Multiple Myeloma. Hemasphere 2021;5(6):e575.
97. Da Via MC, Dietrich O, Truger M, et al. Homozygous BCMA gene deletion in response to anti-BCMA CAR T cells in a patient with multiple myeloma. Nat Med 2021;27(4):616–9.
98. Samur MK, Fulciniti M, Aktas Samur A, et al. Biallelic loss of BCMA as a resistance mechanism to CAR T cell therapy in a patient with multiple myeloma. Nat Commun 2021;12(1):868.
99. Bannerji R, Allan JN, Arnason JE, et al. Clinical Activity of REGN1979, a Bispecific Human, Anti-CD20 x Anti-CD3 Antibody, in Patients with Relapsed/Refractory (R/R) B-Cell Non-Hodgkin Lymphoma (B-NHL). Blood 2019;134(Supplement_1):762.
100. Bannerji R, Arnason JE, Advani R, et al. Emerging Clinical Activity of REGN1979, an Anti-CD20 x Anti-CD3 Bispecific Antibody, in Patients with Relapsed/Refractory Follicular Lymphoma (FL), Diffuse Large B-Cell Lymphoma (DLBCL), and Other B-Cell Non-Hodgkin Lymphoma (B-NHL) Subtypes. Blood 2018;132(Supplement 1):1690.
101. Verkleij CPM, Broekmans M, Wong A, et al. Mechanisms of Resistance and Determinants of Response of the GPRC5D-Targeting T-Cell Redirecting Bispecific Antibody JNJ-7564 in Multiple Myeloma. Blood 2020;136(Supplement 1):8–9.
102. Truger MS, Duell J, Zhou X, et al. Single- and double-hit events in genes encoding immune targets before and after T cell-engaging antibody therapy in MM. Blood Adv 2021;5(19):3794–8.
103. Lee H, Neri P, Ahn S, et al. Role of TNFRSF17 and GPRC5D Structural and Point Mutations in Resistance to Targeted Immunotherapies in Multiple Myeloma (MM). Blood 2022;140(Supplement 1):252–3.
104. Bahlis N, Lee H, Ahn S, et al. Mechanisms of antigen escape from BCMA- or GPRC5D-targeted immunotherapies in multiple myeloma. Nat Med 2023;29(9):2295–306.
105. Leblay N, Maity R, Barakat E, et al. Cite-Seq Profiling of T Cells in Multiple Myeloma Patients Undergoing BCMA Targeting CAR-T or Bites Immunotherapy. Blood 2020;136(Supplement 1):11–2.

106. Philipp N, Kazerani M, Nicholls A, et al. T-cell exhaustion induced by continuous bispecific molecule exposure is ameliorated by treatment-free intervals. Blood 2022;140(10):1104–18.

107. Karlin L, Benboubker L, Nahi H, et al. Durability of responses with biweekly dosing of teclistamab in patients with relapsed/refractory multiple myeloma achieving a clinical response in the majesTEC-1 study. J Clin Oncol 2023; 41(16_suppl):8034.

108. Neri P, Ahn S, Lee H, et al. Dysfunctional Hyper-Expanded Clonotypes and Lack of TCR Clonal Replacement Predict Resistance to T Cell Engagers in Multiple Myeloma. Blood 2022;140(Supplement 1):2093–4.

109. Friedrich MJ, Neri P, Kehl N, et al. The pre-existing T cell landscape determines the response to bispecific T cell engagers in multiple myeloma patients. Cancer Cell 2023;41(4):711–725 e6.

110. Cho SF, Lin L, Xing L, et al. The immunomodulatory drugs lenalidomide and pomalidomide enhance the potency of AMG 701 in multiple myeloma preclinical models. Blood Adv 2020;4(17):4195–207.

111. Meermeier EW, Welsh SJ, Sharik ME, et al. Tumor burden limits bispecific antibody efficacy through T cell exhaustion averted by concurrent cytotoxic therapy. Blood Cancer Discov 2021;2(4):354–69.

112. Meermeier EW, Welsh SJ, Sharik M, et al. Abstract 5588: PD-1 blockade synergizes with IMiDs to enhance bispecific T cell engager immune responses to Vk*MYChCRBN multiple myeloma by preventing T cell exhaustion. Cancer Res 2022;82(12_Supplement):5588.

113. Ravi G, Costa LJ. Bispecific T-cell engagers for treatment of multiple myeloma. Am J Hematol 2023;98(Suppl 2):S13–21.

Chimeric Antigen Receptor T Cells in the Treatment of Multiple Myeloma

Zainul S. Hasanali, MD, PhD, Beatrice Razzo, MD,
Sandra P. Susanibar-Adaniya, MD, Alfred L. Garfall, MD,
Edward A. Stadtmauer, MD, Adam D. Cohen, MD*

KEYWORDS

- Chimeric antigen receptor Tcells (CARTs) • Multiple myeloma
- B cell maturation antigen (BCMA) • Cytokine release syndrome (CRS)
- Relapsed/refractory multiple myeloma

KEY POINTS

- Data from the clinical trials of the Food and Drug Administration (FDA)-approved B cell maturation antigen (BCMA)-targeted CART therapies idecabtagene vicleucel and ciltacabtagene autoleucel show chimeric antigen receptor T cells (CARTs) to be safe and effective in the treatment of multiply relapsed/refractory multiple myeloma.
- There are additional novel BCMA-targeted CARTs in development with varying degrees of efficacy and innovation, including rapid manufacturing protocols.
- CARTs against novel targets, particularly G protein–coupled receptor, class C, group 5, member D (GPRC5D), are showing early promise.
- Strategies to overcome limitations of CART therapy (T cell dysfunction, target loss, immunogenicity, toxicities, and equity) include earlier line treatment, multitargeted CARTs, less immunogenic CARTs, and community access.

INTRODUCTION

A chimeric antigen receptor (CAR) is a synthetically engineered cell surface receptor that combines an antigen recognition domain, most commonly derived from the scFv portion of an antibody, with hinge and transmembrane regions and intracellular signaling domains designed to activate T cells. Peripheral blood T cells obtained through leukapheresis are transduced with genetic material encoding the CAR, leading to expression on the T cell surface, thereby conferring novel antigen specificity.

Division of Hematology/Oncology, Department of Medicine, Abramson Cancer Center, University of Pennsylvania, 3400 Civic Center Boulevard, 12th Floor South Tower, Philadelphia, PA 19104, USA
* Corresponding author.
E-mail address: Adam.Cohen@pennmedicine.upenn.edu

Hematol Oncol Clin N Am 38 (2024) 383–406
https://doi.org/10.1016/j.hoc.2023.12.004
0889-8588/24/© 2023 Elsevier Inc. All rights reserved.

Although the use of CARs to induce T cell activation was initially described more than 30 years ago,[1] the successful translation of this approach to the clinic during the past decade is due to several recent advances, including incorporation of costimulatory domains such as CD28 or 4-1BB to enhance T cell proliferation and survival, development of improved viral vectors for T cell transduction, advances in ex vivo cellular manufacturing, and addition of lymphodepleting chemotherapy conditioning before CAR T cell (CART) infusion.[2–6] These advances paved the way for clinical trials using CD19-directed CARTs, with significant activity seen against relapsed/refractory acute lymphoblastic leukemia (ALL), chronic lymphocytic leukemia (CLL), and B-cell non-Hodgkin lymphomas,[7–9] followed by the first Food and Drug Administration (FDA) approvals of CART products in Fall 2017. Subsequent studies of CARTs demonstrated unprecedented single-agent activity in relapsed/refractory multiple myeloma (RRMM), with 2 products now FDA-approved—idecabtagene vicleucel (ide-cel) in 2021 and ciltacabtagene autoleucel (cilta-cel) in 2022—and several more in development. In this article, we will review the history of CARTs in myeloma, approved agents, side effects and new therapies in development.

HISTORY OF CHIMERIC ANTIGEN RECEPTOR T CELL THERAPY IN MYELOMA

The first reported use of CART therapy in myeloma was published in 2015,[10] describing a heavily pretreated patient who achieved a durable complete response (CR) after infusion of autologous CD19-directed CARTs 12 days after a salvage melphalan-conditioned autologous stem cell transplant (ASCT). The rationale was that CARTs might target a minor CD19+ component of the malignant clone with stem cell-like properties, perhaps delaying or preventing relapse.[11] Only one additional patient treated with this approach derived incremental benefit,[12] and the role (if any) of targeting CD19 in myeloma remains unclear. However, this initial study, along with other early small CART studies targeting CD138[13] or kappa light chain,[14] demonstrated the feasibility of generating a viable CART product from patients with RRMM, as well as important early safety data.

The first consistent clinical responses in RRMM were obtained with CART products targeting B cell maturation antigen (BCMA). BCMA is a cell surface receptor with expression limited to late-stage B lineage cells, particularly plasma cells, and is expressed consistently on myeloma cells, although intensity of expression can vary from patient to patient.[15] Binding of BCMA to its ligands B cell activating factor (BAFF) and a proliferation inducing ligand (APRIL) provides a proliferation and survival signal to myeloma cells, making it a rational target for immunotherapy. Kochenderfer and colleagues were the first to demonstrate preclinical activity of a BCMA-specific CART against myeloma,[16] leading to a first-in-human trial of this CART product, which opened at the National Cancer Institute in 2015.[17] Subsequently, 3 additional phase 1, dose-escalation studies using BCMA-specific CARTs opened in late 2015-early 2016: a single-institution study at the University of Pennsylvania using the CART-BCMA product,[18] and 2 multicenter trials, one in the United States using bb2121 (Bluebird Biotech, ultimately becoming ide-cel)[19] and one in China using LCAR-B38 M (Legend Biotech, ultimately becoming cilta-cel).[20] All were relatively small studies, using different CAR constructs and different lymphodepletion regimens. The US studies had very heavily treated (median 7 lines) patients with high-risk cytogenetics, whereas the Chinese study patients were less heavily treated (median 3 lines) but still had high-risk features (eg, extramedullary disease). All showed high response rates (64%–90% at optimal doses), including minimal residual disease (MRD)-negative CRs in some patients. They did not demonstrate unexpected/unusual toxicities outside those typically associated with CARTs. Together, these studies demonstrated proof-of-principle that targeting BCMA with CARTs could induce deep responses in highly refractory patients. They laid the groundwork for the pivotal trials of ide-cel and cilta-cel leading to commercial approval, as well as an explosion of trials testing alternative CART products targeting BCMA and other antigens.

IDECABTAGENE VICLEUCEL: KarMMa TRIAL AND OTHER DATA IN LATE LINE MULTIPLE MYELOMA

The first BCMA-targeting CART product to gain access for commercial use was Ide-cel. It received accelerated FDA approval on March 26, 2021, and European Medicines Agency (EMA) authorization on August 18, 2021, for use in patients with RRMM following 4 and 3 prior lines of therapy, respectively. Ide-cel was approved on the basis of the KarMMa registration trial, designed as an open-label phase 2 study of single-agent ide-cel given at 1 of 3 different fixed doses (150, 300, and 450×10^6 cells) after lymphodepletion with fludarabine and cytarabine.[21] One hundred and twenty-eight patients with a median of 6 prior lines of therapy (84% triple-class refractory), Eastern Cooperative Oncology Group (ECOG) performance status < 2 and minimal organ dysfunction were enrolled between 2017 and 2018. Groups with atypical presentations of RRMM (eg, nonsecretory disease, central nervous system [CNS], or leukemic involvement) were not eligible.

Commonly reported adverse events (AEs) were hematologic (neutropenia 91%, anemia 91%, and thrombocytopenia 63%), inflammatory (84% cytokine release syndrome [CRS], 5% grade $\geq$3), and infectious (68.8%), in nature. Neurotoxicity was reported in 18% patients (3% grade 3) with a median onset of 2 days.[21] Neurotoxic events were not specifically addressed as immune effector cell-associated neurotoxicity syndrome (ICANS) vs non-ICANS in the KarMMa publication, although are described as both elsewhere.[22]

The overall response rate (ORR) among KarMMa participants was 73%, and 33% of patients achieved a CR—most of these (26% of participants) were MRD-negative stringent CRs. Responses were sustained for a median duration of 10.7 months (95% CI 5.6–11.6) and the median progression-free survival (PFS) was 8.8 months (95% CI 5.6–11.6) for the entire population, and 12.1 months (95% CI 8.8–12.3) at the recommended 450×10^6 CAR+ cell dose. The PFS curves do not seem to plateau, even for those in CR, indicating that, despite robust initial responses, the vast majority of patients eventually relapsed. Indirect matched comparisons of the KarMMa patients with patients with historical RRMM receiving standard regimens (eg, selinexor, belantamab mafodotin, and standard triplets) show superior outcomes for ide-cel.[23–25]

Real-world reports of the commercially administered product have demonstrated comparable tolerability and efficacy to that reported in KarMMa, despite including a more heavily pretreated patient population, most of whom would not have been trial-eligible.[26–28] This real-world experience also demonstrated that patients with prior anti-BCMA therapy exposure, who were excluded from the KarMMa study, could still respond to ide-cel (ORR 73% vs 87% for BCMA therapy-naïve patients) but that the depth of response (CR rate 29% vs 48%, respectively) and PFS (median 3.2 vs 9.0 months, respectively) were significantly lower with prior anti-BCMA therapy exposure.[28] A phase 3 randomized study of ide-cel versus 6 standard of care (SOC) regimens in earlier refractory disease (2–4 prior lines of therapy) demonstrated greater ORR and longer PFS with ide-cel,[29] as discussed -later-. Many other studies of ide-cel in newly diagnosed, early and late RRMM are ongoing and are likely to further inform patient and disease adapted strategies for using this first-in-class agent.

CILTACABTAGENE AUTOLEUCEL: CARTITUDE-1 AND OTHER DATA IN LATE LINE MULTIPLE MYELOMA

Cilta-cel is an FDA-approved second-in-class CART therapy for RRMM after 4 or more prior lines of therapy, including a proteasome inhibitor, an immunomodulatory agent, and an anti-CD38 monoclonal antibody. Unlike its predecessor, cilta-cel has a CAR that expresses 2 BCMA-targeting single domain variable heavy domain of heavy chain (VHH) camelid antibodies, along with a CD3ζ signaling domain and a 4-1BB costimulatory domain. As mentioned earlier, cilta-cel was first studied as LCAR-B38 M in a Chinese phase 1 trial (LEGEND-2) where it showed strong activity in multiply-relapsed myeloma with ORR of 88% and 74% CR rate.[20] A recent update of this study, now with more than 5 years of follow-up, shows these responses can be durable (median duration of response [DOR] 22.3 months, median PFS 18.0 months), with 21.7% of patients still alive and progression-free at 5 years.[30]

CARTITUDE-1 was the phase 1 b/2 study of cilta-cel in the United States using a construct identical to that of LEGEND-2 and whose results led to FDA approval. CARTITUDE-1 was a single-arm open-label study at 16 centers enrolling 113 patients with median 6 lines (88% triple-class refractory) of prior therapy. Cilta-cel was administered to 97 patients as a single infusion (0.75×10^6 CAR+ cells/kg) 5 to 7 days after fludarabine and cyclophosphamide lymphodepletion. As of the first clinical cutoff with a median follow-up of 12.4 months, ORR was 97% with 67% CR rate. The 12-month PFS rate was 77%, and OS was 89%. Patient surveyed health-related quality of life on CARTITUDE-1 was also significantly improved, with increases in physical and emotional scales over time and a concurrent decrease in symptom score.[31] Common grade 3 to 4 adverse event (AE) were neutropenia (95%), anemia (68%), leukopenia (61%), and thrombocytopenia (60%). CRS occurred in 95% of patients, with all but one case resolving (death secondary to hemophagocytic lymphohistiocytosis [HLH]). Neurotoxicity occurred in 21% of patients, including both traditional ICANS as well as delayed neurotoxicity such as cranial nerve palsies and Parkinsonism. Fourteen deaths occurred, 6 due to treatment-related AE, 5 secondary to disease progression, and 3 due to treatment-unrelated events.[32] Most recent analysis at median 33 months of follow-up showed ORR 98%, CR rate 83%, median DOR 33.9 months, median PFS 34.9 months, and median OS not reached, indicating deep and durable responses.[33] Longer follow-up is needed to see if there will be a plateau on this PFS curve but, so far, even patients with sustained MRD-negative CRs are relapsing, suggesting that similar to ide-cel, cilta-cel is likely not curative in the very late-line setting.

Although far from perfect, comparative efficacy analyses have sought to contrast the effectiveness of cilta-cel versus ide-cel and other SOC therapies used in RRMM. Including patients who would have been eligible for ide-cel under clinical trial, there was a significantly improved odds ratio favoring cilta-cel in ORR, CR rate, DOR and PFS, although OS showed no difference.[34] Similarly, using patients who met inclusion criteria for CARTITUDE-1 from the POLLUX, CASTOR and EQUULEUS trials for daratumumab-based triplets as a simulated control arm, odds ratios favored cilta-cel in ORR, CR rate, PFS, and OS, suggesting the use of cilta-cel may be superior to noncellular therapies in the fourth line,[35] although no definitive conclusions can be drawn without head-to-head trials. In addition, a retrospective consortium study of real-world use of cilta-cel found similar ORR (89%) and rates of CRS and ICANS to that seen in CARTITUDE-1, despite 57% of patients being ineligible for trial inclusion. CR rates (56%) were somewhat lower in the real world, although follow-up was less than 6 months, and PFS/OS data were immature. Out-of-specification products were used in 22% (31/143) of patients, reflecting the real-world manufacturing issues that can occur with cilta-cel.[36]

Finally, the safety and efficacy of cilta-cel after prior BCMA-directed therapy (either belantamab mafodotin or a bispecific antibody) was examined in a small prospective study (CARTITUDE-2, cohort C). Similar to ide-cel, cilta-cel can generate responses (ORR 60%) even in these highly-refractory patients but the depth (CR rate 30%) and durability of these responses (median DOR 11.5 months, median PFS 9.1 months) is lower than that seen in BCMA therapy-naïve patients.[37] This suggests that this very late stage is not the optimal time to maximize the potential of these CART products in myeloma.

CHIMERIC ANTIGEN RECEPTOR T CELLS IN EARLIER LINES AND ROLE OF MAINTENANCE

There are several rationales for the use of CARTs in earlier lines of multiple myeloma (MM) therapy: (1) T cells harvested from patients with less prior exposure to lymphotoxic myeloma therapy and lower disease burden may be healthier and therefore yield a more consistently effective product with higher potential for long-lived functional persistence; (2) less-aggressive disease and more options for bridging therapy in early-line patients would reduce the risk of disease-related complications while awaiting manufacturing and allow better myeloma control before infusion, which would potentially reduce the risk of severe CART toxicities that have been associated with high disease burden.

The most notable clinical experiences with CARTs in early-line therapy are 2 randomized phase 3 trials published in the last year comparing ide-cel (KarMMa-3, 2–4 prior regimens)[29] and cilta-cel (CARTITUDE-4, 1–3 prior regimens),[38] to SOC MM therapies. Results of both studies alongside results of the pivotal phase 2 studies of ide-cel and cilta-cel in late-line patients are summarized in **Table 1**. Both studies demonstrated significant improvement in response rate and PFS compared with standard alternative regimens. For KarMMa-3, median PFS was 13.3 months versus 4.4 months (HR 0.49, $P < .001$) for ide-cel versus SOC, respectively. For CARTITUDE-4, median PFS was

Table 1
Comparison of registration trials of cilta-cel and ide-cel

| | Cilta-cel Studies[a] | | | Ide-cel Studies[b] | | |
| | CARTITUDE-4 | | CARTITUDE-1 | KarMMa-3 | | KarMMa |
	cilta-cel	SOC[d]	cilta-cel	ide-cel	SOC[d]	ide-cel
Median lines	2	2	6	3	3	6
Triple-class refractory (%)	14	16	88	65	67	86
ORR[c] (%)	85	67	83	71	42	67
12m PFS (%)	76	49	~75[e]	55	30	~30[e]
G3+ CRS (%)	1	N/A	4	5	N/A	5
G3+ NT (%)	2	N/A	9	3	N/A	3

Abbreviations: CRS, cytokine release syndrome; NT, neurotoxicity; ORR, overall response rate; PFS, progression-free survival.

a 32,53

b 21,29

c Overall response rate in the intent-to-treat population for each study.

d SOC, standard of care. For CARTITUDE-4 this was choice of daratumumab, pomalidomide, dexamethasone (DPd) or bortezomib, pomalidomide, dexamethasone (VPd). For KarMMA-3, this was choice of DPd, DVd (daratumumab, bortezomib, and dexamethasone), IRd (ixazomib, lenalidomide, and dexamethasone), EPd (elotuzumab, pomalidomide, and dexamethasone), or Kd (carfilzomib and dexamethasone)

e Visually estimated from Kaplan–Meier curves for the "as treated" populations.

not reached versus 11.8 months (HR 0.26, $P < .0001$) for cilta-cel versus SOC, respectively. OS data were immature at time of analysis. Incidence of high-grade toxicity, particularly neurotoxicity, with cilta-cel seemed more favorable in early-line usage; only one low-grade episode of the Parkinsonian-like movement and neurocognitive toxicity observed on CARTITUDE-1 was observed on CARTITUDE-4. Collectively, these results support the safety and superior efficacy of CARTs over standard myeloma therapies in patients who have received 1 to 4 prior lines of therapy.

A somewhat surprising finding from these phase 3 trials is that ORR and 12-month PFS after CART therapy when used earlier (CARTITUDE-4[39] and KarMMa-3[29]) seem similar to the later line evaluations (CARTITUDE-1[32] and KarMMa[21]). Although this somewhat undercuts the efficacy rationale for earlier use of CARTs, longer follow-up, particularly with cilta-cel, may be required to appreciate differences in the proportion of long-term survivors. It is also possible that even earlier use is required to realize efficacy gains from fitter T cells since even 1 to 4 prior lines of therapy in the setting of disease progression may be sufficient to compromise T cell fitness.

Several ongoing studies are evaluating CART therapy as a component of first-line MM therapy, typically as a consolidation after response to standard induction therapy with or without ASCT (**Table 2**). We recently published an initial experience with CARTs as consolidation of standard therapy in either the first or the intermediate line-of-therapy.[40] Our findings were reassuring regarding the potential for CARTs to proliferate in vivo and exert antimyeloma activity even in settings of low target antigen burden. The safety profile in this setting was similarly reassuring, and we found that maintenance therapy with lenalidomide or pomalidomide was safe and feasible and associated in some patients with modest CART reexpansion and late-onset clinical responses. Several ongoing studies are also exploring the safety and tolerability of maintenance lenalidomide after BCMA CART therapy (eg, BMT-CTN1902, CARTITUDE-6; see **Table 2**), with the hope that incorporation of CARTs into first-line treatment will improve the frequency of sustained MRD-negative CRs, allowing for a fixed duration of lenalidomide and eliminating the need for indefinite maintenance.

OTHER B CELL MATURATION ANTIGEN-DIRECTED CHIMERIC ANTIGEN RECEPTOR T CELLS IN CLINICAL DEVELOPMENT

In addition to the 2 commercially available BCMA CART products, there are several others undergoing clinical trials. **Table 3** summarizes those with clinical data available for at least 10 patients with a minimum follow-up of more than 90 days. Several autologous CART products are attempting to reduce CAR immunogenicity and perhaps prolong persistence by using either fully human (CT053, CT103 A) or synthetic (CART-ddBCMA) antigen-binding domains. These have shown promising response rates of 90% to 100% in early studies in RRMM[41–43] and are moving toward registrational trials. Several other products (eg, bb21217, P-BCMA-101, and JCARH125/orvacel) used novel transduction and/or manufacturing modifications to generate CAR T cells enriched for a central memory and/or stem cell memory phenotype, also hoping to improve CART persistence but lack of convincing improvement in outcomes led to discontinuation of these programs.[44–46] Perhaps more promising are recent products (eg, GC012 F, PHE885, and CC-98633) that use rapid manufacturing protocols (2–5 days) to limit in vitro activation of CART cells, relying more on in vivo expansion in the patient. This has several potential advantages, including shorter vein-to-vein time with less need for bridging therapy, less induction within the CART cells of a terminally differentiated and/or exhausted state, and greater proliferative capacity of the infused cells. Early clinical data show high response rates (93%–100%) at low

Table 2
Myeloma chimeric antigen receptor T therapy trials in first-line treatment

NCT Number	Study Title	Sponsor/Collaborators	Results
NCT03455972	Study of T Cells Targeting CD19/BCMA (CART-19/BCMA) for High Risk Multiple Myeloma Followed With Auto-HSCT	The First Affiliated Hospital of Soochow University	PMID 35114022
NCT03549442	Up-front CART-BCMA With or Without huCART19 in High-risk Multiple Myeloma	University of Pennsylvania, Novartis	PMID 36413381
NCT04617704	BCMA and CD19 Targeted Fast Dual CART for Chromosomal Abnomalities High-risk BCMA+ Multiple Myeloma	Shanghai Changzheng Hospital, Gracell Biotechnology Shanghai Co., Ltd.	
NCT05712083	A Study of BCMA CAR-T Cell Therapy for Newly Diagnosed Multiple Myeloma	Zhejiang University, Yake Biotechnology Ltd.	
NCT05846737	BCMA CAR-T Cell Therapy in High-risk NDMM Patients With Positive MRD After First-line ASCT	Institute of Hematology & Blood Diseases Hospital	
NCT05032820	MM CAR-T to Upgrade Response BMTCTN1902	Blood and Marrow Transplant Clinical Trials Network, NHLBI, NCI, Bristol Myers Squibb	
NCT05860036	A Study of Bortezomib, Lenalidomide and Dexamethasone (VRd) Followed by BCMA CAR-T Therapy in Transplant-Ineligible Patients With New-diagnosed Multiple Myeloma	Institute of Hematology & Blood Diseases Hospital	
NCT05870917	A Study of Ve-VRD or S-VRD Combined With CART-ASCT-CART2 Treatment in Patients With Primary Plasma Cell Leukemia	Institute of Hematology & Blood Diseases Hospital	
NCT05632380	ASCT in Combination With C-CAR038 for Treating Patients With Ultra High-risk Multiple Myeloma (MM)	Institute of Hematology & Blood Diseases Hospital, Cellular Biomedicine Group Ltd.	

(continued on next page)

Table 2
(continued)

NCT Number	Study Title	Sponsor/Collaborators	Results
NCT04923893	A Study of Bortezomib, Lenalidomide and Dexamethasone (VRd) Followed by Cilta-cel, a CAR-T Therapy Directed Against BCMA vs VRd Followed by Lenalidomide and Dexamethasone (Rd) Therapy in Participants With Newly Diagnosed Multiple Myeloma for Whom ASCT is Not Planned as Initial Therapy	Janssen Research & Development, LLC	
NCT04935580	Study of FasT CAR-T GC012 F Injection in High Risk TE NDMM Patients	Shanghai Changzheng Hospital, Gracell Biotechnology Shanghai Co., Ltd.	https://doi.org/10.1182/blood-2022-162295
NCT05840107	Study of FasT CAR-T GC012 F Injection NDMM Patients	Shanghai Changzheng Hospital, Gracell Biotechnology Shanghai Co., Ltd.	
NCT04196491	A Study to Evaluate the Safety of bb2121 in Subjects With High Risk, Newly Diagnosed Multiple Myeloma (NDMM)	Celgene	
NCT05257083	A Study of Daratumumab, Bortezomib, Lenalidomide and Dexamethasone (DVRd) Followed by Ciltacabtagene Autoleucel vs Daratumumab, Bortezomib, Lenalidomide and Dexamethasone (DVRd) Followed by Autologous Stem Cell Transplant (ASCT) in Participants With Newly Diagnosed Multiple Myeloma (CARTITUDE-6)	Janssen Research & Development, LLC, European Myeloma Network	

Table 3
Novel B cell maturation antigen-targeted chimeric antigen receptor T therapies in early-stage clinical trials

	CT053[41] Zevorcabtagene (Zevor-Cel)	CT103 A[42]	BB21217[44,93]	P-BCMA-101[45]	JCARH125[46] Orvacabtagene Autoleucel (Orva-Cel)	CC-98633[47]	PHE885[48]	ALLO-715[50]	CART-ddBCMA[43]
Product	Fully humanized scFv (25C2) and 4-1BB costimulatory domain	Fully humanized scFv	Ide-cel cocultured with PI3K inhibitor bb007	Nonviral piggyBac DNA mod system using transposons and rimiducid safety switch	Fully human scFv, equal CD4:CD8 ratio enriched for central memory	Orva-cel with NEX-T 5 day manufacturing	Fully humanized 2 day manufacturing with T-charge platform	Second gen scFv with TALEN knockout of T cell receptor alpha constant and CD52 with rituximab safety switch	Synthetic antigen-binding domain with reduced immunogenicity and improved CAR stability
Study	LUMMICAR (NCT03975907)	FUMANBA-1 (NCT05066646)	CRB-042 (NCT03274219)	PRIME/POSEIDA (NCT03288493)	EVOLVE (NCT03430011)	CC-98633/BMS-986354 (NCT04394650)	PHE885 (NCT04318327)	UNIVERSAL (NCT04093596)	iMMagine-1 (NCT05396885)
Trial Phase	2	1 b/2	1	1	1/2	1	1	1	2
Patient population	RRMM ≥3	RRMM ≥3	RRMM ≥3	RRMM ≥3	RRMM ≥3	RRMM ≥3	RRMM ≥2	RRMM ≥3	RRMM ≥3
Patients enrolled	102	103	72	90	44	54	46	43	12
ORR (%)	93	95	69	57	95, 94, 75	98	98, 100 for highest doses	56 (71 at highest dose)	100
CR/sCR (%)	42	74	28	N/A	26, 50, 43	30	42	N/A	75
VGPR or better (%)	82	91	58	N/A	68, 67, 43	57	N/A	N/A	75
mPFS (mo)	NR	NR	14	N/A	N/A	N/A	N/A	N/A	NR
mDOR (mo)	NR	N/A	17	N/A	N/A	N/A	N/A	8	NR
MRD neg rate (%)	CR-95.2, VGPR+ - 88	all-95, CR/sCR-100	93	N/A	N/A	N/A	all-60%	N/A	N/A
total CRS (G3+) (%)	90 (7)	93 (1)	75(2)	25 (0)	70 (2)	80 (2)	96 (11)	56 (2)	100 (17)

(continued on next page)

Table 3
(continued)

	CT053[41] Zevorcabtagene (Zevor-Cel)	CT103 A[42]	BB21217[44,93]	P-BCMA-101[45]	JCARH125[46] Orvacabtagene Autoleucel (Orva-Cel)	CC-98633[47]	PHE885[48]	ALLO-715[50]	CART-ddBCMA[43]
ICANS (G3+) (%)	2	2(0)	15(20)	7 (2)	25 (4)	11 (2)	22 (7)	14 (0)	17 (0)
Prior BCMA treatment allowed	No	yes	No	Yes	No	No	Prior BCMA CART excluded	No	No
Notes		~20% prior BCMA CART treated		25% outpatient administration	3 different doses	3 different doses, median follow-up 4.9 mo	5 different doses, time from apheresis to lymphodepletion 16 d	4 different CART doses, conditioned with ALLO-657 (anti-CD52), infection (53.5% G3+ 23.3%)	2 different doses, 1 death noted later and trial on hold as of June 2023

Abbreviations: BCMA, B cell maturation antigen; CR/sCR, complete response/stringent complete response; CRS, cytokine release syndrome; ICANS, immune effector cell-associated neurotoxicity syndrome; mDOR, median duration of response; mPFS, median progression-free survival; MRD, minimal residual disease; N/A, not applicable (not reported); NR, not reached; ORR, overall response rate; RRMM, relapsed/refractory multiple myeloma; scFv, single-chain variable fragment; VGPR, very good partial response.

cell doses,[47–49] although longer follow-up is needed to determine if response durability will be improved over currently available products. Finally, ALLO-715 is the first allogeneic BCMA CART to demonstrate activity in RRMM, with ORR of 56% (71% at highest dose), and no graft-versus-host-disease seen.[50] Although this product has the obvious advantages of being off-the-shelf and generated from healthy donor T cells, the need for augmented immunosuppression with an anti-CD52 antibody and increased risk of infection are drawbacks, and additional improvements to this approach are likely needed before it supplants autologous CARTs.

TOXICITIES OF CHIMERIC ANTIGEN RECEPTOR T CELL THERAPIES

In line with other CARTs, the main AEs from BCMA CARTs are CRS, neurotoxicity, fatigue, cytopenias, hypogammaglobulinemia, and infections.[51] The most mature data regarding AEs continue to be from ide-cel and cilta-cel and are described here to represent the myeloma CART class. In KarMMa, CRS occurred in 84% of treated patients with 79% of cases either grade 1 or grade 2.[21] CRS rates were higher in CARTITUDE-1 (95%) but again 95% of cases were grade 2 or lower.[32] One major difference between ide-cel and cilta-cel is the median onset of CRS, ranging between 1 and 2 days in the former and 7 days in the latter. In most cases, CRS responds promptly to standard measures such as tocilizumab and/or steroids, although rare cases of refractory CRS and/or development of immune effector cell-associated HLH have been seen with both products, which may require alternative immunosuppressive strategies such as anakinra,[52] and rarely can be fatal.

A second difference between the 2 products is the rate, onset, and severity of ICANS and neurotoxicity. KarMMa had 18% of ide-cel-treated patients experiencing ICANS with only 3% grade 3 or greater, and median onset of 2 days.[21] Comparatively, in the initial report of CARTITUDE-1, 21% of cilta-cel-treated patients developed neurotoxicity, with median onset of 8 days, and 9% had grade 3 or greater. This included ICANS in 17% (2% grade ≥3), and other neurotoxicities in 12% (8% grade ≥3). Eight patients had both ICANS and other neurotoxicities, which could include cranial nerve palsies, peripheral neuropathies, and a Parkinsonism-like movement and neurocognitive disorder.[32] This latter AE ultimately developed in 6 patients in CARTITUDE-1, with median onset of 27 days (range 3–914). It did not improve with carbidopa-levodopa or aggressive immunosuppression. Risk factors included high tumor burden, grade 2 or higher CRS, ICANS after infusion, and/or high CART-cell expansion and persistence.[53,54] Decreasing disease burden before CART administration, continued monitoring with writing tests past day 100 postinfusion and earlier intervention with steroids and tocilizumab to prevent high-grade CRS and ICANS may have reduced the risk of this complication to less than 1% in subsequent cilta-cel studies.[54] Of note, Parkinsonism has been described following ide-cel infusion as well,[55] and has been hypothesized to be an on-target effect of BCMA-directed CART therapy against basal ganglia neurons aberrantly expressing BCMA,[56] although this requires further validation. Optimal management remains unclear.

High-grade cytopenias are expected and near-universal following CART therapy, due to both lymphodepleting chemotherapy and cytokine-mediated effects on the bone marrow. Although most patients recover, prolonged neutropenia and thrombocytopenia beyond 1 to 3 months were seen in 12% to 20% and 41% to 47%, respectively, of late-line RRMM patients with grade 3 or higher cytopenias in the KarMMa and CARTITUDE-1 studies.[21,32] Management includes growth factor and transfusion support, as well as evaluation to rule out viral infections (eg, cytomegalovirus [CMV] and Epstein-Barr virus [EBV]) and secondary myelodysplasia. Patients with prolonged transfusion-dependent cytopenias may benefit from stem cell boost, if available.[57]

Hypogammaglobulinemia and infections remain the most common late risk following BCMA CART therapy, with highest incidence in the first 3 to 6 months, although the risk can persist up to a year. Respiratory viruses and bacterial infections predominate, although pneumocystis pneumonia and more rare viral and fungal infections can occur as well.[58] Recommendations for prevention include antibacterial and antifungal prophylaxis until neutrophil recovery, as well as antiviral and antipneumocystis therapy and intravenous immunoglobulin (IVIG) replacement for 6 to 12 months, along with vaccinations against influenza, coronavirus disease 2019 (COVID-19), and pneumococcus.[59] Finally, secondary malignancies have been commonly seen post-CART therapy in late-line RRMM (eg, 20 out of 97 patients in CARTITUDE-1),[33] including several cases of myelodysplastic syndrome and acute myeloid leukemia, necessitating ongoing vigilance and age-appropriate surveillance.

NON-B CELL MATURATION ANTIGEN-DIRECTED CHIMERIC ANTIGEN RECEPTOR T CELLS FOR MYELOMA

In addition to the development of novel BCMA-targeted CARTs, there have been several strategies aimed at developing CARTs to other myeloma targets, including CD19, GPRC5D, and CS1/SLAMF7. **Table 4** summarizes those with clinical data available for at least 10 patients with a minimum follow-up of more than 90 days.

CD19

Minor subsets of the MM clone with less-differentiated plasma cell phenotypes or B cell phenotypes that are CD19+ can be identified in patients.[60] To target these putative myeloma-propagating cells, Garfall and colleagues clinically evaluated autologous T cells transduced with a CAR against CD19 (CTL019) in patients with RRMM undergoing salvage ASCT (see **Table 4**).[12] Two of 10 evaluable subjects exhibited significantly longer PFS after ASCT+ CTL019 compared with their prior ASCT (479 vs 181 days; 249 vs 127 days). Ex vivo treatment of primary myeloma samples with a combination of CTL019 and CARTs against BCMA reliably inhibited myeloma colony formation in vitro, whereas treatment with either CART alone inhibited colony formation inconsistently.[12] Thus in a follow-up study, they explored the combination of CTL019 and BCMA-targeted CAR T cells (CART-BCMA) in relapsed patients responding to current therapy (n = 10), and also randomized newly-diagnosed high-risk patients with MM responding to induction therapy to CART-BCMA alone or CART-BCMA + CTL019 (n = 10 each). Administration of both CART products did not lead to increased CRS, ICANS or other toxicities, and both products expanded well despite low antigen burden. Although the study was not powered for direct efficacy comparisons between the arms, the addition of CD19-targeting CARTs did not seem to provide additional clinical benefit.[40]

In contrast, 2 trials from Wang and colleagues[61] and Du and colleagues[62] exploring CARTs targeting both CD19 and BCMA had impressive clinical activity (see **Table 4**). In particular, the GC012 F bispecific CART product with rapid manufacturing had an ORR of 93% and median DOR of 37 months in 28 patients with RRMM.[62] It is difficult, however, in these single-arm trials to determine the contribution of the CD19-targeting component versus the BCMA-targeting component and/or other unique attributes of each product, so for now, the benefit of targeting CD19 in MM remains unproven.

G Protein–Coupled Receptor, Class C, Group 5, Member D

G protein–coupled receptor, class C, group 5, member D (GPRC5D) is a cell surface receptor expressed highly on myeloma cells, with lower levels of expression on normal

Table 4
Non-B cell maturation antigen-targeted chimeric antigen receptor T therapies in early-stage clinical trials

CART/Study	Target							
	CD19[12]	CD19[94]	CD19[62]	GPRC5D[67]	GPRC5D[66]	GPRC5D[64]	GPRC5D[65]	CS1/SLAMF7[72]
	CTL019 (NCT02135406)	BCMA + CD19 CART(ChiCTR-OIC-17011272)	BCMA/CD19 dual targeting CART (NCT04236011)	BMS-986393 (NCT04674813)	Anti-GPRC5D CART (ChiCTR2100048888)	MCARH109 (NCT04555551)	POLARIS-OriCar-017 (NCT05016778)	CS1-BCMA dual targeting CART (NCT04662099)
Trial Phase	1	2	1	1	2	1	1	1
Patient population	RRMM getting salvage ASCT	RRMM	RRMM	RRMM	RRMM	RRMM	RRMM	RRMM
Patients enrolled	12	69	28	67	33	17	10	16
ORR (%)	67	92	93	87	91	71	100	81
CR/sCR (%)	0	60		39	63	35	60	38
VGPR or better (%)	50		90	71	75	10	100	56
mPFS (mo)	N/A	18	N/A	N/A	N/A	N/A	N/A	N/A
mDOR (mo)	N/A	20	37	N/A	N/A	N/A	N/A	N/A
MRD neg rate (%)	N/A	N/A	100	N/A	79	N/A	N/A	N/A
Total CRS (G3+) (%)	8(0)	95 (10)	86 (7)	87 (5)	76 (0)	88 (6)	100 (0)	38 (6)

(continued on next page)

**Table 4
(continued)**

				Target				
	CD19[12]	CD19[94]	CD19[62]	GPRC5D[67]	GPRC5D[66]	GPRC5D[64]	GPRC5D[65]	CS1/SLAMF7[72]
ICANS (G3+) (%)	0(0)	11 (3)	0 (0)	10 (3)	6 (3)	6 (6); 12% cerebellar toxicity	0	0
Notes	2 patients with longer PFS with ASCT + CTL019 c/w prior ASCT alone	2 separate CART products	Bispecific CAR	Multicenter, updated data from EHA 2023. 76% ORR if prior BCMA therapy		70% ORR if prior BCMA therapy		Bispecific CAR

Abbreviations: ASCT, autologous stem cell transplant; BCMA, B cell maturation antigen; CR/sCR, complete response/stringent complete response; CRS, cytokine release syndrome; ICANS, immune effector cell-associated neurotoxicity syndrome; mDOR, median duration of response; mPFS, median progression-free survival; MRD, minimal residual disease; N/A, not applicable (not reported); ORR, overall response rate; RRMM, relapsed/refractory multiple myeloma; VGPR, very good partial response.

plasma cells and keratinized tissues (eg, skin, nail beds, and tongue papillae). Talque-tamab, a T-Cell–redirecting GPRC5D bispecific antibody has demonstrated substantial antitumor effects in patients with heavily pretreated RRMM,[63] and GPRC5D is emerging as a highly promising CART target as well. In a phase 1 proof-of-concept study, a GPRC5D-targeted CART therapy (MCARH109) was administered at four dose levels to 17 patients with heavily pretreated MM, including patients with relapse after BCMA CART therapy.[64] One patient had grade 4 CRS and ICANS, and 2 patients had a grade 3 cerebellar disorder of unclear cause. ORR was 71% in the entire cohort and was 70% (7 out of 10) in those who had received previous BCMA therapies. Three additional trials of GPRC5D-targeted CAR T cells have reported preliminary clinical data (see **Table 4**), with ORR's of 86% to 100%, including patients with prior BCMA-therapy exposure.[65–67] Rates of CRS and ICANS are similar to that seen with BCMA CARTs, and GPRC5D-specific toxicities such as rash, nail changes, and dysgeusia are generally low-grade and manageable. Additional cerebellar toxicities have not been reported in these studies. Similar to BCMA, GPRC5D loss may be a resistance mechanism that requires further development.[68] Longer follow-up is needed to assess how durable these responses will be but these preliminary data demonstrate that GPRC5D is an active target for CART therapy in MM.

CS1/SLAMF7

High CS1 (SLAMF7) expression on myeloma cells and the successful use of the CS1/SLAMF7-directed monoclonal antibody, elotuzumab,[69] makes it a promising target for CART therapy, although upregulation of CS1 on activated CD8+ T cells has raised concerns about fratricide during manufacturing. Several investigators have demonstrated preclinical activity of CS1-specific CART cells,[70,71] leading to the initiation of multiple trials in the United States, Europe, and China testing various CS1-specific CART products. To date, only 1 of these has reported preliminary clinical data, a phase 1 Chinese study of a bispecific CS1/BCMA CART, with ORR of 81% in 16 patients with RRMM, and a 12-month DOR of 69% (see **Table 4**).[72]

Other Targets

The Baylor team generated a CAR that is specific for the κ light chain and therefore recognizes κ-restricted cells and spares normal B cells expressing the nontargeted λ light chain, potentially minimizing humoral immunity impairment. In a phase 1 trial including relapsed/refractory NHL, CLL, and MM, 7 patients with RRMM were treated, with 4 having stable disease lasting 2 to 17 months.[14] CYAD-01 is an autologous CART product expressing the natural killer group 2D (NKG2D) receptor, which binds 8 ligands that are overexpressed in a wide range of hematological malignancies but are largely absent on nonneoplastic cells. CYAD-01 was tested in the phase 1 THINK trial in RRMM, relapsed/refractory acute myeloid leukemia (AML) and myelodysplastic syndrome (MDS) (see **Table 4**). However, no patients with MM responded.[73] CD38 is a rational CAR target in myeloma, based on the success of anti-CD38 antibodies[74] but it also is found on the surface of many lymphoid cells, including progenitors, activated CD4+ and CD8+ T lymphocytes, B lymphocytes, and NK cells. Despite concerns about fratricide similar to that seen with CARTs against CS1, CD38-specific CARTs could be generated from patients with MM and demonstrated significant preclinical activity.[75] CAR2 anti-CD38 A2 CAR-T cells are being tested in the phase 1 SOR-CART-MM-001 trial (NCT03464916), although results have not yet been published. CD138, or Syndecan-1, is a heparan-sulfate coated glycoprotein, which is highly expressed on the surface of myeloma cells and is important for adhesion and accumulating survival signals, although it also is expressed on normal epithelial cells. Guo and colleagues reported on 5 patients with RRMM treated with CD138-specific CARTs with good tolerability, with 4 out of 5 having stable disease lasting 3 to 7 months.[13] The group at the University of North Carolina, Chapel Hill demonstrated preclinical anti-MM activity of CD138-targeted CAR T cells without cytotoxicity toward epithelial cells,[76] leading to an ongoing phase 1 study in patients with RRMM (NCT03672318). Other approaches with promising preclinical activity include CAR T cells targeting FcRH5[77] and CD229,[78] as well as a BAFF-ligand based CAR, which binds the 3 receptors BAFF-R, BCMA, and transmembrane activator and CAML interactor (TACI), allowing for targeting of multiple B cell malignancies, including MM.[79]

ONGOING CHALLENGES AND POTENTIAL SOLUTIONS

Despite the remarkable activity of CARTs, they still do not seem curative in late-line myeloma, and certain subsets of patients have lower depth or duration of response. These include patients with high-risk cytogenetics, extramedullary disease, high marrow tumor burden, and/or International Scoring System (ISS) stage 3,[53,80] as well those with recent use of alkylators, proteasome inhibitors, or topoisomerase inhibitors before T cell collection.[81] In addition to these clinical characteristics, lack of durable response has been associated in some studies with certain T cell characteristics, including lower premanufacturing CD4/CD8 ratio, lower frequency of CD8+ cells with a naïve or stem cell memory phenotype, and a higher baseline proportion of hyperexpanded CD8+ clones expressing multiple checkpoint molecules,[18,82] a finding also recently implicated in worse outcomes following T cell-engaging bispecific antibody therapy for myeloma.[83]

There are several potential ways to overcome these negative prognostic factors. More aggressive bridging therapy during manufacturing or using CARTs as consolidation in responding patients[40] can lower tumor burden. Moving CART therapy earlier in the treatment course of myeloma may lead to improved outcomes both through improved T cell quality,[84] as well as lower tumor burden/less aggressive disease biology. Novel rapid manufacturing approaches with less in vitro activation and expansion may also improve the quality of the CART product, leading to enhanced in vivo proliferation and persistence.[48] Off-the-shelf allogeneic products, including CAR-T or CAR-NK cells, may also help overcome the limitation of poor T cell fitness. These latter approaches will also help address another unmet need, namely manufacturing-related issues including access, manufacturing failures or out-of-specification products, and disease progression during manufacturing.

Adaptive resistance by tumor cells is another challenge to navigate. BCMA expression is dynamic, and residual myeloma cells after CART therapy (and perhaps even after standard agents) may have low BCMA expression,[17,18,40] serving as a reservoir for relapse. Permanent biallelic genomic loss of BCMA has also been described,[85,86] although this seems to be relatively uncommon so far, with most patients retaining BCMA expression on progression.[21,29] This persistent BCMA expression, as well as availability of multiple BCMA-targeting agents, has led to another challenge in the field, namely how best to sequence BCMA-directed therapies. As previously mentioned, giving ide-cel or cilta-cel after a prior BCMA-directed therapy can induce responses in the majority of patients but response depth and duration tends to be significantly lower than that seen in BCMA therapy-naïve patients.[28,37] This may reflect not just alterations in BCMA antigen expression but worsening tumor biology in general in these heavily-pretreated patients.[82]

Antigen downregulation potentially could be overcome by using a gamma secretase inhibitor (GSI) to block BCMA shedding, as demonstrated in a study combining BCMA

CARTs with the GSI crenigacestat.[87] Giving more time between BCMA-directed therapies may also help, based on small studies of CARTs in patients with a prior BCMA-directed therapy, in which responding patients on average had a longer duration from prior BCMA therapy than nonresponders.[28,37] This suggests that switching to a non-BCMA-targeted therapy (eg, a GPRC5D or FcRH5-targeted therapy) in next line, and then coming back to target BCMA later may be more effective, although this needs to be confirmed prospectively. Another promising approach now in the clinic is dual-antigen targeting, either simultaneously (eg, with a bispecific CAR)[72,88] or sequentially

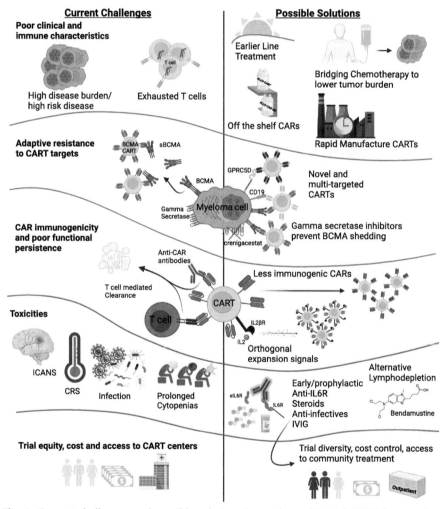

Fig. 1. Current challenges and possible solutions in myeloma-directed CART therapy. Current problems (Left) are grouped into 5 main categories: poor clinical and immune characteristics, adaptive resistance to CART targets, CAR immunogenicity and poor functional persistence, toxicities, and trial equity/cost/access. Solutions to these challenges are depicted in the right-hand column. CRS, cytokine release syndrome; ICANS, immune effector cell-associated neurotoxicity syndrome; IL2βR, interleukin2 receptor beta; sBCMA, soluble B cell maturation antigen; sIL6R, soluble IL6 receptor. (Created with biorender.com.)

(eg, CARTs followed by consolidation with a bispecific antibody against a different antigen) (NCT05801939).

Additional challenges include optimizing lymphodepletion, ideally replacing (eg, bendamustine[89]) or eliminating (eg, through use of novel CARTs using orthogonal IL2/IL2RB in vivo expansion approaches[90]) fludarabine, which can increase the risk of prolonged cytopenias and secondary myelodysplasia; mitigating toxicities such as CRS and neurotoxicity; expanding access to CARTs, particularly in resource-limited regions; and treating patient populations excluded from the clinical trials (eg, those with renal failure, CNS disease, or amyloidosis).

Finally, as has been seen with other classes of novel agents, there is a major imbalance in which groups can participate in clinical trials for and receive commercial CART in MM. Imbach and colleagues describe this problem in insightful detail in regards to CD19 directed CART for B cell lymphomas.[91] All the same principles and arguments apply to CART in MM. Mainly, MM disproportionately affects Blacks compared to Whites; yet, Blacks and other minorities make up a very small percentage of clinical trial participants. The same translates to those who receive commercial CART for the reasons given above and inherent imbalances in affordability and access to therapy. Although the high price tags of these therapies have been accepted because of the benefit gained, they require medical literacy, access, and ability to participate in treatment and good insurance to afford administration. In order for CART to be more equitable, strides in pricing, outpatient administration, and active engagement by CART treatment centers will be required. Greater attention is being paid to this equity and inclusion issue[92], but more progress is needed to be able to truly realize the power of CART in MM. A summary of challenges and potential solutions is depicted in **Fig. 1**.

SUMMARY

The rapid development of CART therapy for myeloma from a few small studies in 2015 to the approval of 2 BCMA-directed CART therapies, ide-cel and cilta-cel, is nothing short of remarkable. Subsequently, as these initial CART products move toward earlier lines of therapy, there has been a boom in other BCMA-directed CARTs as well as those against other targets. Different groups are exploring improvements in design and administration, including dual targeting, rapid expansion, T-cell subclonal selection, allogeneic approaches, and exhaustion avoidance. Unfortunately, although CART represents one of the few therapies in MM that can yield long responses without the need for continuous therapy, cure remains elusive. Perhaps, one or more of the CARTs in clinical or preclinical development today will eventually be able to overcome this last and most important hurdle. For the time being, the fight goes on with CART at the forefront.

CLINICS CARE POINTS

- Lower tumor burden may be associated with less severe toxicity, so give effective bridging therapy during manufacturing, and consider using CAR T cells when patients are responding to current line of therapy.
- Early use of tocilizumab and/or steroids should be considered when CRS or neurotoxicity is suspected.
- Patients should be monitored for prolonged cytopenias and hypogammaglobulinemia and treated with prophylactic antimicrobials and IVIG when necessary.

DISCLOSURE

Z.S. Hasanali, B. Razzo and S.P. Susanibar-Adaniya have nothing to disclose. A.L. Garfall: Consulting: BMS, Janssen, Novartis, GSK, Legend; Research funding: Novartis, Switzerland, Janssen, United States, Tmunity, CRISPR therapeutics; Patents in CAR T cell therapy: Novartis. E.A. Stadtmauer: Consultant for Janssen and BMS and grant funding from Sorrento and Abbvie. A.D. Cohen: Consulting: Janssen, GSK, BMS/Celgene, Genentech/Roche, Pfizer, Abbvie, Arcellx, Ichnos, Takeda; Research Funding: Novartis, GSK, Genentech, United States; Patents in CAR T cell therapy: Novartis.

REFERENCES

1. Eshhar Z, Waks T, Gross G, et al. Specific activation and targeting of cytotoxic lymphocytes through chimeric single chains consisting of antibody-binding domains and the gamma or zeta subunits of the immunoglobulin and T-cell receptors. Proc Natl Acad Sci USA 1993;90:720–4.
2. Milone MC, Fish JD, Carpenito C, et al. Chimeric receptors containing CD137 signal transduction domains mediate enhanced survival of T cells and increased antileukemic efficacy in vivo. Mol Ther 2009;17:1453–64.
3. Savoldo B, Ramos CA, Liu E, et al. CD28 costimulation improves expansion and persistence of chimeric antigen receptor-modified T cells in lymphoma patients. J Clin Invest 2011;121:1822–6.
4. Scholler J, Brady TL, Binder-Scholl G, et al. Decade-long safety and function of retroviral-modified chimeric antigen receptor T cells. Sci Transl Med 2012;4: 132ra53.
5. Levine BL, Humeau LM, Boyer J, et al. Gene transfer in humans using a conditionally replicating lentiviral vector. Proc Natl Acad Sci USA 2006;103:17372–7.
6. Turtle CJ, Hanafi LA, Berger C, et al. Immunotherapy of non-Hodgkin's lymphoma with a defined ratio of CD8+ and CD4+ CD19-specific chimeric antigen receptor-modified T cells. Sci Transl Med 2016;8:355ra116.
7. Porter DL, Hwang WT, Frey NV, et al. Chimeric antigen receptor T cells persist and induce sustained remissions in relapsed refractory chronic lymphocytic leukemia. Sci Transl Med 2015;7:303ra139.
8. Maude SL, Laetsch TW, Buechner J, et al. Tisagenlecleucel in Children and Young Adults with B-Cell Lymphoblastic Leukemia. N Engl J Med 2018;378: 439–48.
9. Neelapu SS, Locke FL, Bartlett NL, et al. Axicabtagene Ciloleucel CAR T-Cell Therapy in Refractory Large B-Cell Lymphoma. N Engl J Med 2017;377:2531–44.
10. Garfall AL, Maus MV, Hwang WT, et al. Chimeric Antigen Receptor T Cells against CD19 for Multiple Myeloma. N Engl J Med 2015;373:1040–7.
11. Matsui W, Wang Q, Barber JP, et al. Clonogenic multiple myeloma progenitors, stem cell properties, and drug resistance. Cancer Res 2008;68:190–7.
12. Garfall AL, Stadtmauer EA, Hwang WT, et al. Anti-CD19 CAR T cells with high-dose melphalan and autologous stem cell transplantation for refractory multiple myeloma. JCI insight 2018;3:e120505.
13. Guo B, Chen M, Han Q, et al. CD138-directed adoptive immunotherapy of chimeric antigen receptor (CAR)-modified T cells for multiple myeloma. J Cell Immunother 2016;2:28–35.
14. Ramos CA, Savoldo B, Torrano V, et al. Clinical responses with T lymphocytes targeting malignancy-associated κ light chains. J Clin Invest 2016;126:2588–96.

15. Salem DA, Maric I, Yuan CM, et al. Quantification of B-cell maturation antigen, a target for novel chimeric antigen receptor T-cell therapy in Myeloma. Leuk Res 2018;71:106–11.

16. Carpenter RO, Evbuomwan MO, Pittaluga S, et al. B-cell maturation antigen is a promising target for adoptive T-cell therapy of multiple myeloma. Clin Cancer Res 2013;19:2048–60.

17. Brudno JN, Maric I, Hartman SD, et al. T Cells Genetically Modified to Express an Anti-B-Cell Maturation Antigen Chimeric Antigen Receptor Cause Remissions of Poor-Prognosis Relapsed Multiple Myeloma. J Clin Oncol 2018;36:2267–80.

18. Cohen AD, Garfall AL, Stadtmauer EA, et al. B cell maturation antigen-specific CAR T cells are clinically active in multiple myeloma. J Clin Invest 2019;129:2210–21.

19. Raje N, Berdeja J, Lin Y, et al. Anti-BCMA CAR T-Cell Therapy bb2121 in Relapsed or Refractory Multiple Myeloma. N Engl J Med 2019;380:1726–37.

20. Zhao W-H, Liu J, Wang BY, et al. A phase 1, open-label study of LCAR-B38M, a chimeric antigen receptor T cell therapy directed against B cell maturation antigen, in patients with relapsed or refractory multiple myeloma. J Hematol Oncol 2018;11:141.

21. Munshi NC, Anderson LD Jr, Shah N, et al. Idecabtagene Vicleucel in Relapsed and Refractory Multiple Myeloma. N Engl J Med 2021;384:705–16.

22. Manier S, Kansagra AJ, Anderson, Jr LD, et al. Characteristics of neurotoxicity associated with idecabtagene vicleucel (ide-cel, bb2121) in patients with relapsed and refractory multiple myeloma (RRMM) in the pivotal phase II KarMMa study. J Clin Oncol 2021;39:8036.

23. Shah N, Mojebi A, Ayers D, et al. Indirect treatment comparison of idecabtagene vicleucel versus conventional care in triple-class exposed multiple myeloma. J Comp Eff Res 2022;11:737–49.

24. Rodriguez-Otero P, Ayers D, Cope S, et al. Matching adjusted indirect comparisons of efficacy outcomes for idecabtagene vicleucel (ide-cel, bb2121) versus selinexor + dexamethasone and belantamab mafodotin in relapsed and refractory multiple myeloma. Leuk Lymphoma 2021;62:2482–91.

25. Jagannath S, Lin Y, Goldschmidt H, et al. KarMMa-RW: comparison of idecabtagene vicleucel with real-world outcomes in relapsed and refractory multiple myeloma. Blood Cancer J 2021;11:116.

26. Sanoyan DA, Seipel K, Bacher U, et al. Real-life experiences with CAR T-cell therapy with idecabtagene vicleucel (ide-cel) for triple-class exposed relapsed/refractory multiple myeloma patients. BMC Cancer 2023;23:345.

27. Hansen DK, Sidana S, Peres LC, et al. Idecabtagene Vicleucel for Relapsed/Refractory Multiple Myeloma: Real-World Experience From the Myeloma CAR T Consortium. J Clin Oncol 2023;41:2087–97.

28. Ferreri CJ, Hildebrandt MA, Hashmi H, et al. Idecabtagene Vicleucel (Ide-cel) Chimeric Antigen Receptor (CAR) T-Cell Therapy in Patients with Relapsed/Refractory Multiple Myeloma (RRMM) Who Have Received a Prior BCMA-Targeted Therapy: Real World, Multi-Institutional Experience. Blood 2022;140:1856–8.

29. Rodriguez-Otero P, Ailawadhi S, Arnulf B, et al. Ide-cel or Standard Regimens in Relapsed and Refractory Multiple Myeloma. N Engl J Med 2023;388:1002–14.

30. Mi J-Q, Zhao WH, Chen LJ, et al. Long-term remission and survival in patients with relapsed or refractory multiple myeloma after treatment of LCAR-B38M CAR-T: At least 5-year follow-up in LEGEND-2. J Clin Oncol 2023;41:8010.

31. Martin T, Lin Y, Agha M, et al. Health-related quality of life in patients given cilta-cabtagene autoleucel for relapsed or refractory multiple myeloma (CARTITUDE-1): a phase 1b-2, open-label study. Lancet Haematol 2022;9:e897–905.
32. Berdeja JG, Madduri D, Usmani SZ, et al. Ciltacabtagene autoleucel, a B-cell maturation antigen-directed chimeric antigen receptor T-cell therapy in patients with relapsed or refractory multiple myeloma (CARTITUDE-1): a phase 1b/2 open-label study. Lancet (London, England) 2021;398:314–24.
33. Lin Y, Martin TG, Usmani SZ, et al. CARTITUDE-1 final results: Phase 1b/2 study of ciltacabtagene autoleucel in heavily pretreated patients with relapsed/refractory multiple myeloma. J Clin Oncol 2023;41:8009.
34. Martin T, Usmani SZ, Schecter JM, et al. Matching-adjusted indirect comparison of efficacy outcomes for ciltacabtagene autoleucel in CARTITUDE-1 versus ide-cabtagene vicleucel in KarMMa for the treatment of patients with relapsed or re-fractory multiple myeloma. Curr Med Res Opin 2021;37:1779–88.
35. Weisel K, Martin T, Krishnan A, et al. Comparative Efficacy of Ciltacabtagene Au-toleucel in CARTITUDE-1 vs Physician's Choice of Therapy in the Long-Term Follow-Up of POLLUX, CASTOR, and EQUULEUS Clinical Trials for the Treatment of Patients with Relapsed or Refractory Multiple Myeloma. Clin Drug Investig 2022;42:29–41.
36. Hansen DK, Patel KK, Peres LC, et al. Safety and efficacy of standard of care (SOC) ciltacabtagene autoleucel (Cilta-cel) for relapsed/refractory multiple myeloma (RRMM). J Clin Oncol 2023;41:8012.
37. Cohen AD, Mateos MV, Cohen YC, et al. Efficacy and safety of cilta-cel in patients with progressive multiple myeloma after exposure to other BCMA-targeting agents. Blood 2023;141:219–30.
38. San-Miguel J, Dhakal B, Yong K, et al. Cilta-cel or Standard Care in Lenalidomide-Refractory Multiple Myeloma. N Engl J Med 2023. https://doi.org/10.1056/NEJMoa2303379.
39. Dhakal B, Yong K, Harrison SJ, et al. First phase 3 results from CARTITUDE-4: Cilta-cel versus standard of care (PVd or DPd) in lenalidomide-refractory multiple myeloma. J Clin Oncol 2023;41:LBA106.
40. Garfall AL, Cohen AD, Susanibar-Adaniya SP, et al. Anti-BCMA/CD19 CAR T Cells with Early Immunomodulatory Maintenance for Multiple Myeloma Responding to Initial or Later-l ine Therapy. Blood cancer Discov 2023;4:118–33.
41. Chen W, Fu C, Fang B, et al. Phase II Study of Fully Human BCMA-Targeting CAR-T Cells (Zevorcabtagene Autoleucel) in Patients with Relapsed/Refractory Multiple Myeloma. Blood 2022;140:4564–5.
42. Li C, Wang D, Song Y, et al. CT103A, a novel fully human BCMA-targeting CAR-T cells, in patients with relapsed/refractory multiple myeloma: Updated results of phase 1b/2 study (FUMANBA-1). J Clin Oncol 2023;41:8025.
43. Frigault MJ, Bishop MR, Rosenblatt J, et al. Phase 1 study of CART-ddBCMA for the treatment of subjects with relapsed and refractory multiple myeloma. Blood Adv 2023;7:768–77.
44. Raje NS, Shah N, Jagannath S, et al. Updated Clinical and Correlative Results from the Phase I CRB-402 Study of the BCMA-Targeted CAR T Cell Therapy bb21217 in Patients with Relapsed and Refractory Multiple Myeloma. Blood 2021;138:548.
45. Costello CL, Cohen AD, Patel KK, et al. Phase 1/2 Study of the Safety and Response of P-BCMA-101 CAR-T Cells in Patients with Relapsed/Refractory (r/r) Multiple Myeloma (MM) (PRIME) with Novel Therapeutic Strategies. Blood 2020;136:29–30.

46. Mailankody S, Jakubowiak AJ, Htut M, et al. Orvacabtagene autoleucel (orvacel), a B-cell maturation antigen (BCMA)-directed CAR T cell therapy for patients (pts) with relapsed/refractory multiple myeloma (RRMM): update of the phase 1/2 EVOLVE study (NCT03430011). J Clin Oncol 2020;38:8504.

47. Costa LJ, Kumar SK, Atrash S, et al. Results from the First Phase 1 Clinical Study of the B-Cell Maturation Antigen (BCMA) Nex T Chimeric Antigen Receptor (CAR) T Cell Therapy CC-98633/BMS-986354 in Patients (pts) with Relapsed/Refractory Multiple Myeloma (RRMM). Blood 2022;140:1360–2.

48. Sperling AS, Derman BA, Nikiforow S, et al. Updated phase I study results of PHE885, a T-Charge manufactured BCMA-directed CAR-T cell therapy, for patients (pts) with r/r multiple myeloma (RRMM). J Clin Oncol 2023;41:8004.

49. Du J, Fu WJ, Jiang H, et al. Updated results of a phase I, open-label study of BCMA/CD19 dual-targeting fast CAR-T GC012F for patients with relapsed/refractory multiple myeloma (RRMM). J Clin Oncol 2023;41:8005.

50. Mailankody S, Matous JV, Chhabra S, et al. Allogeneic BCMA-targeting CAR T cells in relapsed/refractory multiple myeloma: phase 1 UNIVERSAL trial interim results. Nat Med 2023;29:422–9.

51. Frey N, Porter D. Cytokine release syndrome with chimeric antigen receptor T cell therapy. J Am Soc Blood Marrow Transplant 2019;25:e123–7.

52. Hines MR, Knight TE, McNerney KO, et al. Immune Effector Cell-Associated Hemophagocytic Lymphohistiocytosis-Like Syndrome. Transplant Cell Ther 2023; 29:438.e1–16.

53. Martin T, Usmani SZ, Berdeja JG, et al. Ciltacabtagene Autoleucel, an Anti-B-cell Maturation Antigen Chimeric Antigen Receptor T-Cell Therapy, for Relapsed/Refractory Multiple Myeloma: CARTITUDE-1 2-Year Follow-Up. J Clin Oncol 2023; 41:1265–74.

54. Cohen AD, Parekh S, Santomasso BD, et al. Incidence and management of CAR-T neurotoxicity in patients with multiple myeloma treated with ciltacabtagene autoleucel in CARTITUDE studies. Blood Cancer J 2022;12:32.

55. Karschnia P, Miller KC, Yee AJ, et al. Neurologic toxicities following adoptive immunotherapy with BCMA-directed CAR T-cells. Blood 2023;2023020571. https://doi.org/10.1182/blood.2023020571.

56. Van Oekelen O, Aleman A, Upadhyaya B, et al. Neurocognitive and hypokinetic movement disorder with features of parkinsonism after BCMA-targeting CAR-T cell therapy. Nat Med 2021;27:2099–103.

57. Davis JA, Sborov DW, Wesson W, et al. Efficacy and Safety of CD34+ Stem Cell Boost for Delayed Hematopoietic Recovery After BCMA Directed CAR T-cell Therapy. Transplant Cell Ther 2023. https://doi.org/10.1016/j.jtct.2023.05.012.

58. Kambhampati S, Sheng Y, Huang CY, et al. Infectious complications in patients with relapsed refractory multiple myeloma after BCMA CAR T-cell therapy. Blood Adv 2022;6:2045–54.

59. Mohan M, Chakraborty R, Bal S, et al. Recommendations on prevention of infections during chimeric antigen receptor T-cell and bispecific antibody therapy in multiple myeloma. Br J Haematol 2023;203(5):736–46.

60. Billadeau D, Ahmann G, Greipp P, et al. The bone marrow of multiple myeloma patients contains B cell populations at different stages of differentiation that are clonally related to the malignant plasma cell. J Exp Med 1993;178:1023–31.

61. Wang Y, Cao J, Gu W, et al. Long-Term Follow-Up of Combination of B-Cell Maturation Antigen and CD19 Chimeric Antigen Receptor T Cells in Multiple Myeloma. J Clin Oncol 2022;40:2246–56.

62. Du J, Jiang H, Dong B, et al. Updated results of a multicenter first-in-human study of BCMA/CD19 dual-targeting fast CAR-T GC012F for patients with relapsed/refractory multiple myeloma (RRMM). J Clin Oncol 2022;40:8005.
63. Chari A, Minnema MC, Berdeja JG, et al. Talquetamab, a T-Cell–Redirecting GPRC5D Bispecific Antibody for Multiple Myeloma. N Engl J Med 2022;387: 2232–44.
64. Mailankody S, Devlin SM, Landa J, et al. GPRC5D-Targeted CAR T Cells for Myeloma. N Engl J Med 2022;387:1196–206.
65. Zhang M, Wei G, Zhou L, et al. GPRC5D CAR T cells (OriCAR-017) in patients with relapsed or refractory multiple myeloma (POLARIS): a first-in-human, single-centre, single-arm, phase 1 trial. Lancet Haematol 2023;10:e107–16.
66. Xia J, Li H, Yan Z, et al. Anti-G Protein-Coupled Receptor, Class C Group 5 Member D Chimeric Antigen Receptor T Cells in Patients With Relapsed or Refractory Multiple Myeloma: A Single-Arm, Phase II Trial. J Clin Oncol 2023;41:2583–93.
67. Bal, S. et al. BMS-986393 (CC-95266), a G protein–coupled receptor class C group5 member D (GPRC5D)–targeted CAR T-cell therapy for relapsed/refractory multiple myeloma (RRMM): results from a phase 1 study. EHA Libr. (2023).
68. Bahlis, N. et al. Tumor Intrinsic Mechanisms of Antigen Escape to Anti-BCMA and Anti-GPRC5D Targeted Immunotherapies in Multiple Myeloma. (2023) doi:10.21203/rs.3.rs-2657360/v1.
69. Dimopoulos MA, Dytfeld D, Grosicki S, et al. Elotuzumab plus Pomalidomide and Dexamethasone for Multiple Myeloma. N Engl J Med 2018;379:1811–22.
70. O'Neal J, Ritchey JK, Cooper ML, et al. CS1 CAR-T targeting the distal domain of CS1 (SLAMF7) shows efficacy in high tumor burden myeloma model despite fratricide of CD8+CS1 expressing CAR-T cells. Leukemia 2022;36:1625–34.
71. Wang X, Walter M, Urak R, et al. Lenalidomide Enhances the Function of CS1 Chimeric Antigen Receptor-Redirected T Cells Against Multiple Myeloma. Clin Cancer Res 2018;24:106–19.
72. Li C, Wang X, Wu Z, et al. Bispecific CS1-BCMA CAR-T Cells Are Clinically Active in Relapsed or Refractory Multiple Myeloma: An Updated Clinical Study. Blood 2022;140:4573–4.
73. Sallman DA, Kerre T, Havelange V, et al. CYAD-01, an autologous NKG2D-based CAR T-cell therapy, in relapsed or refractory acute myeloid leukaemia and myelodysplastic syndromes or multiple myeloma (THINK): haematological cohorts of the dose escalation segment of a phase 1 trial. Lancet Haematol 2023;10: e191–202.
74. Lonial S, Weiss BM, Usmani SZ, et al. Daratumumab monotherapy in patients with treatment-refractory multiple myeloma (SIRIUS): an open-label, randomised, phase 2 trial. Lancet 2016;387:1551–60.
75. Drent E, Themeli M, Poels R, et al. A Rational Strategy for Reducing On-Target Off-Tumor Effects of CD38-Chimeric Antigen Receptors by Affinity Optimization. Mol Ther 2017;25:1946–58.
76. Sun C, Mahendravada A, Ballard B, et al. Safety and efficacy of targeting CD138 with a chimeric antigen receptor for the treatment of multiple myeloma. Oncotarget 2019;10:2369–83.
77. Jiang D, Huang H, Qin H, et al. Chimeric antigen receptor T cells targeting FcRH5 provide robust tumour-specific responses in murine xenograft models of multiple myeloma. Nat Commun 2023;14:3642.
78. Radhakrishnan SV, Luetkens T, Scherer SD, et al. CD229 CAR T cells eliminate multiple myeloma and tumor propagating cells without fratricide. Nat Commun 2020;11:798.

79. Wong DP, Roy NK, Zhang K, et al. A BAFF ligand-based CAR-T cell targeting three receptors and multiple B cell cancers. Nat Commun 2022;13:217.

80. Shah N, Munshi NC, Berdeja JG, et al. Baseline Correlates of Complete Response to Idecabtagene Vicleucel (ide-cel, bb2121), a BCMA-Directed CAR T Cell Therapy in Patients with Relapsed and Refractory Multiple Myeloma: Subanalysis of the KarMMa Trial. Blood 2021;138:1739.

81. Rytlewski J, Fuller J, Mertz DR, et al. Correlative analysis to define patient profiles associated with manufacturing and clinical endpoints in relapsed/refractory multiple myeloma (RRMM) patients treated with idecabtagene vicleucel (ide-cel; bb2121), an anti-BCMA CAR T cell therapy. J Clin Oncol 2022;40:8021.

82. Dhodapkar KM, Cohen AD, Kaushal A, et al. Changes in Bone Marrow Tumor and Immune Cells Correlate with Durability of Remissions Following BCMA CAR T Therapy in Myeloma. Blood cancer Discov 2022;3:490–501.

83. Friedrich MJ, Neri P, Kehl N, et al. The pre-existing T cell landscape determines the response to bispecific T cell engagers in multiple myeloma patients. Cancer Cell 2023;41:711–25.e6.

84. Garfall AL, Dancy EK, Cohen AD, et al. T-cell phenotypes associated with effective CAR T-cell therapy in postinduction vs relapsed multiple myeloma. Blood Adv 2019;3:2812–5.

85. Samur MK, Fulciniti M, Aktas Samur A, et al. Biallelic loss of BCMA as a resistance mechanism to CAR T cell therapy in a patient with multiple myeloma. Nat Commun 2021;12:868.

86. Da Vià MC, Dietrich O, Truger M, et al. Homozygous BCMA gene deletion in response to anti-BCMA CAR T cells in a patient with multiple myeloma. Nat Med 2021;27:616–9.

87. Cowan AJ, Pont MJ, Sather BD, et al. γ-Secretase inhibitor in combination with BCMA chimeric antigen receptor T-cell immunotherapy for individuals with relapsed or refractory multiple myeloma: a phase 1, first-in-human trial. Lancet Oncol 2023;24:811–22.

88. Fernández de Larrea C, Staehr M, Lopez AV, et al. Defining an Optimal Dual-Targeted CAR T-cell Therapy Approach Simultaneously Targeting BCMA and GPRC5D to Prevent BCMA Escape-Driven Relapse in Multiple Myeloma. Blood cancer Discov 2020;1:146–54.

89. Chong EA, Gerson JN, Nasta SD, et al. Outcomes with bendamustine lymphodepletion prior to brexucabtagene autoleucel for mantle cell lymphoma. J Clin Oncol 2023;41:e19540.

90. Zhang Q, Hresko ME, Picton LK, et al. A human orthogonal IL-2 and IL-2Rβ system enhances CAR T cell expansion and antitumor activity in a murine model of leukemia. Sci Transl Med 2023;13:eabg6986.

91. Imbach KJ, Patel A, Levine AD. Ethical Considerations in the Translation of CAR-T Cell Therapies. Cell Gene Ther Insights 2018;4:295–307.

92. Derman BA, Parker WF. Fair Allocation of Scarce CAR T-Cell Therapies for Relapsed/Refractory Multiple Myeloma. JAMA 2023. https://doi.org/10.1001/jama.2023.11846.

93. Petersen CT, Hassan M, Morris AB, et al. Improving T-cell expansion and function for adoptive T-cell therapy using ex vivo treatment with PI3Kδ inhibitors and VIP antagonists. Blood Adv 2018;2:210–23.

94. Yan Z, Cao J, Cheng H, et al. A combination of humanised anti-CD19 and anti-BCMA CAR T cells in patients with relapsed or refractory multiple myeloma: a single-arm, phase 2 trial. Lancet Haematol 2019;6:e521–9.

Is There Still a Role for Stem Cell Transplantation in Multiple Myeloma?

Morie A. Gertz, MD, MACP

KEYWORDS

- Multiple myeloma • Stem cell transplantation • High-dose chemotherapy

KEY POINTS

- Stem cell transplantation remains the standard of care for the management of eligible patients outside a clinical trial.
- Stem cell transplant transiently reduces quality of life for approximately 3 months and produces an improvement in progression-free survival but not overall survival.
- Patient's selected for stem cell transplant should have an anticipated therapy-related mortality well under 1%. If this is not the case, nontransplant therapy should be used for consolidation.

INTRODUCTION

No therapy in multiple myeloma (MM) has been as extensively investigated as stem cell transplantation following high-dose chemotherapy. A search of the national library of medicine in February 2023 revealed over 27,000 publications covering stem cell transplantation. However, given the rapid advances seen in the treatment of (MM), it is legitimate to ask whether the technique first introduced in 1983 by Thomas McElwain still has relevance. In 1984, Barlogie introduced infusional vincristine, doxorubicin, and dexamethasone and in 1986 published a first series on high-dose therapy with autologous marrow-derived stem cells. At this point, the only available therapies were melphalan, prednisone, other intensive steroids such as methylprednisolone, and interferon. Cyclophosphamide was used both orally and parenterally. Vincrstine Carmustine melphalan cyclophosphamide prednisone was introduced as a combination therapy at Memorial Hospital subsequently shown not to be superior to melphalan and prednisone.

With the introduction of thalidomide and its derivatives, proteasome inhibitors, antibodies to CD38, the utilization of routine maintenance therapy, and the availability of car T therapy as well as by functional T-cell engagers, it is fair to ask whether the

Mayo Clinic, 200 SW First street, Rochester, MN 55905, USA
E-mail address: gertz.morie@mayo.edu

Hematol Oncol Clin N Am 38 (2024) 407–420
https://doi.org/10.1016/j.hoc.2023.12.005
0889-8588/24/© 2023 Elsevier Inc. All rights reserved.

technology of stem cell transplantation now at 40 years still has relevance in the current treatment of MM. In this manuscript, the author will review outcomes for transplant, its use single, and in tandem. Its use in consolidation in newly diagnosed patients as well as in salvage. The role of patient selection in the current myeloma environment will all be reviewed. In countries where access to novel agents is restricted by health care economics, stem cell transplant is more cost effective than newer agents. As a consequence, the continued use of stem cell transplant is virtually certain until widespread availability of inexpensive novel agents becomes a reality.[1]

What Constitutes a Transplant Eligible Population?

Comparisons of transplant-eligible and non-transplant-eligible populations of myeloma patients are inherently biased. Patients who are transplant eligible will be younger, have a better performance status, better renal function, and well-maintained cardiac function.[2] Therefore, transplant-eligible populations will always do better than non-transplant eligible so these comparisons should not be made. There is considerable variability, however, as to what constitutes a transplant-eligible patient. In many of the early European trials, this was done based on age only, where age over 65 years was considered not eligible. This does not conform to current practice where frailty index is used as a qualifying criterion.[3] At Mayo Clinic, patients up to the age of 79 have been successfully transplanted if they have normal cardiopulmonary reserve and a performance status of 0 or 1.[4] Outcomes of patients over the age of 75 are identical to younger patients although the former undergoes significant selection for eligibility. Melphalan conditioning dose appears to have little impact on outcomes, and it is unclear that transplant at doses of melphalan 140 mg per m^2 are inferior to traditional dosing.[5]

Renal impairment is not an exclusion criterion from safe autologous stem cell transplantation. In a review of 34 patients transplanted with a creatinine clearance less than 60 mL/minute, grade 1 to 2 mucositis was seen in 62%, grade 3 mucositis seen in 12%, and 48% had a grade 3 infection. Grade 4 infection was reported in 8% and half the patients had a grade 1 increase in serum creatinine. Engraftment syndrome was seen in 12% and cardiac adverse events were seen in 15%. One patient died and one patient had secondary platelet graft failure. At a median follow-up of 26.2 months following transplantation median, progression-free and overall survival (OS) was not reached. Patients on dialysis can be safely transplanted with reduction in the melphalan dose to 140 mg per m^2. Patients with renal insufficiency can be safely transplanted without concern regarding further decline in renal function.[6] An analysis of 370 patients with chronic kidney disease undergoing first transplant showed no differences in transplant-related mortality, progression-free, or overall survival compared to the patient's with normal renal function.[7] A total of 110 patients who were dialysis dependent prior to stem cell transplantation were reported. All of them were on dialysis pretransplant. Seventy-one of the 110 received bortezomib-based induction. A very good partial response was reported in 39%. A total of 82% received 140 mg melphalan per m^2 or less; the progression-free survival (PFS) was 35 months and the median overall survival was 102 months. Patients achieving dialysis independence did have a better survival. Dialysis independence occurred more frequently in the group that achieved at least a very good partial response following induction before transplant. This suggests that the deeper remission following high-dose chemotherapy and stem cell transplant contributed to dialysis independence.[8] In screening patients for safe transplant, a diffusing capacity of the lungs for carbon monoxide (DLCO)<60% is associated with poor outcomes. Median OS (mOS) was significantly shorter in the DLCOc $\leq$ 60% group irrespective of relapse, with mOS of 27.3 versus 77.2 months ($P = .0002$) in relapsed patients with DLCOc $\leq$ 60% (n = 22) and DLCOc > 60% (n = 193), respectively.[9] Survival outcomes in men and women appeared to be identical.[10]

Stem Cell Mobilization

Collection failure has significantly decreased with changes in induction therapy. At the beginning of transplantation, oral melphalan was commonly used and cumulative doses more than 500 mg resulted in poor collections. Lenalidomide has been reported inconsistently to reduce stem cell yields at apheresis. Since the introduction of plerixafor, mobilization failures are uncommon.[11] In a review of 330 patients receiving induction with either daratumimab carfilzomib lenalidomide dexamethasone (d-KRd), daratumumab bortezomib lenalidomide dexamethasone (D-VRd), or bortezomib lenalidomide dexamethasone (VRd), the percentage of patients not meeting criteria for stem cell yield were 7%, 2%, and 6%, respectively. On remobilization, nearly all collected enough stem cells. Ultimately 98%, 99%, and 98%, respectively proceed with transplantation. Four cycles of daratumumab and lenalidomide-based quadruplet induction therapy had a minimal impact on mobilization.[12] The fact that the addition of daratumumab has no impact on the yield of stem cells or the number of collection days has been reconfirmed.[13]

Motixafortide is a CXCR4 inhibitor with extended activity. In a prospective phase 3 double-blind placebo controlled multicenter trial, this agent combined with granulocyte colonysstimulating factor(G-CSF) mobilized significantly greater CD34 cells within 2 apheresis procedures compared to placebo.[14]

Conditioning

For 40 years, the standard is melphalan as a single agent in doses of 200 mg per m^2 although adjustments are made for renal insufficiency and age. Other regimens have been investigated including bendamustine and melphalan the former given a dose of 225 mg per m^2 and found to be safe and tolerable.[15] Melphalan at 140 mg per m^2 has been combined with escalated total marrow radiation at a dose of 12 Gy. After a median follow-up of 55 months, 70% of participants were alive. Four of 13 patients remained in complete response.[16] Recovery of platelets following stem cell reinfusion occurs at a median of 14 days but may be delayed in patients that have clonal hematopoiesis of indeterminate potential.[17] In an open label study, the use of romiplostim starting day 1 after stem cell infusion resulted in an enhanced platelet recovery to normal values beginning at approximately day +15. It did not reduce the number of days requiring platelet transfusions or the time to platelet engraftment.[18]

Timing of Stem Cell Transplantation

Traditionally stem cell collection and transplantation were performed after approximately 4 cycles of induction chemotherapy. The number of induction cycles appears to have very little impact on overall outcome. There are centers that will collect stem cells and cryopreserve them for later use in transplantation as a salvage therapy. Unfortunately, as many as 25% of patients with cryopreserved stem cells never come to transplant due to issues such as aggressive relapse, rapid decline in performance status, and patient preference. In addition, when transplant is used as a salvage therapy, many of these patients have had a decline in performance status due to progressive disease making the morbidity associated with transplant and the requirement for hospitalization substantially greater. Early autologous stem cell transplantation (ASCT) cohort had a benefit of 1.96 quality-adjusted life years (QALYs), 0.23 QALYs more than delayed ASCT.[19] Early ASCT maintains quality of life better than those patients who receive delayed stem cell transplantation.[20] A randomized open label phase 2 trial conducted in the United Kingdom enrolled 281 patients. One hundred nine ultimately went to ASCT and 109 were alternatively randomized to carfilzomib-cyclophosphamide-dexamethasone consolidation in place of transplantation; the 2-year progression-free survival was 75% in the transplant group and 68% in the consolidation group. This did not meet the criteria for noninferiority suggesting that autologous transplantation was superior to chemotherapy consolidation. Upfront autologous stem cell transplant was concluded to be the preferred treatment.[21]

ASCT in first relapse was associated with superior PFS (HR 0.63, $P = .03$) and OS (HR 0.59, $P = .04$) compared to later lines of therapy. Ninety-five patients underwent delayed transplant at first relapse; median PFS and OS from the start of therapy were 30 and 69 months, and median OS from diagnosis was 106 months, suggesting that a salvage transplant can play an important role in prolonging PFS in myeloma patients.[22] A total of 57 patients who had a salvage second stem cell transplant achieved a very good partial response or better (80%) with median PFS and OS of 1.6 and 3.6 years, respectively.[23] Eighty-three patients with relapsed myeloma were induced with daratumumab-pomalidomide-dexamethasone. Twenty-one out of the 83 patients proceeded to autologous stem cell transplant. The remaining 60 continued with daratumumab-pomalidomide-dexamethasone. Stringent complete responses were seen in 57% of the transplanted patients compared to 16% of the nontransplant cohort, $P = .006$. Survival in the transplant group was not reached compared to 38.1 months in the nontransplant group. Relapsed patients undergoing stem cell transplantation demonstrated superior depth and duration of remission compared to the chemotherapy-only group.[24] Early SCT has been associated with prolonged PFS, but this did not consequently translate into prolonged OS in patients with newly diagnosed MM. The benefit of early SCT in terms of OS is less clear in the era of novel agents.[25] A total of 106 patients were assessed to determine the outcome of salvage stem cell transplantation. With a second stem cell transplant, the response rate was 98% and therapy-related mortality was 1.8%. Median overall survival estimated at 80 months and median PFS after the second transplant was 24 months comparable to many salvage chemotherapy regimens. Predictors of the second progression-free survival included progression on immunomodulatory drug-based maintenance. These are acceptable outcomes and are a valuable salvage therapy for relapsed MM.[26]

In the myeloma X trials, patients who relapsed after transplant received bortezomib, doxorubicin, and dexamethasone followed by randomization to a second transplant or weekly oral cyclophosphamide. Patients in this stem cell transplant arm had a PFS of 19 versus 11 months and OS of 67 versus 52 months both of which achieved statistical significance. The complete response rate for transplant was 39% compared to 22% for weekly cyclophosphamide.[27] In a German trial, at relapse, patients received lenalidomide-dexamethasone and were then randomized to stem cell transplant followed by lenalidomide maintenance compared to lenalidomide-dexamethasone without stem cell transplant to progression. In this trial, there were no statistical differences in overall response rate, PFS, and OS.[28] This may be related to the choice of cyclophosphamide in the British trial as opposed to lenalidomide in the German trial.

Stem Cell Transplant Outcomes

In the largest phase 3 randomized trial, 722 patients were randomized to induction with bortezomib-lenalidomide-dexamethasone followed by stem cell transplantation with melphalan or bortezomib-lenalidomide-dexamethasone followed by stem cell collection, deferred stem cell transplant, and consolidation with bortezomib-lenalidomide-dexamethasone. This trial was limited to patients less than or equal to

65 years of age. Lenalidomide maintenance was given to both groups through progression. At a median follow-up of 76 months, median PFS was 46.2 months and 67.5 months, respectively, for the nontransplant and transplant arms. There was no difference in response depth or OS between the 2 groups. This was an intent to treat analysis. Fifty-five of 365 patients assigned to transplantation did not have transplantation performed (15%). Treatment-related death in the transplantation group was seen in 1.4%. There was no difference in second primary cancers between the groups (10.4% and 10.7%, respectively). Although patients in the RVD alone arm had the option for stem cell transplantation and delayed transplant, this occurred in only 28% so the benefit of delayed stem cell transplant could not be adequately assessed.[29]

The STAMINA trial investigated 3 arms. Arm 1 was single autologous stem cell transplant followed by lenalidomide maintenance, the second arm was tandem autologous stem cell transplant followed by lenalidomide maintenance, and the third was single autologous stem cell transplant followed by consolidation followed by lenalidomide maintenance. This trial had multiple weakness including different induction regimens permitted, up to 2 induction regimens, and up to 1 year before randomization. Dropout rates were quite high. Patients could be up to 70 years old. The primary endpoint was 38-month PFS. There was no difference in PFS between the 3 arms and no difference in the complete response rate. They concluded that consolidation posttransplant or a second transplant in tandem did not improve outcomes. Their conclusion was that the standard of care was single autologous transplant with lenalidomide maintenance therapy.[30] The failure of consolidation or a second stem cell transplant to benefit this patient population was seen in both standard risk and high-risk populations. Predictors of improved PFS and OS included measurable residual disease (MRD) negativity and mass fix negativity for absence of the monoclonal protein.[31] Other groups have reported benefit from post stem cell transplantation consolidation. Forty-five patients failing to achieve a complete response following autologous stem cell transplantation received consolidation with cyclophosphamide, bortezomib, and dexamethasone. A total of 52.4% improved their response depth following consolidation.[32]

A well-recognized high-risk feature of MM is plasma cell leukemia. A retrospective analysis compared single autologous transplant, single allogeneic transplant, tandem autologous followed by allogeneic transplant, and tandem autologous transplant in patients with plasma cell leukemia. Allogeneic transplant had a lower relapse rate but a higher nonrelapse mortality (27%). Patients undergoing tandem autologous allogeneic transplant had a significant benefit in PFS at day 100 compared to single autologous transplant with a hazard ratio of 0.69. Tandem autologous transplant was effective for patients achieving complete remission prior to the first transplant. Although allogeneic transplant provides more durable response, the significant mortality risk within the first 100 days remains a major drawback in widespread implementation.[33] A single-center study of 36 patients, median age 52, reported a median PFS of 15 months. Only 8.3% were alive in a complete remission. Treatment-related mortality was 35%. Given the availability of multiple novel drugs, the utility of allogeneic transplant is in decline and would be reserved for patients where novel drug availability is limited.[34]

The Forte trial was a 3-arm phase 2 comparison of carfilzomib-lenalidomide-dexamethasone plus transplant, 12 cycles of carfilzomib- lenalidomide-dexamethasone without transplant, or carfilzomib-cyclophosphamide-dexamethasone followed by transplant. Maintenance was carfilzomib-lenalidomide or lenalidomide alone. Carfilzomib-lenalidomide-dexamethasone with autologous stem cell transplant showed superiority with improved responses compared to the other 2 treatment arms.[35] In a recent meta-analysis reviewing 7 randomized clinical trials and nonobservational studies, stem cell transplant showed an advantage in achieving complete response with an odds ratio of 1.24 with a survival advantage with a hazard ratio of 0.58. The advantage of transplant was greater in older individuals, males, international stage III disease, and high-risk genetic features.[36]

Other groups suggest that the need for autologous stem cell transplant in the management of MM is in decline. A retrospective review of 55 patients aged 65 to 74 revealed no significant differences in the 3 year OS or PFS between those receiving stem cell transplantation and those not receiving stem cell transplantation. MRD rates were identical between the 2 groups. Multivariable analysis showed that complete response was the only independent predictor of PFS.[37]

Using flow cytometry, it is possible to detect clonal plasma cells in the apheresis product that is reinfused into the patient. The presence of plasma cells in the peripheral blood product independently predicts a worse PFS and OS and was found in 18% of autografts. This does not mean that the circulating cells are the source of relapsed disease but may reflect chemotherapy resistance following induction manifest by persistent circulating cells.[38]

Flourescent in situ hybridization genetics are predictive of outcomes. As demonstrated in the FORTE trial, PFS and OS declines among patient groups that have no cytogenetic abnormalities those with 1 and those with more than 1. The most common high-risk cytogenetic abnormality detected in myeloma is t(4;14). Recently, 79 patients were reported. Forty-four of the 79 had a second high-risk cytogenetic abnormality (56%). Fifty patients (63%) achieved a very good partial response or better. Twenty of the 50 achieved MRD negativity in the bone marrow. Median progression-free and overall survival were 22.9 months and 60.4 months, respectively. Patients achieving MRD negativity had improved PFS and OS on multi variable analysis. Additional high-risk cytogenetic abnormalities in addition to t(4;14) did not adversely impact outcomes. Lenalidomide maintenance improved overall survival. The outcome for patients with high-risk cytogenetic abnormalities remains inferior post-transplantation.[39] Reported phase 3 trials and their outcomes are given in **table 1**.

Toxicities Associated with Stem Cell Transplantation

At Mayo Clinic, stem cell transplantation is an outpatient procedure. Patients are monitored as outpatients daily and only hospitalized if they have a significant decline in performance status triggered by infection, mucositis, or atrial fibrillations which are the 3 most common causes for admission. Ultimately, 45% of patients require hospitalization. The median duration of hospitalization is 7 days. The only predictor of hospitalization is age. Therapy-related mortality all cause at day 100 at Mayo Clinic is

Table 1
Selected stem cell transplant outcomes

	≥PR, %	≥CR	PFS, mo	OS, mo
Determination[29]	97.5	46.8	67.5 median	46.8%@5 y
STAMmINA[30]	93	27	53.9%@38 mo	83.7%@38 mo
Forte,KRd arm 0 HRCA[35]		46%MRD-	71%@4 yr	94%@4 yr
1 HRCA		50%MRD-	60%@4 yr	83%@4 yr
2+ HRCA		38%MRD-	39@@4 y	63%@4 yr

Abbreviations: HRCA, high-risk cytogenetic abnormalities; KRd, carfilzomib lenalidomide dexamethasone; MRD, measurable residual disease.

0.3% only 25% of patients require a hospital stay of 5 days or greater.[40] Opportunistic infection remains a major risk factor in stem cell transplantation for multiple myeloma. The cumulative incidence rate in multiple myeloma transplants were 6.3%, 19.1%, 4.2%, and 5.6%, respectively, for fungal, varicella zoster virus, cytomegalovirus, and pneumocystis. These unusually high numbers underscore the need for pre transplant prophylaxis with acyclovir or valacyclovir, sulfamethoxazole-trimethoprim, and fluconazole since most of these infections should be prevented with appropriate prophylaxis.[41] As an example, the hazard ratio for patients receiving varicella zoster virus (VZV) prophylaxis was 0.096. Quality of life is significantly decreased immediately after stem cell transplantation, myeloma survivors who achieve disease control after transplant have excellent recovery of quality of life and scores return to population norms by 1-year posttransplant. This transient decline in quality of life is important for patients to recognize before agreeing to the procedure.[42] Compared with autologous transplant recipients without myeloma those with multiple myeloma are more likely to have high fatigue scores 48% versus 36% $P<.01$. This symptom can have a significant impact on quality of life.[43] High-dose melphalan significantly increases the mutational burden on plasma cells that remain following transplantation. The newly acquired mutations are associated with DNA damage and double-stranded breaks. All patients treated with high-dose melphalan have clonal selection. Those transplanted patients who achieve a complete response have significantly more mutations at relapse. Ultimately, this increases the complexity of residual clones.[44] Our approach to Stem Cell transplantation is given in **Box 1**.

Box 1
Procedure used at mayo for stem cell transplantation

Discontinue induction chemotherapy 2 weeks prior to pretransplant evaluation. This includes lenalidomide and daratumumab.

Stem cell mobilization is done with G-CSF 10 μg/kg subcutaneous once daily. The collection of stem cells may be done without a central line if vascular access is adequate.

For patients with a goal of 1 intended transplant–If Day 4 pCD34+ is < 10, begin plerixafor that evening and initiate collections following morning.

For patients with a goal of more than 1 intended transplant–If Day 4 pCD34+ is < 20, begin plerixafor that evening and initiate collections following morning.

Plerixafor Dosing
    For patients with normal renal function (CrCl >50), calculate dose at 0.24 mg/kg.
    For patients with renal impairment (estimated CrCl < 50 mL/min), reduce the dose to 0.16 mg/kg.
    Maximum dose is 24 mg (1 vial).

The goal for 1 transplant is 3×10^6/kg; for 2 transplants 6×10^6/kg.

Chemo mobilization is used for patients with circulating plasma cells by flow at the time of proposed collection. Patients who failed to achieve a partial response to induction chemotherapy are also candidate for chemo mobilization.

Cyclophosphamide 1.5 g/M2 for 2 consecutive days. Initiate G-CSF on day 5. Begin collections when the total white blood cell count exceeds 1000. No uroprophylaxis is required for cyclophosphamide at this dose.

Growth factor is not administered after day 0 stem cell infusion. Patients are monitored daily as an outpatient and are hospitalized for uncontrolled infection, uncontrolled mucositis impeding oral medication administration, severe decline in performance status, or atrial fibrillation.

One Transplant or Two?

In the original studies of total therapy from the University of Arkansas, tandem transplantation was a routine part of successive total therapy trials. The introduction of tandem transplantation was done in the absence of a comparative trial, so its actual value remained unclear for decades. In a recent update, steady improvements in OS were found, with patients treated in 2014 or later having superior OS (hazard ratio, 0.35) and reduced excess risk for MM death (relative excess risk, 0.30) compared with patients treated in 1997 or earlier. A total of 10.0% to 18.6% of patients achieved their normal life expectancy across multiple periods.[45] There has been a movement in recent years to restrict application of tandem stem cell transplantation to those patients with high-risk disease usually defined by adverse FISH genetics. In a report with bortezomib-lenalidomide-dexamethasone, induction followed by tandem stem cell transplantation 2 year PFS and OS was significantly improved in patients with multiple adverse genetic abnormalities 77.8 and 83.3 months, respectively (double hit myeloma).[46] In 1 study, the major predictor of benefit from tandem stem cell transplantation was response improvement after the first stem cell transplant with a hazard ratio of 0.64. The actual depth of response after the first transplant did not influence survival from tandem transplant.[47] A non inferiority trial was performed comparing single versus tandem stem cell transplantation. Event-free survival and OS were not different between the 2 groups. However, the rates of complete response increased from first to second stem cell transplant. Although no differences were seen, patients were not stratified based on cytogenetic risk[48]

The European myeloma network enrolled 1503 patients. Patients were randomized to bortezomib-lenalidomide-dexamethasone consolidation or no consolidation. Seven hundred two were assigned to autologous stem cell transplantation and 495 to bortezomib- melphalan-prednisone. Median progression-free survival was significantly improved with autologous stem cell transplant compared to bortezomib-melphalan-prednisone, 56.7 months compared to 41.9 months, respectively. In addition, consolidation significantly improved median progression-free survival compared to no consolidation, 58.9 compared to 45.5 months. This study supported the use of autologous stem cell transplantation as intensification as well as the use of consolidation therapy.[49] Current practice in Europe is to proceed with tandem stem cell transplantation in patients who achieve less than a near complete response after the first transplant.[50]

Maintenance Therapy Following Autologous Stem Cell Transplantation

A total of 180 patients were randomly assigned to post-transplant maintenance with carfilzomib, lenalidomide, and dexamethasone or lenalidomide alone. Both groups received treatment for up to 3 years (36 cycles). Patients randomized to carfilzomib-lenalidomide maintenance who were MRD negative with standard risk genetics received lenalidomide alone after 8 cycles of the triplet. Median progression-free survival was 59.1 months in the carfilzomib group versus 41.4 months in the lenalidomide group; hazard ratio 0.51. There was 1 treatment-related adverse event leading to death, pneumonia, in the carfilzomib group. Lower respiratory infections were more severe in the carfilzomib maintenance group, 8% versus 1%. This supports carfilzomib-lenalidomide-dexamethasone maintenance therapy following autologous stem cell transplantation.[51]

Future Strategies to Improve Outcomes

The neutrophil to lymphocyte ratio was investigated as a predictor PFS and OS in myeloma transplantation. The neutrophil to lymphocyte ratio was an independent factor influencing progression-free survival. Predictors for overall survival included the neutrophil lymphocyte ratio, pretransplant bortezomib, and age. Patients with a high neutrophil to lymphocyte ratio may obtain less benefit for transplant and could be considered a target group for alternate interventions that are non transplant.[52]

There is increasing evidence that the gut microbiology impacts outcomes following autologous stem cell transplant. Loss of bacterial diversity in the bowel at engraftment appears to be associated with impaired response to stem cell transplant in MM.[53] These changes occurred due to intravenous antibiotic exposure. The gut microbiome may serve as a biomarker for outcome and a target for dietary intervention in a transplant population. Lower diversity of the gut microbial environment has been reported to lead to adverse outcomes in other hematologic malignancies.[53]

Lenalidomide remains the standard of care for post-transplantation maintenance. In the Cassiopeia trial, the addition of daratumumab to lenalidomide improved progression-free survival but only in patients who did not receive daratumumab with induction therapy. For those patients who received daratumumab induction, the addition of daratumumab as maintenance did not improve outcomes compared to lenalidomide alone.[54] The addition of daratumumab to lenalidomide improved PFS in the Griffin trial.[55] PERSEUS and AURIGA will be informative on the role of 2 drug maintenance daratumumab and lenalidomide as posttransplant maintenance. The myeloma XI trial has performed a landmark analysis suggesting that the benefit of lenalidomide maintenance could not be demonstrated beyond 4 years. This is not randomized evidence but suggests that the benefit of lenalidomide maintenance may decline over time[56]

The Role of Measurable Residual Disease

They are now several clinical trials underway where post induction assessment of MRD negativity at 10^{-6} will be performed in patients who will then be randomized to transplant or no transplant. This is an effort to determine if in patients who have achieved a maximal depth response whether intensification with transplant will be beneficial. The primary concern is the risk of second primary malignancies associated with stem cell transplantation and post-transplantation lenalidomide maintenance. Currently, the risk of a second primary hematologic malignancy is approximately 2% and tends to be genetically unfavorable with poor outcomes following allogeneic transplantation for these therapy-related myeloid neoplasms.

SUMMARY

The evidence is mixed. However, most thought leaders in the field believe that stem cell transplantation remains the standard of care for eligible patients for the time being. It would be inappropriate to subject the patient to stem cell transplantation if comorbidities predict a therapy-related mortality of 2% or greater. Trials are currently underway that replace stem cell transplantation with car T intervention. New maintenance trials are also underway using multiple agents to prolong PFS. It remains to be seen whether these interventions will make autologous stem cell transplantation unnecessary. However, currently, it remains the standard of care for patients with MM outside of clinical trial participation.

CLINICS CARE POINTS

- Stem cell transplantation remains the standard of care for eligible myeloma patients because of its significant improvement in PFS and higher rate of MRD negativity.

- With appropriately selected patients, stem cell transplantation should carry an all cause day 100 mortality of less than 0.5%.
- Full-dose melphalan at 200 mg per m^2 is recommended for all patients with the exception of those who have a serum creatinine> 2 mg/dL or are frail.
- Post-transplantation growth factor does not reduce hospitalization or infections.
- Transplantation has been sufficiently standardized to be performed as an outpatient.

REFERENCES

1. Singh S, Sharma R, Singh J, et al. Autologous stem cell transplantation for multiple myeloma in the novel agent era: Systematic review of Indian data and implications for resource constrained settings. J Cancer Res Ther 2023; 19(Supplement): S12–s19.
2. Lamm W, Wohlfarth P, Bojic M, et al. Outcome in Multiple Myeloma Patients Eligible for Stem Cell Transplantation: A Single-Center Experience. Oncology 2015;89(4):196–204.
3. Belotti A, Ribolla R, Cancelli V, et al. Transplant eligibility in elderly multiple myeloma patients: Prospective external validation of the international myeloma working group frailty score and comparison with clinical judgment and other co-morbidity scores in unselected patients aged 65-75 years. Am J Hematol 2020; 95(7):759–65.
4. Vaxman I, Visram A, Kumar S, et al. Autologous stem cell transplantation for multiple myeloma patients aged ≥ 75 treated with novel agents. Bone Marrow Transplant 2021;56(5):1144–50.
5. Kumar L, Sahoo RK, Kumar S, et al. Autologous stem cell transplant for multiple myeloma: Impact of melphalan dose on the transplant outcome. Leuk Lymphoma 2023;64(2):378–87.
6. Zhai Y, Yan L, Jin S, et al. Autologous stem cell transplantation in multiple myeloma patients with renal impairment. Ann Hematol 2023;102(3):621–8.
7. Lazana I, Floro L, Christmas T, et al. Autologous stem cell transplantation for multiple myeloma patients with chronic kidney disease: a safe and effective option. Bone Marrow Transplant 2022;57(6):959–65.
8. Waszczuk-Gajda A, Gras L, de Wreede LC, et al. Safety and efficacy of autologous stem cell transplantation in dialysis-dependent myeloma patients-The DIADEM study from the chronic malignancies working party of the EBMT. Bone Marrow Transplant 2023;58(4):424–9.
9. Awada H, Hajj Ali A, Ali MF, et al. Validation of the role of corrected DLCO in predicting outcomes post autologous hematopoietic cell transplant for multiple myeloma. Eur J Haematol 2023;110(6):780–3.
10. Pasvolsky O, Saliba RM, Masood A, et al. Impact of gender on outcomes of patients with multiple myeloma undergoing autologous Haematopoietic stem cell transplant. Br J Haematol 2023;201(4):e37–41.
11. Prakash VS, Malik PS, Sahoo RK, et al. Multiple myeloma: risk adapted use of plerixafor for stem cell mobilization prior to autologous stem cell transplantation is effective and cost efficient. Clin Lymphoma Myeloma Leuk 2022;22(1):44–51.
12. Chhabra S, Callander N, Watts NL, et al. Stem cell mobilization yields with daratumumab- and lenalidomide-containing quadruplet induction therapy in newly diagnosed multiple myeloma: findings from the MASTER and GRIFFIN trials. Transplant Cell Ther 2022;06:06.

13. Thurlapati A, Roubal K, Davis JA, et al. Stem cell mobilization for multiple myeloma patients receiving daratumumab-based induction therapy: a real- world experience. Transplant Cell Ther 2023;29(5):340.e341–4.

14. Crees ZD, Rettig MP, Jayasinghe RG, et al. Motixafortide and G-CSF to mobilize hematopoietic stem cells for autologous transplantation in multiple myeloma: a randomized phase 3 trial. Nat Med 2023;29(4):869–79.

15. Gomez-Arteaga A, Mark TM, Guarneri D, et al. High-dose bendamustine and melphalan conditioning for autologous stem cell transplantation for patients with multiple myeloma. Bone Marrow Transplant 2019;54(12):2027–38.

16. Cailleteau A, Maingon P, Choquet S, et al. Phase 1 study of the combination of escalated total marrow irradiation using helical tomotherapy and fixed high-dose melphalan (140 mg/m^2) followed by autologous stem cell transplantation at first relapse in multiple myeloma. Int J Radiat Oncol Biol Phys 2023;115(3): 677–85.

17. Li N, Liang L, Xiang P, et al. Clonal haematopoiesis of indeterminate potential predicts delayed platelet engraftment after autologous stem cell transplantation for multiple myeloma. Br J Haematol 2023;201(3):577–80.

18. Scordo M, Gilbert LJ, Hanley DM, et al. Open-label pilot study of romiplostim for thrombocytopenia after autologous hematopoietic cell transplantation. Blood Adv 2023;7(8):1536–44.

19. Pandya C, Hashmi S, Khera N, et al. Cost-effectiveness analysis of early vs. late autologous stem cell transplantation in multiple myeloma. Clin Transplant 2014; 28(10):1084–91.

20. Asrar MM, Lad DP, Bansal D, et al. Health-related quality of life in transplant eligible multiple myeloma patients with or without early ASCT in the real-world setting. Leuk Lymphoma 2021;62(13):3271–7.

21. Yong K, Wilson W, de Tute RM, et al. Upfront autologous haematopoietic stem-cell transplantation versus carfilzomib-cyclophosphamide-dexamethasone consolidation with carfilzomib maintenance in patients with newly diagnosed multiple myeloma in England and Wales (CARDAMON): a randomised, phase 2, non-inferiority trial. Lancet Haematol 2023;10(2):e93–106.

22. Lemieux C, Muffly LS, Iberri DJ, et al. Outcomes after delayed and second autologous stem cell transplant in patients with relapsed multiple myeloma. Bone Marrow Transplant 2021;56(11):2664–71.

23. Khan AM, Ozga M, Bhatt H, et al. Outcomes after salvage autologous hematopoietic cell transplant for patients with relapsed/refractory multiple myeloma: a single-institution experience. Clin Lymphoma Myeloma Leuk 2022;05:05.

24. Hashmi H, Atrash S, Jain J, et al. Daratumumab, pomalidomide, and dexamethasone (DPd) followed by high dose chemotherapy-Autologous Stem Cell Transplantation leads to superior outcomes when compared to DPd-alone for patients with Relapsed Refractory Multiple Myeloma. Transplant Cell Ther 2023; 20:20.

25. Jain T, Sonbol MB, Firwana B, et al. High-dose chemotherapy with early autologous stem cell transplantation compared to standard dose chemotherapy or delayed transplantation in patients with newly diagnosed multiple myeloma: a systematic review and meta-analysis. Biol Blood Marrow Transplant 2019;25(2): 239–47.

26. Khan S, Reece D, Atenafu EG, et al. Post salvage therapy autologous transplant for relapsed myeloma, ongoing relevance within modern treatment paradigms? Clin Lymphoma Myeloma Leuk 2023;23(2):e97–106.

27. Cook G, Ashcroft AJ, Cairns DA, et al. The effect of salvage autologous stem-cell transplantation on overall survival in patients with relapsed multiple myeloma (final results from BSBMT/UKMF Myeloma X Relapse [Intensive]): a randomised, open-label, phase 3 trial. Lancet Haematol 2016;3(7):e340–51.
28. Goldschmidt H, Baertsch MA, Schlenzka J, et al. Salvage autologous transplant and lenalidomide maintenance vs. lenalidomide/dexamethasone for relapsed multiple myeloma: the randomized GMMG phase III trial ReLApsE. Leukemia 2021;35(4):1134–44.
29. Richardson PG, Jacobus SJ, Weller EA, et al. Triplet therapy, transplantation, and maintenance until progression in myeloma. N Engl J Med 2022;387(2):132–47.
30. Stadtmauer EA, Pasquini MC, Blackwell B, et al. Autologous transplantation, consolidation, and maintenance therapy in multiple myeloma: results of the BMT CTN 0702 Trial. J Clin Oncol 2019;37(7):589–97.
31. Dispenzieri A, Krishnan A, Arendt B, et al. Mass-fix better predicts for PFS and OS than standard methods among multiple myeloma patients participating on the STAMINA trial (BMT CTN 0702/07LT). Blood Cancer J 2022;12(2):27.
32. Jung J, Kim K, Jung SH, et al. Cyclophosphamide, Bortezomib, and Dexamethasone Consolidation in Patients with Multiple Myeloma after Stem Cell Transplantation: The KMM130 Study. Cancer Res Treat 2023;55(2):693–703.
33. Lawless S, Iacobelli S, Knelange NS, et al. Comparison of autologous and allogeneic hematopoietic cell transplantation strategies in patients with primary plasma cell leukemia, with dynamic prediction modelling. Haematologica 2022;30:30.
34. Kriz T, Jungova A, Lysak D, et al. Allogeneic stem cell transplantation in patients with multiple myeloma-single center experience. Neoplasma 2023;23:23.
35. Gay F, Musto P, Rota-Scalabrini D, et al. Carfilzomib with cyclophosphamide and dexamethasone or lenalidomide and dexamethasone plus autologous transplantation or carfilzomib plus lenalidomide and dexamethasone, followed by maintenance with carfilzomib plus lenalidomide or lenalidomide alone for patients with newly diagnosed multiple myeloma (FORTE): a randomised, open-label, phase 2 trial. Lancet Oncol 2021;22(12):1705–20.
36. Lin CM, Chang LC, Shau WY, et al. Treatment benefit of upfront autologous stem cell transplantation for newly diagnosed multiple myeloma: a systematic review and meta-analysis. BMC Cancer 2023;23(1):446.
37. Sato S, Tsunoda S, Kawahigashi T, et al. Clinical significance of high-dose chemotherapy with autologous stem cell transplantation in the era of novel agents in patients older than 65 years with multiple myeloma. Ann Hematol 2023;102(5):1185–91.
38. Pasvolsky O, Milton DR, Rauf M, et al. Impact of clonal plasma cells in autografts on outcomes in high-risk multiple myeloma patients. Blood Cancer J 2023;13(1):68.
39. Pasvolsky O, Gaballa MR, Milton DR, et al. Autologous Stem Cell Transplantation for Patients with Multiple Myeloma with Translocation (4;14): The MD Anderson Cancer Center Experience. Transplant Cell Ther 2023;29(4):260.e1-6.
40. Gertz MA, Buadi FK, Hayman SR, et al. Safety Outcomes for Autologous Stem Cell Transplant in Multiple Myeloma. Mayo Clin Proc 2018;93(1):56–8.
41. Kim DJ, Jeong S, Kong SG, et al. Incidence and risk factors of opportunistic infections after autologous stem cell transplantation: a nationwide, population-based cohort study in Korea. Sci Rep 2023;13(1):2551.

42. D'Souza A, Brazauskas R, Stadtmauer EA, et al. Trajectories of quality of life recovery and symptom burden after autologous hematopoietic cell transplantation in multiple myeloma. Am J Hematol 2023;98(1):140–7.
43. Ullrich CK, Baker KK, Carpenter PA, et al. Fatigue in Hematopoietic Cell Transplantation Survivors: Correlates, Care Team Communication, and Patient-Identified Mitigation Strategies. Transplant Cell Ther 2023;29(3):200.e1-8.
44. Samur MK, Roncador M, Aktas Samur A, et al. High-dose melphalan treatment significantly increases mutational burden at relapse in multiple myeloma. Blood 2023;141(14):1724–36.
45. Nishimura KK, Barlogie B, van Rhee F, et al. Long-term outcomes after autologous stem cell transplantation for multiple myeloma. Blood Adv 2020;4(2):422–31.
46. Tang S, Lu Y, Zhang P, et al. Lenalidomide, bortezomib and dexamethasone followed by tandem- autologous stem cell transplantation is an effective treatment modality for multi-hit multiple myeloma. Leuk Res 2021;110:106710.
47. Blocka J, Hielscher T, Goldschmidt H, et al. Response Improvement Rather than Response Status after First Autologous Stem Cell Transplantation Is a Significant Prognostic Factor for Survival Benefit from Tandem Compared with Single Transplantation in Multiple Myeloma Patients. Biol Blood Marrow Transplant 2020; 26(7):1280–7.
48. Mai EK, Benner A, Bertsch U, et al. Single versus tandem high-dose melphalan followed by autologous blood stem cell transplantation in multiple myeloma: long-term results from the phase III GMMG-HD2 trial. Br J Haematol 2016; 173(5):731–41.
49. Cavo M, Gay F, Beksac M, et al. Autologous haematopoietic stem-cell transplantation versus bortezomib-melphalan-prednisone, with or without bortezomib-lenalidomide-dexamethasone consolidation therapy, and lenalidomide maintenance for newly diagnosed multiple myeloma (EMN02/HO95): a multicentre, randomised, open-label, phase 3 study. Lancet Haematol 2020; 7(6):e456–68.
50. Baertsch M-A, Mai EK, Hielscher T, et al. Lenalidomide versus bortezomib maintenance after frontline autologous stem cell transplantation for multiple myeloma. Blood Cancer J 2021;11(1):1.
51. Dytfeld D, Wrobel T, Jamroziak K, et al. Carfilzomib, lenalidomide, and dexamethasone or lenalidomide alone as maintenance therapy after autologous stem-cell transplantation in patients with multiple myeloma (ATLAS): interim analysis of a randomised, open-label, phase 3 trial. Lancet Oncol 2023; 24(2):139–50.
52. Mikulski D, Kościelny K, Nowicki M, et al. Neutrophil to lymphocyte ratio (NLR) impact on the progression-free survival and overall survival of multiple myeloma patients treated with high-dose chemotherapy and autologous stem cell transplantation. Leuk Lymphoma 2023;64(1):98–106.
53. D'Angelo C, Sudakaran S, Asimakopoulos F, et al. Perturbation of the gut microbiome and association with outcomes following autologous stem cell transplantation in patients with multiple myeloma. Leuk Lymphoma 2023;64(1): 87–97.
54. Moreau P, Hulin C, Perrot A, et al. Maintenance with daratumumab or observation following treatment with bortezomib, thalidomide, and dexamethasone with or without daratumumab and autologous stem-cell transplant in patients with newly diagnosed multiple myeloma (CASSIOPEIA): an open-label, randomised, phase 3 trial. Lancet Oncol 2021;22(10):1378–90.

55. Voorhees PM, Kaufman JL, Laubach J, et al. Daratumumab, lenalidomide, borte-zomib, and dexamethasone for transplant-eligible newly diagnosed multiple myeloma: the GRIFFIN trial. Blood 2020;136(8):936–45.

56. Jenner MW, Pawlyn C, Davies FE, et al. The addition of vorinostat to lenalidomide maintenance for patients with newly diagnosed multiple myeloma of all ages: results from 'Myeloma XI', a multicentre, open-label, randomised, phase III trial. Br J Haematol 2022;201(2):267–79.

Role of Consolidation and Maintenance

Anupama D. Kumar, MD*, Ajai Chari, MD

KEYWORDS

- Multiple myeloma • Consolidation • Maintenance • Minimal residual disease
- High-risk

KEY POINTS

- Consolidation therapy after transplant: After a stem cell transplant in multiple myeloma, there is a short-term treatment called consolidation therapy. It is like a boost to the transplant.
- Mixed results from trials: Some important tests about consolidation therapy had different outcomes. This made doctors unsure if it is always needed after a transplant, so they have different ways of treating patients.
- Maintenance therapy for long term: After the transplant, there is also long-term treatment called maintenance therapy. It can last for a fixed time or even longer.
- Different treatments for different risks: Patients with a regular risk usually get one medicine, whereas those with higher risk might need two or more medicines together.
- Side effects and quality of life: Doctors need to think about side effects and how patients feel during treatment. They are still studying to find out the best time for patients to stop maintenance therapy.

INTRODUCTION

Consolidation in multiple myeloma refers to a limited duration of systemic therapy given after autologous stem cell transplant (ASCT) and before maintenance therapy. The goal of consolidation therapy is to improve the frequency and depth of response without unacceptable toxicity.[1] Modern consolidation therapy typically consists of a triplet or even quadruplet regimen, often but not always identical to the regimen used during induction therapy. Clinical trials often include consolidation in their study schema, but trials specifically examining the role of consolidation have shown mixed results, which may be explained by variable drugs and duration of induction ahead of ASCT. As a result, clinical practice on the use of consolidation post-ASCT is not standardized. Here, the authors review the existing evidence on the role of consolidation therapy after ASCT.

University of California, San Francisco, 400 Parnassus Avenue, ACC Building, 4th Floor, San Francisco, CA 94143, USA
* Corresponding author.
E-mail address: anupama.kumar@ucsf.edu

Hematol Oncol Clin N Am 38 (2024) 421–440
https://doi.org/10.1016/j.hoc.2023.12.006
0889-8588/24/© 2023 Elsevier Inc. All rights reserved.

Although some definitions include ASCT within the category of consolidation, this topic is discussed in depth in our previous article titled, "Is There Still a Role for Stem Cell Transplant in Multiple Myeloma?" However, it is important to note here that ASCT itself extends progression-free survival (PFS) and, variably, overall survival (OS). The Intergroupe Francophone du Myélome (IFM) published in 1996 the first randomized trial comparing conventional chemotherapy alone to ASCT in myeloma and demonstrated improved OS in the ASCT arm (not reached in ASCT arm after median follow-up of 41 months vs 37.4 months in the chemotherapy arm after median follow-up of 37 months).[2] A subsequent trial by the British Medical Research Council similarly demonstrated that ASCT improved survival by nearly 1 year compared with conventional chemotherapy alone.[3] These trials provide historical perspective on the benefit of ASCT without consolidation as we include some phase 2 consolidation trials without a comparator arm.

Maintenance therapy involves long-term therapy after the completion of upfront induction, ASCT in eligible patients, and consolidation. The single-agent maintenance therapy is typically used in standard-risk disease, whereas a doublet is considered in higher risk individuals. Given the anticipated prolonged duration of maintenance therapy over years, factors such as adverse events (AEs) (including the dreaded long-term risk of secondary malignancy), quality of life, route of administration, and cost must be considered. Here, the authors highlight pivotal trials examining the evidence behind various maintenance strategies.

DISCUSSION
Consolidation

Various consolidation strategies have been studied in multiple myeloma; here, the authors discuss key phase 2 and 3 trials and summarize study regimens and outcomes (**Table 1**). The first of such trials is the 2013 Nordic Myeloma Study, a phase 3 trial in 370 patients that assessed the efficacy of single-agent bortezomib consolidation in bortezomib-naïve patients.[4] Patients received variable induction, most commonly cyclophosphamide and dexamethasone (89%), with others receiving thalidomide and steroids or vincristine, doxorubicin, and dexamethasone (VAD). Data on duration of induction were not provided. Bortezomib-exposed individuals were excluded from the trial. Patients underwent ASCT and then were randomized 1:1 to receive 20 doses of single-agent bortezomib consolidation or no consolidation. The bortezomib consolidation arm experienced longer PFS (27 months vs 20 months, $P = .05$), increased rate of very good partial response (VGPR) or better (71% vs 57%, $P<.01$), and a trend toward increased complete response (CR) or near CR (45% vs 35%, $P = .055$). OS and health-related quality of life were unchanged between the treatment arms. Not surprisingly, peripheral neuropathy rates were increased in the bortezomib consolidation group (57% vs 24%). Although this trial is not applicable in the era of novel therapies as most patients are bortezomib-exposed during induction, it sets the groundwork for further consolidation trials in the subsequent decade.

The Italian PETHEMA/GEM2012 trial was a randomized phase 3 clinical trial comparing bortezomib, thalidomide, and dexamethasone (VTd) induction and consolidation to thalidomide, dexamethasone (Td) induction and consolidation in 408 participants with newly diagnosed multiple myeloma (NDMM).[5] All participants received double ASCT after induction and dexamethasone maintenance after consolidation. The trial demonstrated a PFS advantage at 3 years (60% vs 48%, $P = .042$) favoring the VTd group. The investigators note that the CR and near-CR rates were equivalent in both arms after induction but significantly improved after consolidation in the VTd

Table 1
Clinical trials examining the role of consolidation therapy in multiple myeloma

Year	Study	N	Treatment Regimen	Outcome
2011	IFM 2008[7]	31	I: VRd × 3 cycles q21 days → ASCT → C: VRd × 2 cycles q21 days → M: lenalidomide 15 mg × 1 year	Non-randomized, but promising ORR (94%) and sCR (39%)
2013	Mellqvist et al[4]	370	I: variable (bortezomib not permitted) → ASCT → C: bortezomib × 4 cycles (two 21 day cycles, four 28 days cycles), vs none → M: None	Improved PFS, VGPR rate in bortezomib arm, trend toward significance for CR/near-CR, OS unchanged
2017	IFM 2009[8]	700	I: VRd × 3 cycles q21 days → ASCT + VRd × 2 cycles q21 days vs VRd × 5 cycles q21 days → M: lenalidomide 10 mg daily × 3 months, followed by possible increase to 15 mg daily; maximum duration of maintenance: 1 year	Improved PFS, CR rate, MRD negativity with ASCT arm; no change in OS
2012	PETHEMA/GEM2012[5]	480	I: VTd × 3 cycles q21 days vs Td × 3 cycles q21 days → double ASCT (Td between transplants) → C: VTd × 2 cycles q35 days (in VTd-induced) vs Td × 2 cycles q35 days (in Td induced) → M: dexamethasone 40 mg d1-4/28 until PD	Improved CR/near-CR rate post-consolidation with VTd compared with Td

(continued on next page)

Table 1
(continued)

Year	Study	N	Treatment Regimen	Outcome
2018	BMT CTN 0702 (StaMINA)[10]	758	*I:* Variable ASCT vs double ASCT → vs ASCT + VRd × 4 cycles q21 days → *M:* lenalidomide 10 mg daily × 3 months then 15 mg daily until PD	No difference in PFS and OS in ASCT vs double ASCT vs ASCT + VRd
2019	CASSOPEIA[17]	1085	*First randomization, I:* DVTd × 4 cycles q28 days vs VTd × 4 cycles q28 days → ASCT → *C:* DVTd × 2 cycles q28 days (in DVTd-induced) vs VTd × 2 cycles q28 days (in VTd-induced) → *Second randomization, M:* daratumumab × 2 years vs observation	Improved PFS, response, MRD negativity with DVTd, deepened response in each after consolidation
2020	GRIFFIN[16]	207	*I:* DRVd × 4 q21 days vs VRd × 4 q21 days → ASCT → *C:* DRVd × 2 cycles q21 days (in DRVd-induced) vs VRd × 2 cycles q21 days(in VRd-induced) → *M:* DR (in DRVd-induced) vs lenalidomide 10 mg d1-21/28 × 3 cycles then 15 mg d1-21/28 (in VRd-induced); maximum duration of either maintenance treatment: 2 year	Improved PFS, response, MRD negativity with DRVd, deepened response in both arms after consolidation

| 2021 | EMN02/HOVON95[11] | 878 | I: VCd × 3–4 cycles q21 days
→
First randomization: VMP × 4 cycles q6weeks vs single ASCT
vs double ASCT (in participating centers)
→
Second randomization, C: VRd × 2 cycles q28 days vs no consolidation
→
M: Lenalidomide 10 mg d1-21/28 until PD | Improved PFS, CR + rate with VRd consolidation compared with no consolidation in lenalidomide-naïve patients |
| 2021 | IFM KRd[14] | 46 | I: KRd × 4 cycles q28 days
→
ASCT
→
C: KRd × 4 cycles q28 days
→
M: Lenalidomide 10 mg d1-21/28 × 13 cycles | Improved ORR, VGPR + rate, CR + rate, sCR rate, MRD rate from post-ASCT to post-consolidation |

Abbreviations: ASCT, autologous stem cell transplant; C, consolidation; CR, complete response; I, induction; M, maintenance; MRD, minimal residual disease; ORR, overall response rate; PD, progressive disease; sCR, s:ringent complete response.

arm only, supporting the added benefit of VTd consolidation. Like in the 2013 Nordic Myeloma Study, an increased rate of peripheral neuropathy (8.1% vs 2.4%) was seen in the participants treated with bortezomib consolidation. This was the first phase 3 clinical trial to compare a triplet vs doublet regimen in both induction and consolidation. There were no arms without consolidation therapy altogether.

The single-arm phase 2 IFM 2008 trial evaluated the combination of bortezomib, lenalidomide, and dexamethasone (VRd), a regimen then known to be effective in the induction setting, as consolidation therapy.[6,7] Thirty-one symptomatic NDMM patients were treated with VRd for 3 cycles, followed by ASCT, 2 cycles of VRd consolidation, and ultimately 1 year of lenalidomide maintenance. The trial demonstrated that the overall response rate (ORR) was 91% after the completion of ASCT and 94% after VRd consolidation and that the stringent CR rate deepened from 36% after ASCT to 39% after VRd consolidation. Expected toxicities including peripheral neuropathy (23%), grade 3 to 4 neutropenia (17%), and thrombocytopenia (10%) were observed, and no treatment-related mortalities occurred. The subsequent IFM 2009 trial, which sought to evaluate the necessity of ASCT in the era of modern therapies, also used VRd consolidation.[8] Patients were randomized after VRd induction to ASCT with 2 cycles of VRd or no ASCT and 5 cycles of VRd. Although no OS difference was detected, transplant followed by consolidation was associated with a PFS advantage and a higher CR and minimal residual disease (MRD) negativity, at the cost of increased toxicity.

The BMT CTN 0702 (STaMINA)[9] trial was a phase 3 clinical trial across 54 centers in the United States. Patients undergoing induction were enrolled on trial, and any induction regimen was permitted. Bortezomib, lenalidomide, dexamethasone (VRd) was most commonly used, composing 57% of the study populations, but others received cyclophosphamide, bortezomib, and dexamethasone; lenalidomide and dexamethasone; bortezomib and dexamethasone; or other regimens. Patients were required to receive at least 2 cycles of any systemic therapy without progression and to be within 2 to 12 months of first dose of initial therapy, resulting in considerable variation in therapy duration before trial enrollment. Participants were randomized to single transplant, single transplant followed by 4 cycles of VRd consolidation, or double transplant. All participants then received maintenance lenalidomide. There was no PFS or OS benefit at 38 months with the addition of VRd consolidation or second ASCT, leading the investigators to conclude that single ASCT without consolidation followed by lenalidomide maintenance should remain the standard of care to avoid unnecessary toxicities. Six-year follow-up data showed similar PFS and OS across all three arms in the intention-to-treat analysis ($P = .6$ for PFS, $P = .8$ for OS).[10] In high-risk patients using as-treated analysis, 6-year PFS was prolonged in the double ASCT arm (43.6%) compared with single ASCT without consolidation ($P = .03$); 6-year PFS for high-risk patients in the ASCT with VRd consolidation arm was not provided.

The European Myeloma Network (EMN) conducted the prospective, open-label phase 3 EMN02/HOVON95 clinical trial to understand the utility of VRd consolidation.[11] They enrolled 1197 participants with untreated multiple myeloma. All patients received induction with vincristine, cyclophosphamide, and dexamethasone (VCd) for 3 to 4 cycles. Importantly, lenalidomide, which was later used in consolidation and maintenance, was absent from the induction regimen. Patients were first randomized to ASCT vs bortezomib, melphalan, and prednisone (VMP) intensification. ASCT demonstrated a PFS benefit over VMP.[12] A second randomization was done for 878 eligible participants to VRd consolidation for 2 cycles followed by maintenance lenalidomide vs maintenance lenalidomide alone. There was a PFS benefit (59.3 months vs 42.9 months, hazard ratio [HR] = 0.81, $P = .016$) favoring the VRd consolidation arm at a median follow-up of 74.8 months. This result was upheld in most subgroups, except in the high-risk deletion *17p* patients. There was also an improvement in CR or better (59% vs 46%, *P*<.001) in the VRd consolidation arm. This trial established the benefit of VRd consolidation in NDMM who are lenalidomide naïve and received 3 to 4 cycles of VCd. OS was not reached in either arm, indicating the need for longer follow-up.

Given that the STaMINA trial and the EMN02/HOVON95 trial yielded contradictory results on the role of VRd consolidation, it is important to highlight key differences. Of note, in the STaMINA trial, the induction regimen was heterogenous and patients were predominantly lenalidomide-exposed, whereas all patients received VCd induction in the EMN02/HOVON95 trial and were not exposed to lenalidomide until consolidation. The STaMINA investigators suggest that VRd induction, an accepted standard in the United States, is superior to VCd, obviating the need of consolidation or double ASCT. The STaMINA trial had a high rate of nonadherence (up to 32%) with the second intervention, although this may be in line with natural patterns of patient behavior. Another possible interpretation of STaMINA is that the heterogeneity in the drugs and cycles before induction therapy blunted the ability of post-SCT therapies to show a difference.

In more recent years, carfilzomib, a second-generation proteosome inhibitor, has been studied in combination with carfilzomib, lenalidomide, and dexamethasone (KRd), initially in the relapsed/refractory setting and now in the upfront NDMM setting.[13–15] The phase II IFM KRd study administered 4 cycles of KRd induction and ASCT, 4 cycles of KRd consolidation, and 1 year of lenalidomide maintenance to 46 participants.[14] Responses deepened at every step in the treatment regimen, with CR+ rate improving from 41.5% post-ASCT to 64.3% post-consolidation. Notable AEs include two cases of heart failure: a toxicity associated with carfilzomib and five pulmonary embolisms/deep vein thromboses, which may be due to lenalidomide. The most common grade 3 and 4 AEs were cytopenias (74%) and infection (22%). The FORTE trial done across 42 centers in Italy also included an arm with KRd consolidation after KRd induction and ASCT; the comparator arms were 12 cycles of KRd without ASCT and carfilzomib, cyclophosphamide, and dexamethasone (KCd) induction/ASCT/KCd consolidation.[15] The KRd/ASCT/KRd arm had superior responses overall (4-year PFS 69%, compared with 56% in the KRd12 arm and 51% in the KCd/ASCT/KCd arm). In all arms, responses deepened after consolidation. For example, in the KRd/ASCT/KRd arm, VGPR+ rate improved from 82% to 89% and sCR improved from 25% to 46%.

In the ever-evolving field of myeloma, quadruplet regimens have recently been studied in the front line in NDMM; both the GRIFFIN and CASSOPEIA trials included consolidation post-ASCT in their study schema.[16,17] The GRIFFIN trial randomized patients to daratumumab, lenalidomide, bortezomib, and dexamethasone (DRVd) vs RVd. Patients received 4 induction cycles of their assigned regimen, ASCT, then 2 consolidation cycles, followed by maintenance daratumumab and lenalidomide (DR) in the DRVd arm vs lenalidomide alone in the RVD arm for up to 2 years. DRVd proved to have better PFS, response, and MRD negativity rate. With regard to consolidation, response deepened after consolidation therapy in both arms (sCR improved from 21.2% to 42.4% and VGPR+ improved from 86.9% to 90.9% in the DRVd arm; sCR improved from 14.4% to 32%; and VGPR+ improved from 66% to 73.2% in the RVd arm). The CASSOPEIA trial similarly randomized 1085 patients to a quadruplet of daratumumab VTd (DVTd) or VTd induction, followed by ASCT, then DVTd or VTd consolidation. DVTd improved PFS, depth of response, and MRD negativity much like the GRIFFIN trial; consolidation deepened responses in both arms (sCR 13.4% to 28.9% and VGPR+ 76.7% to 83.% in the DVTd arm; sCR 9.4% to 20.3%; and

VGPR+ 67.4% to 78% in the VTd arm). Both trials did not include treatment arms without consolidation, making it difficult to make definitive conclusions about the added utility of consolidation.

A novel approach in recent trials has been using a response-adapted fixed treatment duration strategy to administer consolidation to certain patients. The MASTER trial treated patients with daratumumab KRd (DKRd), ASCT, followed by 0, 4, or 8 cycles of KRd consolidation based on MRD status (assessed after induction, after ASCT, and every 4 weeks during consolidation).[18] Once MRD negativity was attained for two consecutive time points, all therapy was discontinued. Eighty percent of patients were able to reach MRD negativity with this approach, and 2-year PFS was 87%. Extended follow-up data demonstrated that patients with two or more high-risk cytogenetic abnormalities (HRCAs) had worse 3-year PFS (51% compared with 91% and 97% in individuals with 0 or 1 high-cytogenetic features, $P < .001$) and OS (75% compared with 96% and 91%, $P = .004$), suggesting that alternative strategies are necessary for ultra-high-risk patients.[19] The ongoing open-label, single-arm CONPET trial (NCT03314636) instead uses an imaging-guided approach and aims to administer KRd consolidation to PET-CT positive patients after induction (VRd, VTd, or VCd) and ASCT.[20]

Maintenance

Numerous maintenance trials have investigated different maintenance regimens, as single-agent therapy or multi-agent combinations and as fixed-duration, indefinite, or response-adapted. The authors review here pivotal trials and provide details on study drugs, therapy duration, and adverse effects (**Table 2**).

Thalidomide, an immunomodulatory agent (IMiD), is rarely used in the United States since the advent of lenalidomide. However, thalidomide is still widely used in many parts of the world and has been studied at doses of 50 to 200 mg.[21] The MMC Myeloma IX trial compared indefinite thalidomide maintenance at up to 100 mg if tolerated to observation after induction (with either intensive therapy including transplant or non-intensive therapy based on patient performance status).[22] Thalidomide maintenance prolonged PFS (23 vs 15 months, HR = 1.45, log-rank $P < .001$) but did not impact OS. Fifty-two percent of patients discontinued the trial early due to AEs, including paresthesias, drowsiness, constipation, skin conditions, hematological events, infection, thrombosis, and tremor. Owing to the early discontinuation of maintenance, median time on therapy was only 7 months despite intended indefinite therapy until progression. There was an equal rate of secondary malignancy between the maintenance and observation arms. The investigators conducted a meta-analysis of five existing thalidomide maintenance trials including their own, when pooling data, thalidomide significantly prolonged OS ($P = .047$) and had a late survival benefit (4% survival benefit at 3 years and 12.3% survival benefit at 7 years).

Single-agent lenalidomide is a mainstay of maintenance therapy in the United States and increasingly around the world and has been evaluated in numerous trials. The IFM investigators evaluated 614 patients treated with lenalidomide, administered as consolidation 25 mg on day 1 to 21 (out of a 28 day cycle) for 2 cycles followed by maintenance 10 mg daily for 3 months with dose escalation to 15 mg, vs placebo for a fixed duration of 2 years.[23] The trial demonstrated an improvement in PFS in the lenalidomide arm (41 vs 23 months, HR = 0.50, $P < .001$) with no difference in OS at long-term 5 year follow-up.[23,24] Thromboembolic events (6% vs 2%, $P = .01$), grade 3 to 4 cytopenias, and secondary malignancy (3.1 vs 1.2 per 100 patient-year, $P = .002$) were more common in the lenalidomide group. Lenalidomide was stopped early in January 2011 after a median duration of 27 months in 119

Table 2
Clinical trials examining the maintenance therapies in multiple myeloma

Year	N	Study	Maintenance	Induction, ASCT, Consolidation	Outcomes	AEs
THALIDOMIDE						
2012	820	MMC Myeloma IX[22]	Thalidomide 50 mg × 4 weeks, then 100 mg until PD vs observation	*If intensive pathway:* I: CVAD × 4–6 cycles q28 days vs CTD × 4–6 cycles q28 days → ASCT *If non-intensive pathway:* I: MP q28 days vs attenuated CTD q28 days	Maintenance prolonged PFS, no change in OS	Increased infection in thalidomide maintenance arm (intensive pathway), increased rate of any serious AE in thalidomide maintenance arm (both intensive and non-intensive pathway)
LENALIDOMIDE						
2012	614	IFM 2005–02[23,24]	Lenalidomide 10 mg daily × 3 months, then 15 mg vs placebo. Stopped early in 119 participants, after median 27 months) due to increased secondary cancers	I: variable → ASCT → C: Lenalidomide 25 mg d1-21/ 28 × 2 cycles	Maintenance prolonged PFS, 5-year OS unchanged	Increased cytopenias, thromboembolic events, and secondary malignancy in lenalidomide maintenance arm
2014	251	RV-MM-209[26]	Lenalidomide 10 mg d1-21/28 until PD vs observation	I: Rd × 4 cycles q28 days → C: MP × 6 cycles q28 days vs ASCT (with melphalan 200 mg/m² monthly × 4 doses prior)	Maintenance prolonged PFS, OS improvement not statistically significant	Increased rate of neutropenia and skin reactions in lenalidomide maintenance arm

(continued on next page)

Table 2
(continued)

Year	N	Study	Maintenance	Induction, ASCT, Consolidation	Outcomes	AEs
2017	460	CALGB 100104[25]	Lenalidomide 10 mg daily × 3 months, then 15 mg daily until PD vs placebo	I: Variable → ASCT	Maintenance prolonged time to progression, OS	Increased cytopenias and secondary cancers in lenalidomide maintenance arm
2019	1917	Myeloma XI[28]	Lenalidomide 10 mg d1-21/28, until PD vs observation	*If intensive pathway:* I: CTD × 4+ cycles vs CRD × 4+ cycles vs KCRd × 4+ cycles → ASCT *If non-intensive pathway:* I: attenuated CTD × 6+ cycles vs attenuated CRD × 6+ cycles	Maintenance prolonged PFS, 3-year OS improvement was not statistically significant	Most common grade 3–4 AE in maintenance arm were neutropenia (33%), thrombocytopenia (7%), and anemia (4%)
BORTEZOMIB						
2012	827	HOVON-65/GMM-HD4[32]	Bortezomib 1.3 mg/m² every 2 weeks in PAD arm vs thalidomide 50 mg daily in VAD arm	I: PAD × 3 cycles q28 days vs VAD × 3 cycles q28 days → ASCT	CR, PFS, OS prolonged in bortezomib arm	Peripheral neuropathy increased (40% vs 18%) in bortezomib arm
IXAZOMIB						
2018	656	TOURMALINE-MM3[33]	Ixazomib 3 mg d1, 8, 15/28 × 5 cycles, then 4 mg vs placebo. Maintenance up to 2 years	I: Variable, must include PI or IMiD → ASCT	5.2 month PFS benefit with ixazomib	Equal rate of secondary malignancy

	Year	N	Study	Intervention	Treatment	Outcomes	Toxicity/Notes
CARFILZOMIB							
	2022	168	CARFI[34]	Carfilzomib 27 mg/m² every other weeks × 4 weeks, then 56 mg/m² 20 mg every other week vs observation	I: KCd × 4 cycles q28 days → ASCT	Improved PFS with maintenance, OS benefit not statistically significant	Increased thrombocytopenia anemia, dyspnea, and bacterial infection in the Kd maintenance arm
DARATUMUMAB							
	2021	886	CASSOPEIA	Daratumumab 16 mg/kg q8 weeks × 2 years vs observation	First randomization, I: DVTd × 4 cycles q28 days vs VTd × 4 cycles q28 days → ASCT → C: DVTd × 2 cycles q28 days (in DVTd-induced) vs VTd × 2 cycles q28 days (in VTd-induced)	Improved PFS in daratumumab-naïve patients	Increased lymphopenia in daratumumab maintenance arm, 2 fatalities (sepsis, NK-lymphoblastic leukemia) due to daratumumab
LENALIDOMIDE + BORTEZOMIB							
	2013	45, high-risk	Nooka et al[37]	Lenalidomide 10 mg d1-21/28, bortezomib 1.3 mg/m² weekly, dexamethasone 40 mg weekly (VRd) × 3 years followed by lenalidomide maintenance	I: Variable → ASCT	PFS 32 months, 3-year OS 93%	Dose modification in 40% patients, no early cessation of therapy due to AE, no new grade 3–4 neuropathy
	2020	1000	Joseph et al[38]	Variable; 1000 patients with RVD induction followed, 107 received IMiD + PI	I: RVD → Non-randomized: Upfront or deferred ASCT	PFS 40.3, OS 78.2 in IMiD + PI group	Not described in article

(continued on next page)

Table 2
(continued)

Year	N	Study	Maintenance	Induction, ASCT, Consolidation	Outcomes	AEs
LENALIDOMIDE + DARATUMUMAB						
2020	207	GRIFFIN[16]	Daratumumab 16 mg/kg IV q4–8 weeks + lenalidomide 10 mg d1-21/28 × 3 cycles then 15 mg vs lenalidomide alone. DR or R up to 2 years	*I:* DRVd × 4 q21 days vs VRd × 4 q21 days → ASCT → *C:* DRVd × 2 cycles q21 days (in DRVd-induced) vs VRd × 2 cycles q21 days (in VRd-induced)	Improved PFS, response, MRD negativity with DRVd, deepened response at each stage of therapy	Increased grade 3–4 hematological AE and infections with DRVd vs RVd, similar grade 3–4 infection in both arms
LENALIDOMIDE + CARFILZOMIB						
2021	356	FORTE[15]	Lenalidomide 10 mg d1-21/28 + carfilzomib 70 mg IV d1, 15 vs lenalidomide alone. Carfilzomib up to 2 years, lenalidomide until progression	*First randomization:* *I:* KRd × 4 cycles[a] → ASCT → *C:* KRd × 4 cycles[a] vs *I:* KRd × 12 cycles[a] vs *I:* KCd × 4 cycles[a] → ASCT → *C:* KCd × 4 cycles[a] [a]All cycles q28 days	Improved 3-year PFS, MRD conversion in doublet arm	Most common grade 3–4 AEs were neutropenia (20% in KR vs 23% in R), infection (5% vs 7%), and vascular events (7% vs 1%)
2023	180	ATLAS[42]	Carfilzomib 36 mg/m² d1, 2, 8, 9, 15, 16/28 during cycle 1–4, then carfilzomib 36 mg/m² on d1, 2, 15, 16/28 from cycle 5–36, lenalidomide 25 mg d1-21/28, dexamethasone 20 weekly (KRd) × 36 cycles then lenalidomide alone until PD vs lenalidomide 10 mg daily for 3 cycles, then 15 mg daily until PD	*I:* Variable → ASCT	Improved PFS in triplet maintenance arm	Most common grade 3–4 AE were neutropenia (48% in KRd vs 60% in R), thrombocytopenia (13% vs 7%), and lower respiratory tract infection (8% vs 1%)

Abbreviations: IMiD, immunomodulatory agent; NK, natural killer; PI, proteosome inhibitor.

patients due to the signal for increased secondary malignancy. The CALGB 100104 trial randomized 460 post-ASCT participants to indefinite lenalidomide 10 mg daily (with dose escalation permitted at 3 months to 15 mg) vs placebo.[25] Time to progression was prolonged in the lenalidomide group (57.3 months vs 28.9 months, HR = 0.57, $P < .001$) as was median OS (113.8 months vs 84.1 months, HR = 0.61, $P < .004$). Cytopenias and secondary malignancies were increased in the maintenance arm (7.8% hematological malignancies, 6.1% solid tumors in lenalidomide arm vs 1.3% hematological malignancies, and 3.9% solid tumor in the placebo arm). The Italian RV-MM-209 used a 2-by-2 factorial design; after induction lenalidomide and dexamethasone, patients underwent first randomization to melphalan SCT or melphalan, prednisone, and lenalidomide consolidation.[26] The trial then performed a second randomization to lenalidomide 10 mg on day 1 to 21 (out of a 28 day cycle) until progression vs observation and demonstrated a PFS advantage (41.9 vs 21.6 months, HR = 0.47, $P < .001$) without a statistically significant OS benefit at 3 years (88% vs 79.2%, HR = 0.62, $P = .14$).[26] There was an increased rate of neutropenia (23.3% vs 0%) and skin reactions (4.3% vs 0%) in the lenalidomide arm. Of note, a meta-analysis of IFM 2005 to 02, CALGB 100104, and RV-MM-209 did in fact show both a PFS and OS benefit (not reached in lenalidomide maintenance vs 86.0 months in placebo/observation group, at median follow-up of 79.5 months).[27]

The Myeloma XI trial, which had not completed accrual at the time of the above meta-analysis, used an adaptive design with three potential randomizations at induction, intensification, and maintenance.[28] At the maintenance stage, the trial randomized participants to indefinite lenalidomide 10 mg on day 1 to 21 (out of a 28 day cycle) or observation and demonstrated a statistically significant PFS benefit (39 vs 20 months, HR = 0.46, $P < .001$) and 3-year OS increase (78.6% vs 75.8%, HR = 0.87, $P = .15$) that was not statistically significant. Updated long-term follow-up data indicated that the benefit of lenalidomide persisted beyond 3 years, but the magnitude of benefit diminished after 4 to 5 years in all comers and even earlier in patients who achieved MRD negativity after transplant.[29] However, caution should be used as this was a post-hoc analysis with a diminishing number of patients continued on therapy beyond 4 years.

Although these lenalidomide maintenance trials vary in terms of lenalidomide dose, schedule, duration, and presence of placebo or observation as a comparator arm, they all uniformly show a benefit of either PFS or time to progression and some demonstrate an OS advantage. However, the optimal duration remains unclear. Many patients may be unable to continue the initial maintenance lenalidomide dose of 10 to 15 mg indefinitely, particularly real-world patients that may have comorbidities. Importantly, the dose of lenalidomide during maintenance must be adjusted for renal function as per the prescribing label. The Myeloma XI trial demonstrated that 69% of patients required dose modification, and 594 of 1137 (52%) in the lenalidomide maintenance arm had discontinued therapy after a median follow-up of 31 months, due to disease progression, death, AE, patient preference, or other.[28] The RV-MM-209 trial in contrast demonstrated that 11% of patients discontinued therapy, either due to AE, withdrawal of consent, or investigator's decision after a median follow-up of 51.2 months.[26]

Until prospective, risk-adapted studies are available, physicians should consider a patient's genomic and functional risk (ie, depth of response attained) as well as long-term toxicities of lenalidomide, including cytopenias, rash, venous thromboembolism, and secondary malignancy, when determining optimal dosing and duration for individual patients. Cost is also an important consideration, though there is increasing availability of generic lenalidomide globally.

There are no data to our knowledge evaluating pomalidomide, iberdomide, or mezigdomide as maintenance after front-line SCT. There are existing data evaluating these agents for maintenance of salvage ASCTs, which are beyond the scope of this article.[21,30,31]

Thus far, the authors have discussed IMiDs, but proteasome inhibitors can also be used for maintenance therapy. The HOVON-65/GMM-HD4 trial randomized patients to a regimen VAD induction, ASCT followed by thalidomide 50 mg daily maintenance, or bortezomib, doxorubicin, dexamethasone (PAD) induction followed by ASCT and bortezomib 1.3 mg/m^2 every 2 weeks.[32] Bortezomib maintenance had superior CR/near-CR (49% vs 34%, $P < .001$). At a median follow-up of 41 months, the PAD/ASCT/bortezomib arm outperformed the VAD/ASCT/thalidomide arms in terms of PFS (35 vs 28 months, HR = 0.75, $P = .002$) and OS (per multivariate analysis, HR = 0.77, $P = .49$). This benefit persisted in high-risk patients, including those harboring a 17p deletion. However, owing to the variable induction regimens, it is challenging to attribute the superior responses to bortezomib maintenance alone. The rate of peripheral neuropathy in the first year of therapy was increased in the bortezomib arm compared with thalidomide (40% vs 18%, HR = 1.50, $P < .001$). If considering bortezomib maintenance, providers must keep in mind the potential irreversibility of neuropathy and the fact that it can interfere with balance and ambulation, a consequence that may be particularly devasting in the elderly. Bortezomib in addition requires frequent in-person visits to an infusion center, which poses an inconvenience to patients but may be favorable if compliance is under question with oral medications.

The TOURMALINE-MM3 trial evaluated the effectiveness of ixazomib, a second-generation oral proteosome inhibitor, in 656 participants.[33] Post-ASCT patients were randomized 3:2 to oral ixazomib 3 mg on day 1, 8, 15/28 (with increase to 4 mg at cycle 5 if tolerable) vs placebo, for a duration of 2 years. The trial met its primary endpoints, with a PFS benefit favoring ixazomib (26.5 vs 21.3 months, HR = 0.72, $P = .0023$). The rate of secondary malignancy was equal across both arms (3%), unlike results seen in many lenalidomide trials. Although generally well tolerated, ixazomib has not been taken up widely in clinical practice given that magnitude of PFS benefit is short compared to lenalidomide.

Carfilzomib, an intravenous second-generation proteosome inhibitor has been recently studied in the maintenance setting. The phase 2 CARFI trial enrolled relapsed myeloma patients and administered 4 cycles of KCd followed ASCT.[34] Of 200 patients who were enrolled, 168 patients were then randomized to carfilzomib (27 mg/m^2 every other week, dose escalated to 56 mg/m^2 after 4 weeks) and dexamethasone 20 mg every other week or observation. The median time to progression was 25.1 months in the maintenance arm and 15.7 months in the observation arm (HR = 0.46, $P = .004$). OS was not reached in the maintenance arm compared with 44.5 months in the observation arm, although this difference was not statistically significant (HR = 0.47, $P = .10$). Like other maintenance therapies previously discussed, carfilzomib most commonly caused hematological toxicity (thrombocytopenia in 29% vs 21%, anemia in 58% vs 44%). Notable non-hematological toxicities include dyspnea (24% vs 11%) and bacterial infections (41% vs 26%).

Daratumumab, an anti-CD38 monoclonal antibody now included in many upfront triplet and quadruplet regimens, was studied as maintenance therapy in the CASSO-PEIA trial.[35] As discussed earlier, transplant-eligible patients were randomized to DVTd vs VTd as induction and consolidation. Next, a second randomization was performed to daratumumab maintenance at 16 mg/kg IV every 8 weeks for up to 2 years vs observation. Daratumumab maintenance prolonged PFS (not reached vs 35.4, HR = 0.53, $P < .0001$) and increased conversion to MRD negativity (44% vs 30%, odds ratio = 1.84, nominal P = .004). However, an important caveat is that the PFS benefit only existed in the daratumumab-naïve patients who received VTd (HR = 0.32, nominal P < .001), not in the daratumumab-exposed patients who received DVTd (HR = 1.02, nominal P = .91). In addition, the every 8 week dosing schedule that was used is not standard; pharmacokinetic data shows that the drug should be dosed long-term at an every 4 week schedule after initial weekly then biweekly dosing.[36] Longer follow-up data are required as the highest rates of MRD negativity attained were in patients who received daratumumab before and after SCT. Lymphopenia was increased in the daratumumab arm (4% vs 2%). Two deaths were attributed to the drug (septic shock and natural killer-cell lymphoblastic leukemia).

Ongoing research in recent years has evaluated multi-agent maintenance regimens, particularly in high-risk patients who have worse prognoses. In an observational study, Nooka and colleagues at Emory reported the outcomes of 45 patients with HRCAs (deletion 17p, deletion 1p, t(4;14), t(14;16), or plasma cell leukemia), treated with 3 years of RVd maintenance followed by a de-escalation to lenalidomide mainte-nance.[37] PFS was 32 months, 3-year OS was 93%, and best response was VGPR or better in 96% of patients. No patients terminated therapy early due to AEs. In their larger observational study following 1000 patients induced with RVd, 251 had high-risk cytogenetic features and 107 received a combination of an IMiD+ proteosome inhib-itor (most commonly RVd), with a median PFS of 40.3 months and OS of 78.2 months.[38] The GRIFFIN trial used a DR doublet for 2 years in the DRVd induction arm, after which daratumumab was discontinued and only lenalidomide was continued until progression.[16]

The much-awaited phase 3 AURGIA trial (NCT03901963) will compare head-to-head DR to lenalidomide alone in both standard and high-risk patients who are anti-CD38 naïve and are MRD+ after SCT.[39] The DRAMMATIC trial (NCT04071457) will include both anti-CD38 exposed and naïve patients, randomized to DR or lenalido-mide alone for 2 years, with a second randomization at the 2 year mark of MRD nega-tive patients to discontinuation of therapy or ongoing therapy up to 7 years.[40] The maintenance component of the FORTE trial randomized patients to carfilzomib and lenalidomide for 2 years or lenalidomide alone and demonstrated improved 3-year PFS (75% vs 65%, P = .023) and MRD conversation (46% vs 30%, P = .046), without a statistically significant difference in 3-year OS (94% vs 90%).[15] Preplanned cytoge-netic subgroup analysis showed that patients with more high-risk features had worse 4-year PFS (71% if 0 HRCA, 60% if 1 HRCA, and 39% if 2 or more HRCAs) and 4-year OS (94%, 83%, and 63%, respectively).[41] These findings reiterate the need for refined strategies for ultra-high-risk patients with 2 or more HRCAs. Interim analysis of ATLAS trial, which compares 3 years of KRd maintenance to lenalidomide alone, demon-strated an improved median PFS with triplet therapy (59.1 vs 31.4 months, HR = 0.51, P = .01).[42]

SUMMARY

The authors demonstrate that many consolidation therapies have been used in multiple myeloma, including single-agent bortezomib, VRd, VTd, KRd, KCd, DVRd, and DVTd. As illustrated, many trials include consolidation in their study schema and demonstrate that response and MRD negativity deepen from post-ASCT values to post-consolidation values. However, in these studies, it is difficult to definitely ascertain whether such improvements are directly a result of the consolidation or due to lasting effects of potent induction therapy and ASCT. Two recent pivotal trials that directly compared consolidation to no consolidation were the EMN02/HOVON95 and BMT

CTN 0702 (STaMINA) trials.[10,12] EMN02/HOVON95 found improved PFS and response rates with VRd consolidation compared with no consolidation in lenalidomide-naïve patients but used VCd induction which arguably is inferior to VRd induction. The STaMINA trial did not standardize induction regimens but demonstrated no added benefit to VRd consolidation post-ASCT and risk of added toxicity. In the present day, clinical practice on the routine use of consolidation varies, based on geographic region of practice, patient fitness, and response after induction and ASCT.

The authors show that there are many options for maintenance therapy in multiple myeloma, including single agents which generally are acceptable for standard-risk patients and doublets which are of interest particularly in high-risk patients. The authors demonstrate that maintenance therapy prolongs PFS or time to progression, with mixed results regarding OS. Debate still exists as to the optimal duration of therapy, as the magnitude of benefit seems to diminish with time and maintenance can lead to drug-resistance and long-term toxicities including secondary malignancies.

SUMMARY AND FUTURE DIRECTIONS

Given that high-risk individuals have worse outcomes despite advances in therapy, myeloma researchers need to first refine the definition of high-risk disease. Genomic high risk must be segregated into no risk factors, single-hit, or double-hit characteristics. Functional high risk, defined as patients who relapse within 12 months or have persistent disease based on dynamic assessments MRD testing and imaging, must be considered as well. Although there has been much excitement about MRD testing, currently this test primarily has prognostic and not predictive value. The authors anticipate that this will evolve over the coming years, as trials use MRD and other dynamic assessments to guide treatment intensity and duration.[40]

The authors eagerly await data from randomized prospective genomic and functional risk-stratified studies to guide practice. Until then, if a patient is lenalidomide- or daratumumab-naïve and/or is functionally-high risk with measurable or MRD-positive disease and/or received induction therapy for 3 to 4 cycles without attaining a CR, then 2 cycles of triplet/quadruplet consolidation may be considered. In the absence of these features, the benefit of consolidation is unclear based upon current data. When clinicians use more than single-agent maintenance therapy, they need to consider both AEs and quality of life concerns, including time commitment to receiving IV/SC therapy in an infusion center and cost. Avoiding overtreatment in patients who do not benefit from additional therapy is important. The authors suggest that single-agent maintenance therapy is sufficient in standard-risk MRD-negative myeloma. The longer such patients remain MRD-negative, the more any AEs experienced by the patient should drive a discussion with the patient about the pros/cons of continued therapy. For high-risk patients and possibly standard-risk MRD-positive patients, more-intensified doublet maintenance approaches until progression should be considered.

Drug refractoriness should also be considered when determining the optimal duration of maintenance therapy. Lenalidomide refractoriness has been associated with worse outcomes including OS compared with lenalidomide-exposed non-refractory patients; however, this is offset by the OS benefit even in CALGB 100104 study where lenalidomide was used until progression.[25,43] Now, the long-term impact of anti-CD38 refractoriness is unknown and caution should be used with using these agents in the maintenance setting until progression.

Novel therapies, including bi-specific T-cell engagers and chimeric antigen receptor (CAR) T-cells, have been an exciting new development in relapsed myeloma.

Preliminary data for ciltacabtagene autoleucel in functional high-risk patients are already encouraging.[44] The role of these agents in consolidation and maintenance is an area of active investigation with several trials ongoing, including the following: NCT05846737 BCMA CAR-T Cell Therapy in High-risk NDMM Patients With Positive MRD After First-line ASCT evaluating BCMA-directed CAR-T in MRD positive patients post-ASCT, NCT05632380 ASCT in Combination With C-CAR088 for Treating Patients With Ultra High-risk Multiple Myeloma (MM) investigating a BCMA-directed CAR-T 3 days post-ASCT in ultra-high risk patients, CARTITUDE-5 (NCT04923893) comparing DRVd followed by ASCT and DRVd followed by ciltacabtagene autoleucel, and MagnestisMM-7 (NCT05317416) studying elranatamab monotherapy vs lenalidomide monotherapy as maintenance post-ASCT. Of particular interest will the ability of these highly potent therapies, after a fixed duration of therapy, to provide a treatment-free interval after frontline therapy is completed.

CLINICS CARE POINTS

- Clinical trials evaluating the role of short-duration consolidation therapy after autologous stem cell transplant have shown mixed results. EMN02/HOVON95 showed a progression-free survival (PFS) advantage with bortezomib, lenalidomide, and dexamethasone (VRd) consolidation in lenalidomide-naïve patients, whereas STaMINA did not show an added benefit for VRd consolidation.

- Single-agent lenalidomide is the mainstay for maintenance therapy for standard-risk myeloma in the United States.

- Doublet maintenance strategies are being investigated, particularly for high-risk patients.

- The optimal duration of maintenance therapy is unknown. Adverse events, secondary malignancy, drug resistance, quality of life, cost, PFS and overall survival endpoints need to be considered.

DISCLOSURE

A. Chari: Consulting: Abbvie, Adaptive, Amgen, Antengene, Bristol Myers Squibb, Forus, Genetech/Roche, Glaxo Smith Klein, Janssen, Karyopharm, Millenium/Takeda, Sanofi/Genzyme. Research: Janssen. *A. Kumar*: Research: Janssen, BMS.

REFERENCES

1. Cavo M, Brioli A, Tacchetti P, et al. Role of consolidation therapy in transplant eligible multiple myeloma patients. Semin Oncol 2013;40(5):610–7.
2. Attal M, Harousseau JL, Stoppa AM, et al. A prospective, randomized trial of autologous bone marrow transplantation and chemotherapy in multiple myeloma. N Engl J Med 1996;335(2):91–7.
3. Child JA, Morgan GJ, Davies FE, et al. High-Dose Chemotherapy with Hematopoietic Stem-Cell Rescue for Multiple Myeloma. N Engl J Med 2003;348(19): 1875–83.
4. Mellqvist UH, Gimsing P, Hjertner O, et al. Bortezomib consolidation after autologous stem cell transplantation in multiple myeloma: a Nordic Myeloma Study Group randomized phase 3 trial. Blood 2013;121(23):4647–54.
5. Cavo M, Pantani L, Petrucci MT, et al. Bortezomib-thalidomide-dexamethasone is superior to thalidomide-dexamethasone as consolidation therapy after

autologous hematopoietic stem cell transplantation in patients with newly diagnosed multiple myeloma. Blood 2012;120(1):9–19.

6. Richardson PG, Weller E, Lonial S, et al. Lenalidomide, bortezomib, and dexamethasone combination therapy in patients with newly diagnosed multiple myeloma. Blood 2010;116(5):679–86.

7. Roussel M, Robillard N, Moreau P, et al. Bortezomib, lenalidomide, and dexamethasone (VRD) consolidation and lenalidomide maintenance in frontline multiple myeloma patients: updated results of the IFM 2008 phase II VRD intensive program. Blood 2011;118(21):1872.

8. Attal M, Lauwers-Cances V, Hulin C, et al. Lenalidomide, bortezomib, and dexamethasone with transplantation for myeloma. N Engl J Med 2017;376(14): 1311–20.

9. Stadtmauer EA, Pasquini MC, Blackwell B, et al. Autologous transplantation, consolidation, and maintenance therapy in multiple myeloma: results of the BMT CTN 0702 Trial. J Clin Oncol 2019;37(7):589–97.

10. Hari P, Pasquini MC, Stadtmauer EA, et al. Long-term follow-up of BMT CTN 0702 (STaMINA) of postautologous hematopoietic cell transplantation (autoHCT) strategies in the upfront treatment of multiple myeloma (MM). J Clin Oncol 2020; 38(15_suppl):8506.

11. Sonneveld P, Dimopoulos MA, Beksac M, et al. Consolidation and maintenance in newly diagnosed multiple myeloma. J Clin Oncol 2021;39(32):3613–22.

12. Cavo M, Gay F, Beksac M, et al. Autologous haematopoietic stem-cell transplantation versus bortezomib-melphalan-prednisone, with or without bortezomib-lenalidomide-dexamethasone consolidation therapy, and lenalidomide maintenance for newly diagnosed multiple myeloma (EMN02/HO95): a multicentre, randomised, open-label, phase 3 study. Lancet Haematol 2020;7(6):e456–68.

13. Dimopoulos M, Wang M, Maisnar V, et al. Response and progression-free survival according to planned treatment duration in patients with relapsed multiple myeloma treated with carfilzomib, lenalidomide, and dexamethasone (KRd) versus lenalidomide and dexamethasone (Rd) in the phase III ASPIRE study. J Hematol OncolJ Hematol Oncol 2018;11(1):49.

14. Roussel M, Lauwers-Cances V, Wuilleme S, et al. Up-front carfilzomib, lenalidomide, and dexamethasone with transplant for patients with multiple myeloma: the IFM KRd final results. Blood 2021;138(2):113–21.

15. Gay F, Musto P, Rota-Scalabrini D, et al. Carfilzomib with cyclophosphamide and dexamethasone or lenalidomide and dexamethasone plus autologous transplantation or carfilzomib plus lenalidomide and dexamethasone, followed by maintenance with carfilzomib plus lenalidomide or lenalidomide alone for patients with newly diagnosed multiple myeloma (FORTE): a randomised, open-label, phase 2 trial. Lancet Oncol 2021;22(12):1705–20.

16. Voorhees PM, Kaufman JL, Laubach J, et al. Daratumumab, lenalidomide, bortezomib, and dexamethasone for transplant-eligible newly diagnosed multiple myeloma: the GRIFFIN trial. Blood 2020;136(8):936–45.

17. Moreau P, Attal M, Hulin C, et al. Bortezomib, thalidomide, and dexamethasone with or without daratumumab before and after autologous stem-cell transplantation for newly diagnosed multiple myeloma (CASSIOPEIA): a randomised, open-label, phase 3 study. Lancet 2019;394(10192):29–38.

18. Costa LJ, Chhabra S, Medvedova E, et al. Daratumumab, carfilzomib, lenalidomide, and dexamethasone with minimal residual disease response-adapted therapy in newly diagnosed multiple myeloma. J Clin Oncol 2022;40(25):2901–12.

19. Costa LJ, Chhabra S, Medvedova E, et al. Outcomes of MRD-adapted treatment modulation in patients with newly diagnosed multiple myeloma receiving daratumumab, carfilzomib, lenalidomide and dexamethasone (Dara-KRd) and autologous transplantation: extended follow up of the master trial. Blood 2022; 140(Supplement 1):7275–7.

20. Nørgaard JN, Abildgaard N, Lysén A, et al. Carfilzomib-Lenalidomide-Dexamethasone Consolidation in Myeloma Patients with a Positive FDG PET/CT after Upfront Autologous Stem Cell Transplantation: A Phase II Study (CONPET). Blood 2021;138:3939.

21. Holstein SA, Suman VJ, Hillengass J, et al. Future directions in maintenance therapy in multiple myeloma. J Clin Med 2021;10(11):2261.

22. Morgan GJ, Gregory WM, Davies FE, et al. The role of maintenance thalidomide therapy in multiple myeloma: MRC myeloma IX results and meta-analysis. Blood 2012;119(1):7–15.

23. Attal M, Lauwers-Cances V, Marit G, et al. Lenalidomide maintenance after stem-cell transplantation for multiple myeloma. N Engl J Med 2012;366(19):1782–91.

24. Attal M, Lauwers VC, Marit G, et al. Maintenance treatment with lenalidomide after transplantation for MYELOMA: final analysis of the IFM 2005-02. Blood 2010; 116(21):310.

25. Holstein SA, Jung SH, Richardson PG, et al. Updated analysis of CALGB 100104 (Alliance): a randomised phase III study evaluating lenalidomide vs placebo maintenance after single autologous stem cell transplant for multiple myeloma. Lancet Haematol 2017;4(9):e431–42.

26. Palumbo A, Cavallo F, Gay F, et al. Autologous transplantation and maintenance therapy in multiple myeloma. N Engl J Med 2014;371(10):895–905.

27. McCarthy PL, Holstein SA, Petrucci MT, et al. Lenalidomide maintenance after autologous stem-cell transplantation in newly diagnosed multiple myeloma: a meta-analysis. J Clin Oncol 2017;35(29):3279–89.

28. Jackson GH, Davies FE, Pawlyn C, et al. Lenalidomide maintenance versus observation for patients with newly diagnosed multiple myeloma (Myeloma XI): a multicentre, open-label, randomised, phase 3 trial. Lancet Oncol 2019;20(1): 57–73.

29. Pawlyn C, Menzies T, Davies FE, et al. Defining the optimal duration of lenalidomide maintenance after autologous stem cell transplant - data from the myeloma XI trial. Blood 2022;140(Supplement 1):1371–2.

30. Atieh T, Hubben A, Faiman B, et al. Pomalidomide-based maintenance post-autologous hematopoietic cell transplantation in multiple myeloma: a case series. Ann Hematol 2019;98(10):2457–9.

31. Garderet L, Kuhnowski F, Berge B, et al. Pomalidomide and dexamethasone until progression after first salvage therapy in multiple myeloma. Br J Haematol 2023; 201(6):1103–15.

32. Sonneveld P, Schmidt-Wolf IGH, van der Holt B, et al. Bortezomib induction and maintenance treatment in patients with newly diagnosed multiple myeloma: results of the randomized phase III HOVON-65/GMMG-HD4 trial. J Clin Oncol 2012;30(24):2946–55.

33. Dimopoulos MA, Gay F, Schjesvold F, et al. Oral ixazomib maintenance following autologous stem cell transplantation (TOURMALINE-MM3): a double-blind, randomised, placebo-controlled phase 3 trial. Lancet 2019;393(10168):253–64.

34. Gregersen H, Peceliunas V, Remes K, et al. Carfilzomib and dexamethasone maintenance following salvage ASCT in multiple myeloma: A randomised phase 2 trial by the Nordic Myeloma Study Group. Eur J Haematol 2022;108(1):34–44.

35. Moreau P, Hulin C, Perrot A, et al. Maintenance with daratumumab or observation following treatment with bortezomib, thalidomide, and dexamethasone with or without daratumumab and autologous stem-cell transplant in patients with newly diagnosed multiple myeloma (CASSIOPEIA): an open-label, randomised, phase 3 trial. Lancet Oncol 2021;22(10):1378–90.

36. Clemens PL, Yan X, Lokhorst HM, et al. Pharmacokinetics of daratumumab following intravenous infusion in relapsed or refractory multiple myeloma after prior proteasome inhibitor and immunomodulatory drug treatment. Clin Pharmacokinet 2017;56(8):915–24.

37. Nooka AK, Kaufman JL, Muppidi S, et al. Consolidation and maintenance therapy with lenalidomide, bortezomib and dexamethasone (RVD) in high-risk myeloma patients. Leukemia 2014;28(3):690–3.

38. Joseph NS, Kaufman JL, Dhodapkar MV, et al. Long-term follow-up results of lenalidomide, bortezomib, and dexamethasone induction therapy and risk-adapted maintenance approach in newly diagnosed multiple myeloma. J Clin Oncol 2020;38(17):1928–37.

39. Shah N, Patel S, Pei H, et al. Subcutaneous daratumumab (DARA SC) plus lenalidomide versus lenalidomide alone as maintenance therapy in patients (pts) with newly diagnosed multiple myeloma (NDMM) who are minimal residual disease (MRD) positive after frontline autologous stem cell transplant (ASCT): The phase 3 AURIGA study. J Clin Oncol 2021;39(15_suppl):TPS8054.

40. Krishnan A, Hoering A, Hari P, et al. Phase III Study of daratumumab/rhuph20 (nsc- 810307) + lenalidomide or lenalidomide as post-autologous stem cell transplant maintenance therapy in patients with multiple myeloma (mm) using minimal residual disease todirect therapy duration (DRAMMATIC study): SWOG s1803. Blood 2020;136(Supplement 1):21–2.

41. Mina R, Musto P, Rota-Scalabrini D, et al. Carfilzomib induction, consolidation, and maintenance with or without autologous stem-cell transplantation in patients with newly diagnosed multiple myeloma: pre-planned cytogenetic subgroup analysis of the randomised, phase 2 FORTE trial. Lancet Oncol 2023;24(1):64–76.

42. Dytfeld D, Wróbel T, Jamroziak K, et al. Carfilzomib, lenalidomide, and dexamethasone or lenalidomide alone as maintenance therapy after autologous stem-cell transplantation in patients with multiple myeloma (ATLAS): interim analysis of a randomised, open-label, phase 3 trial. Lancet Oncol 2023;24(2):139–50.

43. Hajek R, Sliwka H, Stork M, et al. Patient characteristics and survival outcomes of lenalidomide exposed non- refractory vs. lenalidomide refractory multiple myeloma patients in the honeur federated data network. Blood 2022; 140(Supplement 1):7200–2.

44. van de Donk NWCJ, Agha ME, Cohen AD, et al. Biological correlative analyses and updated clinical data of ciltacabtagene autoleucel (cilta-cel), a BCMA-directed CAR-T cell therapy, in patients with multiple myeloma (MM) and early relapse after initial therapy: CARTITUDE-2, cohort B. J Clin Oncol 2022; 40(16_suppl):8029.

Management of Newly Diagnosed Multiple Myeloma Today, and in the Future

Anup Joseph Devasia, MBBS, MD, DM,
Guido Sebastian Lancman, MD, Alexander Keith Stewart, MBChB*

KEYWORDS

- Newly diagnosed MM • Quadruplets • Triplets • T cell-directed therapies

KEY POINTS

- Quadruplet therapy incorporating daratumumab has been practice changing in newly diagnosed multiple myeloma.
- Treatment of high-risk myeloma is challenging and difficult.
- Bispecific antibodies and chimeric antigenicT cell therapies as upfront options are expected to produce impressive results.

INTRODUCTION

Treatment options have expanded rapidly and widely in the past 2 decades for patients with multiple myeloma (MM). This has translated to significantly improved responses and survival of patients with this complex and heterogenous plasma cell disorder.[1] The use of triplet novel agent-based induction regimens has led to faster, deeper, and more durable responses and this has been accepted as the standard practice over the last decade both for transplant-eligible (TE) and transplant ineligible (TI) patients. More recently, incorporation of monoclonal antibodies into induction regimens has led to deeper responses and longer progression-free survival (PFS) in both TE[2,3] and TI[1,6] patients, as well as longer overall survival (OS) in TI patients[4,5] with minimal added toxicity.

Response to initial therapy is vital as the first remission tends to be the longest and real-world data show substantial attrition seen with subsequent lines of therapy due to comorbidities, disease factors, and cumulative treatment-related adverse events.[6,7] Given the median age of myeloma patients at diagnosis and the prevalence of comorbidities in this population, the best available treatments should be given upfront rather than reserved for relapse.

Division of Medical Oncology and Haematology, Princess Margaret Cancer Centre, 700 University Avenue, Toronto, Ontario, M5G 1X6 Canada
* Corresponding author.
E-mail address: keith.stewart@uhn.ca

Hematol Oncol Clin N Am 38 (2024) 441–459
https://doi.org/10.1016/j.hoc.2023.12.007
0889-8588/24/© 2023 Elsevier Inc. All rights reserved.

At the current time, eligibility for autologous stem cell transplantation (ASCT) remains a key decision point in the newly diagnosed MM treatment pathway. Multiple clinical trials have shown a consistent PFS benefit for ASCT over standard of care triplets without ASCT.[8-10] Although these studies did not demonstrate an OS benefit for ASCT, it is important to note that this was not the primary endpoint and that OS is confounded by the abundance of salvage therapies available at relapse. In the IFM2009 study using just 1 year of lenalidomide maintenance, 35% of patients receiving ASCT had not relapsed at nearly 8 years of follow-up,[11] while in the DETERMINATION study using lenalidomide until progression, the median PFS of ASCT patients was 67.5 months.[9] To date, no other treatment in MM has shown such a prolonged disease-free interval with minimal medications and excellent quality of life and therefore ASCT remains a mainstay for patients who are fit enough to endure the peri-transplant period. The role of ASCT may continue to evolve with the introduction of immunotherapies in front-line treatment and is discussed in a separate article.

The field of MM is being revolutionized by potent immunotherapies, including chimeric antigen receptor (CAR)- T cells and bispecific antibodies. These immunotherapies have demonstrated unprecedented response rates, minimal residual disease (MRD) negativity, and PFS in heavily relapsed patients. Both modalities are currently being tested in both the TE and TI settings and may prove to be a new standard of care in the future. In anticipation of this potential paradigm shift, opportunities and challenges in the use of immunotherapies in newly diagnosed MM will be discussed.

TRANSPLANT-ELIGIBLE PATIENTS

Recommendations for initial treatment still hinge on whether the patient is considered to be eligible for ASCT. Better patient selection by various frailty scores[12,13] and the predictable toxicity profile of ASCT have helped to better define "transplant-eligible" patients. Nevertheless, identifying the optimal induction strategy prior to ASCT remains a challenge. Although historically triplets have been considered standard of care, these are now being challenged by quadruplets incorporating anti-CD38 monoclonal antibodies.

Triplet Therapy

Triplet novel agent-based induction using immunomodulators (IMiDs) and proteasome inhibitors (PIs) on a steroid backbone was until recently the standard of care approach in newly diagnosed myeloma for both transplant-eligible and transplant- ineligible patients.[14,15] Although there are no prospective randomized control trials comparing lenalidomide-bortezomib-dexamethasone (RVd) and bortezomib-cyclophosphamide-dexamethasone (VCd), several real world studies did not show any significant differences between these 2 regimens in terms of responses, PFS, or OS,[16] while another real-world study from Canada showed a PFS of 58.2 months using predominantly VCd induction followed by transplant and lenalidomide maintenance,[17] which is comparable to real-world studies using RVd induction. There are prospective data demonstrating improved response rates for bortezomib-thalidomide-dexamethasone (VTd) over VCd, however, no PFS data were reported.[18] While RVd has been the preferred triplet induction regimen in the United States, VTd or VCd remains the most used induction before ASCT in many parts of Europe, and Canada, largely due to differences in drug approval and funding policies. The use of VCd or VTd is preferred in patients with renal failure, although these patients can be transitioned to RVd if they experience renal recovery.

Carfilzomib was tested as part of triplet induction in 2 randomized trials. There is no direct comparison between RVd and carfilzomib-lenalidomide-dexamethasone (KRd) in the setting of planned upfront ASCT. The phase 3 ENDURANCE trial[19] comparing KRd to RVd conducted among patients not eligible or not deemed for upfront ASCT did not observe any superiority of KRd, but did show higher rates of renal and cardiopulmonary toxicity in the carfilzomib arm. Although patients were not planned for immediate ASCT, the median age was 65 and most patients had Eastern Cooperative Oncology Group (ECOG) performance status of 0 or 1, indicating most patients would have been transplant-eligible. Given the similar response rates even with prolonged treatment, it is unlikely that 4 to 6 cycles given prior to ASCT would produce a meaningful difference in outcomes. Importantly, this trial did not include patients with high-risk disease. The FORTE trial showed clear superiority for KRd induction and ASCT over KCd (carfilzomib-cyclophosphamide-dexamethasone) followed by ASCT, with similar benefits in both standard and high-risk groups.[10] As both of these arms received carfilzomib, it is not possible to determine the added value of carfilzomib in induction from this study.

Quadruplet Therapy

In order to deepen and prolong responses in frontline therapy, anti-CD38 monoclonal antibodies have been tested in clinical trials as add-ons to standard triplet therapies and are rapidly being integrated as the standard of care where accessible.

The CASSIOPEIA trial was the first to show that the addition of an anti-CD38 monoclonal antibody to induction and consolidation is highly effective without adding significant additional toxicity.[3] This Phase III trial randomized patients to receive daratumumab with VTd versus VTd alone as induction followed by ASCT. While the study met its primary endpoint (median PFS not reached in either arm; HR, 0.47; 95% CI, 0.33–0.67; $P<.0001$), resulting in the Food and Drug Administration (FDA) approval of Dara- VTd, it has not been practice-changing in some countries including the United States and Canada, where thalidomide is no longer routinely used.

The Phase 2 GRIFFIN trial randomized 207 patients (1:1) to Dara-RVd or RVd induction (4 cycles), ASCT, Dara-RVd or RVd consolidation (2 cycles), and lenalidomide or lenalidomide plus Dara maintenance (26 cycles).[2] The primary endpoint was stringent complete response (sCR) rate by the end of post-ASCT consolidation and it favored Dara-RVd (42.4% vs 32.0%) in the first analysis. At longer follow-up (median, 22.1 months), responses deepened; sCR rates improved for D-RVd versus RVd (62.6% vs 45.4%; $P=.0177$), as did minimal residual disease (MRD) negativity (10^{-5} threshold) rates in the intent-to-treat population (51.0% vs 20.4%; $P<.0001$). At a 4 year follow-up, the estimated 4-year PFS favored Dara-VRd, 87.2% versus 70% (HR 0.45; 95% confidence interval 0.21–0.95, $P = .0324$). Higher MRD negativity was also seen with Dara-VRd, 64% versus 30%. Adverse events were manageable and included higher grade 3 to 4 neutropenia (41% vs 22%), grade 3 to 4 thrombocytopenia (16% vs 9%), and all-grade infections (91% vs 62%), although these were primarily grade 1 to 2 respiratory infections and the grade 3 to 4 infection rate did not differ. Infusion reactions occurred in 42%; however, this is much lower now with subcutaneous formulations of daratumumab. Daratumumab did have a slight detrimental effect on stem cell yield, leading to higher plerixafor use (70% vs 56%). This combination is now being tested in the registrational phase III PERSEUS trial, a collaborative study with the European Myeloma Network (NCT03710603). However, due to the impressive efficacy and minimal added toxicity seen in the relatively small phase 2 trial, many centers have begun to adopt this regimen as standard practice for TE patients. Early real-world data further support Dara-VRd over VRd, with improved response rates, depth of response, and PFS.[20]

The Phase II, single-arm, multi-center MASTER trial looked at MRD response-directed finite versus infinite therapy and enrolled predominantly high-risk patients.[21] Treatment consisted of 4 cycles of daratumumab, weekly carfilzomib with lenalidomide and dexamethasone (Dara- KRd) followed by ASCT and up to 2 phases of Dara-KRd consolidation with 4 cycles each. MRD by next-generation sequencing was performed after induction, transplant, and each phase of consolidation, and patients were observed if 2 consecutive MRDs were negative ($<10^{-5}$). Patients completing the 2 phases of consolidation without 2 consecutive MRD less than 10^{-5} were transitioned to lenalidomide maintenance. More than half of the patients in this trial had at least 1 high-risk cytogenetic abnormality (HRCA), which included t(4;14), t(14;16), del(17), as well as gain or amplification (1q) and t(14;20). Post ASCT, 65% and 48% were MRD negative ($<10^{-5}$ and $<10^{-6}$ respectively), and this proportion of MRD negativity incrementally increased with sequential phases. This was seen across the standard risk as well as the high-risk groups. Although MRD rates were similar across the risk groups, patients with 0 or 1 HRCA who discontinued therapy only had 0% to 4% resurgence of MRD positivity or disease progression at 1 year, while for 2+ HRCA it was 27%. The 2 year PFS and OS were an impressive 87% and 94% across the whole patient group which was similar in patients with no (PFS 91%, OS 96%) or 1 HRCA (PFS 97%, OS 100%), but inferior in patients with 2 HRCA (PFS 58%, OS 76%), highlighting the need for intensive treatment and monitoring strategies in these patients.

The ongoing IFM-2018 to 04 trial uses a similar quadruplet (Dara-KRd)-based induction in high-risk myeloma patients followed by tandem ASCT and has shown it to be safe with deep responses.[22] Longer follow-up of this treatment strategy for high-risk patients is eagerly anticipated.

Certain daratumumab-containing quadruplets may prove useful in specific situations. The LYRA study, a single-arm, US multi-center, Phase II trial enrolled newly diagnosed as well as relapsed myeloma patients from 14 community oncology centers.[23] After at least 4 cycles of daratumumab with CyBorD (Cyclophosphamide, Bortezomib, Dexamethasone), eligible patients underwent ASCT followed by daratumumab maintenance for 12 months. Among the 39 patients who underwent ASCT, median PFS and OS were not reached. Very good partial response (VGPR) and above at the end of at least 4 cycles of Dara-CyBorD induction was 44.2%. This may provide an option for patients with renal failure, as lenalidomide can be difficult to tolerate in this population. This regimen has also become the standard of care in patients with newly diagnosed light-chain (AL) amyloidosis based on the landmark Andromeda study.[24,25]

In the phase 2 IFM 2018 to 01 trial, standard risk myeloma patients received 6 cycles of daratumumab with ixazomib-lenalidomide and dexamethasone (D-IRd) followed by ASCT, 4 cycles of D-IRd consolidation followed by lenalidomide maintenance.[26] More than 50% of patients were negative for MRD at levels less than 10^{-6} at the end of consolidation and the 2-year PFS was 95.2%. This regimen allows for an easier administration schedule with fewer treatment visits, and may also be considered in patients with pre-existing neuropathy.

Several trials are also evaluating another anti-CD38 monoclonal antibody, isatuximab, as part of quadruplet induction regimens. The GMMG-HD7 trial is similar to the GRIFFIN study but has isatuximab combined with RVd in induction followed by ASCT and maintenance.[27] The part 1 data have shown improved MRD negativity after induction (50% vs 36%) with no new safety concerns. There is also an ongoing Phase II, single-arm multi-center study CMRG008 by the Canadian Myeloma Research

Group (NCT04786028) of isatuximab added to CyBorD as induction for transplant-eligible patients followed by ASCT and maintenance with isatuximab and lenalidomide. The IsKia trial (NCT04483739) is another similar phase III study by the European myeloma network that will compare the efficacy and safety of adding isatuximab to KRd in induction and post-ASCT consolidation.

Not all monoclonal antibodies have proven effective in quadruplet induction therapy. Elotuzumab, an anti-SLAMF7 monoclonal antibody, was tested with 2 combinations in 2 different trials as upfront quadruplet options in newly diagnosed patients. Neither the phase 3 GMMG-HD6 trial[28] nor the SWOG-1211[29] showed any benefit of adding elotuzumab to the existing VRd triplet. However, preliminary results from an ongoing German phase 3 study have shown significantly improved rates of early, deep (>VGPR), and MRD- negative post-induction responses following induction with Elo-KRd when compared with KRd in TE patients.[30]

While the depth of response is clearly greater with anti-CD38-containing quadruplet regimens compared to the 3-drug combinations, there are many open questions regarding the use of quadruplets. While some studies are showing early benefits for PFS, frontline studies may not show an OS difference due to the abundance of salvage regimens available. Therefore, in determining the optimal treatment sequence, it would be useful to know the PFS2 for these studies and understand how patients were treated at relapse, especially those who progressed on anti-CD38 maintenance. The financial and sequencing implications of these regimens must also be considered, especially in publicly-funded health systems where funders may not be willing to fund the same drug twice. The CASSIOPEIA trial found that the benefit of daratumumab was achieved whether it was used in induction/consolidation or maintenance, and patients who received it in induction did not gain any additional benefit from maintenance.[31] However, the trial used daratumumab maintenance every 8 weeks and without lenalidomide. Therefore, the optimal timing and duration of anti-CD38 therapy in newly diagnosed TE-MM is still unknown.

Optimizing patient selection would be helpful as it is unclear if the PFS benefit would apply to all patients or only to those not achieving a deep response with the 3-drug regimens. Further investigation is needed into MRD-directed escalation or de-escalation of treatment, as well as fixed-duration approaches. As shown in the MASTER trial,[21] high-risk patients continue to relapse despite impressive response rates and MRD-negativity, indicating that novel approaches are needed for these patients. **Table 1** summarizes the various quadruplet regimens in TE patients.

Addressing High-Risk Disease

High-risk MM will be discussed in detail in a separate article; however, the authors will provide a brief overview of alternative strategies to quadruplet inductions plus ASCT for these patients. The UK multi-center OPTIMUM/MUKnine trial[32] included exclusively ultra-high-risk patients—defined as (≥2 high risk lesions: t(4;14), t(14;16), t(14;20), gain(1q), del(1p), del(17p)), or gene expression SKY92 (SkylineDx) profiling, or with PCL (circulating plasma blasts > 20%) and treated them with a combination of daratumumab-cyclophopshamide-bortezomib-lenalidomide-dexamethasone (Dara-CVRd) induction followed by ASCT, 18 months of dara-VRd consolidation, and dara-R maintenance. Response rates were high in this ultra-high-risk patient group and 61% achieved MRD negativity by flow cytometry with a sensitivity of 10^{-5} after SCT with manageable side effects, but early progression still poses a challenge, especially among patients with plasma cell leukemia.

Data from the phase III European multi-center trials[33,34] and the long-term follow-up data from the STAMINA trial[35] have shown PFS benefit of upfront planned tandem

Table 1
Quadruplet induction regimen in transplant eligible, newly diagnosed multiple myeloma

Study	Phase	No of Patients	Induction Regime	Primary Endpoint	ORR/≥VGPR, (%)	sCR/MRD-Ve n(%)	PFS	OS	Ref
GRIFFIN	2	104 : 103	Dara-VRd vs VRd	sCR at end of post consolidation	99 vs 91.8 90.9 vs 73.2	42 vs 32 47.1 vs 16.5	Median NR in both arms 87.2% vs 70% (estimated at 48m) HR 0.45,95% CI, 0.21–0.95	NR	Voorhees et al,[2] 2020
CASSIOPEIA	3	543:542	Dara-VTd vs VTd	sCR at 100 d post ASCT	92.6 vs 89.8 83.4 vs 78	29 vs 20 64 vs 44	Median NR vs 46.7 m (HR 0·53, 95% CI 0·42–0·68)	NR	Moreau et al,[3] 2019
MASTER	2 (single arm)	123	Dara-KRd	MRD negativity at any point	ORR -98	65 (MRD $<10^{-5}$) and 48 ($<10^{-6}$) post ASCT	87% at 2 y	94% at 2 y	Sweeney et al,[20] 2023
OPTIMUM/MUK9	2 (single arm)	107 (ultra-high risk)[a]	Dara-CVRd	MRD negativity post ASCT and PFS	94 80	64 (MRD $<10^{-5}$) post ASCT	NA	NA	Goldschmidt et al,[28] 2021
LYRA (transplant cohort)	2 (single arm)	39	Dara-CyBorD	≥VGPR at end of 4 cycles of induction	≥VGPR 44.2 after 4 cycles of induction	NA	Median NR 69.3% estimated at 36 m (95% CI, 81.0–98.7)	Median NR 94.9% at estimated 36 m (95% CI, 43.0–85.3)	Touzeau et al,[22] 2022
IFM-2018-01	2 (single arm)	45	Ixa-Rd-Dara	MRD negativity after consolidation and before maintenance	ORR-100 ≥VGPR-93.4	39.5 (MRD $<10^{-5}$) 51.4(MRD $<10^{-6}$)	95.2% at 2 y [CI 82.1–98.8].	100% at 2 y	Yimer et al,[23] 2022

Study	Phase	N	Regimen	Primary endpoint	ORR	MRD/Response		Citation
GMMG-HD7	3	331:329	Isa-VRd vs VRd	MRD at end of induction	90 vs 84	50 vs 36 (MRD $<10^{-5}$)	NA	Kastritis et al,[24] 2021
IFM 2018-04	2 (single arm)	50 (all high risk)[b]	wKRc-Dara	Safety and efficacy	96/92	62 (MRD $<10^{-5}$)	NA	Costa et al,[21] 2022
NCT03948035	3	579	Elo-KRd vs KRd	≥VGPR and MRD negativity at end of induction		49.8% vs 35.4%	NA	Usmani et al,[29] 2021

Abbreviations: d, dexamethasone; Dara, daratumumab; Elo, elotuzumab; Isa, isatuximab; K, carfilzomib; MRD, minimal residual disease; NA, not available; NR, not reached; ORR, overall response; OS, overall survival; PFS, progression-free survival; R, lenalidomide; sCR, stringent CR; T, thalidomide; V, bortezomib; VGPR, very good partial response; wK, weekly carfilzomib.

[a] Defined by (≥2 high risk lesions: t(4;14), t(14;16), t(14;20), gain(1q), del(1p), del(17p)) or gene expression SKY92 profiling, or with PCL (circulating plasma blasts > 20%).

[b] Defined by the presence of del17p, t(4;14) and/or t(14;16).

ASCT in the subgroup of high-risk patients. Single-center data have also shown a significant PFS benefit of tandem ASCT in del(17p).[36] The potential benefit of tandem transplants for high-risk disease in the era of quadruplet regimens with high MRD-negative rates is an important unanswered question. The IFM-2018 to 04 trial[22] is evaluating the feasibility of dara-KRD induction, ASCT, dara-KRD consolidation, ASCT, and dara-len maintenance, however, ideally, there would be an MRD-guided randomized trial evaluating a quadruplet plus either 1 or 2 ASCT for high-risk patients.

Lastly, fit patients presenting with primary plasma cell leukemia or other aggressive manifestations including extensive extramedullary disease and/or visceral organ dysfunction may benefit from a more intensive approach upfront. Chemotherapy regimens like (bortezomib, dexamethasone, thalidomide/lenalidomide, cisplatin, doxorubicin, cyclophosphamide, etoposide) (VDT/R-PACE) can provide rapid cytoreduction which can ameliorate or prevent organ dysfunction. Once stabilized, patients can transition to standard outpatient induction, or in the case of highly aggressive disease, stem cells can be collected upon blood count recovery and patients can proceed directly to ASCT.

The role of ASCT is discussed in detail in a separate article. Even with effective quadruplet induction regimens, ASCT still deepens response and remains the mainstay upfront treatment in this group of young and fit patients (**Fig. 1**).

TRANSPLANT-INELIGIBLE PATIENTS

Elderly and frail patients with myeloma are underrepresented in clinical trials and are not well studied despite the fact that most myeloma diagnoses and related mortality occur at this age. Treating elderly adults with myeloma should incorporate the selection of regimen and schedule depending on patient fitness assessment, comorbidities, disease characteristics, patient preferences, and understanding the goals of treatment. Since elderly age is a heterogenous group with existing comorbidities and their treatment-related effects, individual assessment to delineate them as fit, pre-frail, or frail needs to be done before initiation of any therapy. Validated geriatric assessment tools like the International Myeloma Working Group geriatric assessment tool (IMWG

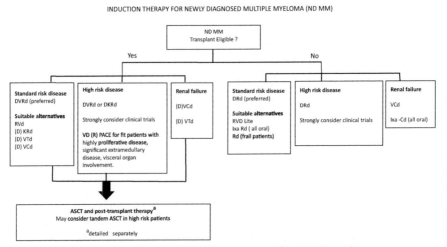

Fig. 1. Current induction approaches for newly diagnosed multiple myeloma.

GAT)[12] and the revised myeloma co-morbidity index (R-MCI)[13] are useful tools for clinical application to tailor therapeutic decisions in this vulnerable group.

The safety and tolerability of daratumumab-based combinations as per the MAIA[4] and the ALCYONE[37] trials are encouraging and represent the most effective treatment options in this population who are not eligible for stem cell transplantation. In situations where daratumumab is not available or not accessible, dose-adjusted VRD lite, or ixazomib-Rd, or Rd is good alternative. Algorithms are in place for personalizing drug dosages based on age[38] and comorbidities[39] and these can help optimize therapy in this vulnerable group.

For TI patients, all the current standard of care regimens and randomized control trials have been built on the backbone of continuous Rd induction which was considered until a few years ago as the standard of care.[40] The SWOG0777 trial showed superiority of RVd triplet over Rd but this was in a predominantly TE group who were not intended for upfront transplant,[14,41] with a median age of 63 years. In addition, many patients discontinued therapy possibly due to the twice weekly intravenous bortezomib schedule, which further hampers any possible cross-trial comparisons of this regimen with other TI regimens. The single-arm phase 2 study looking at a dose-modified RVd lite in an effort to mitigate the drug toxicities in the elder and frail TI population was found to be highly effective with PFS of 41.9 months and 5-year OS of 61%.[42] The use of carfilzomib compared with bortezomib added to an Rd combination for patients not intended for an upfront ASCT not only did not improve the PFS, but also led to more non-hematological toxicity and deaths in the KRd group.[19]

More recently, daratumumab has been approved in combination with Rd and bortezomib-melphalan and prednisolone (VMP) for upfront treatment of patients, who are not eligible for transplant, based on the pivotal phase 3 trials MAIA and ALCYONE. The phase III MAIA trial in particular has set a new standard of care in the TI population. In a population with a median age of 73 years, patients receiving DRd (Daratumumab, Lenalidomide, Dexamethasone) as compared with Rd had significantly longer PFS and OS, with the PFS of 61.9 months being the longest achieved to date in this setting.[4] Patients receiving DRd had higher rates of grade 3/4 neutropenia (54% vs 37%), grade 3/4 infections (43% vs 30%), and grade 3/4 pneumonia (20% vs 11%). It is important to note that although this is a TI-population, patients still had to be fit enough to enroll in a clinical trial, which creates a challenge in interpreting and generalizing the data. In the real world, most patients with myeloma are not eligible for clinical trials, with age and Charlson co-morbidity index ≥ 2 as independent predictors of ineligibility, and these patients have inferior OS.[43] Real-world studies of DRd are urgently needed to better understand toxicities and treatment burden on a wider and more representative patient population. In particular, the increased infection risk requires further study as elderly and frail patients can experience a significant decline in functional status and quality of life after a serious infection. One study found that intravenous immunoglobulin replacement substantially reduced serious infections in a selected group of patients receiving daratumumab in relapsed MM,[44] and this approach could be tested in this population. Other strategies including using a fixed duration of daratumumab, lower doses of lenalidomide, and discontinuation of dexamethasone merit further study.

Other daratumumab-containing regimens have been tested in this setting. The Phase III ALCYONE trial randomized TI newly diagnosed patients to receive either Dara –VMP or VMP with PFS being the primary end point.[5] After a median follow-up of 40.1 months, the median PFS was 36.4 months in the D-VMP group versus 19.3 months in the VMP group (HR = 0.42; P<.0001). As patients in the VMP arm received about 1 year of treatment and no maintenance, the PFS curve sharply declined around this time as compared with patients in the Dara-VMP arm who received daratumumab maintenance. Again, the Dara arm had higher grade 3/4 infections, 23% versus 15%. In the non-transplant cohort of the single-arm LYRA study, which used daratumumab with CyBorD (n = 48), the estimated PFS was 72.6% at 36 months, providing evidence for a dara-based regimen that could be applied to patients with renal insufficiency.[23]

Not all frail patients are able or willing to travel for weekly or biweekly infusions or injections for 6 months as in the daratumumab schedules. The phase 3 TOURMALINE-MM2 trial showed that the addition of oral ixazomib to a combination of lenalidomide and dexamethasone led to a clinically meaningful PFS benefit (35.3 vs 21.8 months, although not statistically significant) with minimal added toxicity, primarily gastrointestinal.[45] For very frail patients and/or those with more indolent disease, the Rd doublet may still be an adequate treatment. **Table 2** summarizes the current therapeutic approaches in the TI population. Choices of currently available induction regimens in treating newly diagnosed MM patients are summarized in **Fig. 2**.

FUTURE DIRECTIONS

The treatment paradigms in multiple myeloma are constantly shifting with the introduction of highly effective therapies. The use of novel agent triplets and quadruplets with anti-CD38 monoclonal antibodies has significantly improved outcomes in both TE and TI newly diagnosed myeloma and will likely remain the standard of care for the foreseeable future. Immunotherapies, including chimeric antigen receptor T cells (CAR-T) and bispecific antibodies (BsAbs), are currently revolutionizing the treatment of relapsed/refractory MM (RRMM) and are already being tested in the newly diagnosed setting.

Currently, there are 2 CAR-T products, idecabtagene vicleucel (Ide-cel) and ciltacabtagene autoleucel (Cilta-cel), as well as 1 BsAb, teclistamab, that are FDA approved for the treatment of RRMM. All of these target B-cell maturation antigen (BCMA), a member of the tumor necrosis factor (TNF) superfamily of receptors that is primarily expressed on mature B-cells as well as benign and malignant plasma cells.

Ide-cel was approved on the basis of the phase II KarMMa trial, which treated 128 patients with a median of 6 prior lines of therapy (LOT) and achieved a 73% overall response (ORR) with 8.8 months median PFS.[46] It was then shown to be superior to the standard of care in the phase III KarMMa-3 trial for patients with 2 to 4 prior LOT, with a median PFS of 13.3 versus 4.4 months.[47] It is now being explored in the single-arm phase I trial KarMMa-4 (NCT04196491) for newly diagnosed patients with R-ISS 3.

Cilta-cel demonstrated impressive efficacy in the phase Ib/II CARTITUDE-1 study, with a 98% ORR and median PFS of 34.9 months, which is unprecedented in patients with 6 prior LOT.[48] In the phase III CARTITUDE-4 trial in RRMM with 1 to 3 prior LOT, Cilta-cel far outperformed standard of care (SOC) treatments, with intention-to-treat analysis demonstrating ORR 85% (99% in the as-treated group) versus 67%, and 12-month PFS 76% versus 49% with an unprecedented hazard ratio of 0.26 for progression or death.[49] There are 2 planned pivotal trials in newly diagnosed MM 1 each in TI and TE. The ongoing CARTITUDE-5 (NCT04923893) will evaluate RVd × 8 cycles plus Cilta-cel versus RVd × 8 cycles followed by Rd maintenance. Although this trial was designed prior to the full results of the MAIA trial that established DRd as the SOC in this population, it may still provide useful information on the tolerability of CAR-T in these patients as well as a first look at its efficacy in the newly diagnosed setting. Importantly, patients with a frailty index of ≥2 on the Myeloma Geriatric Assessment

Table 2
Induction regimen in transplant ineligible, newly diagnosed multiple myeloma

Study	Phase	No of Patients	Induction Regime	Primary Endpoint	ORR/≥vgpr (%)	sCR/MRD-Ve (%)	PFS	OS	Ref
SWOG0777	3	235:225	RVd vs Rd	PFS	ORR-90.2 vs 78.8 vs ≥VGPR -74.9 vs 53.2	NA	41 m vs 29 m HR:0.742 (0.594,0.928)	NR vs 69 m HR:0.709 (0.543, 0.926)	Engelhardt et al,[13] 2017; Mateos et al,[37] 2021
NCT01782963	2	53	RVD lite	ORR	86/66	NA	41.9 m	61% at 5 y	Palumbo et al,[38] 2011
ALCYONE	3	350:356	Dara VMP vs VMP	PFS	90.9 vs 73.9 73 vs 50	14 vs 3 (MRD)	36.4 m vs 19.3 m HR 0.42 [0.34–0.51]	75% vs 62% (estimated at 42m)	Mateos et al,[5] 2020
MAIA	3	368:369	Dara Rd vs Rd	PFS	ORR-93 vs 82	35 vs 15 (sCR) 31 vs 10 (MRD)	NR vs 34.4 m 68% vs 46% (estimated at 36m)	NR in both groups	Facon et al,[4] 2021
TOURMALINE-MM2	3	351:354	Ixa-Rd vs Placebo Rd	PFS	82 vs 80 63 vs 48	26 vs 14 (CR)	35.3 vs 21.8 m HR:0.830 (0.676–1.018)	NR vs 51.8 m HR:0.524 (0.243–1.131)	Durie et al,[41] 2020
LYRA (non-transplant cohort)	2 (single arm)	48	Dara VCd	≥VGPR at end of 4 cycles of induction	≥VGPR 64% at end of induction	NA	Median NR 72.6% estimated at 36m (95% CI, 54.0–84.7)	Median NR 84.3 estimated at 36m (95% CI, 69.8–92.2)	Touzeau et al,[22] 2022

Abbreviations: d, dexamethasone; Dara, daratumumab; Ixa, ixazomib; K, carfilzomib; MRD, minimal residual disease; NA, not available; NR, not reached; ORR, overall response; OS, overall survival; PFS, progression-free survival; R, lenalidomide; sCR, stringent CR; T, thalidomide; V, bortezomib; VGPR, very good partial response; wK, weekly Carfilzomib.

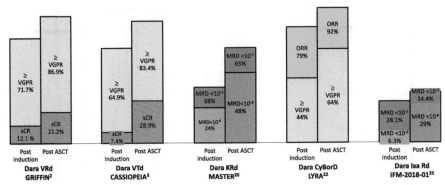

Fig. 2. Deepening response with autologous stem cell transplantation after quadruplet induction.

Score are excluded from this trial, which will limit its generalizability to a significant proportion of the older myeloma population. In the TE setting, the highly anticipated CARTITUDE-6 study (NCT05257083) will for the first time directly compare CAR-T to ASCT, in patients after they receive SOC Dara-RVd induction.

Teclistamab was the first BsAb to be FDA approved in MM in 2022, on the basis of the MajesTEC-1 trial.[50] Patients with RRMM and a median of 5 prior LOT experienced a 63% ORR and 11.3-month median PFS, while those who achieved a CR had a 26.7-month median duration of response (DOR).

There are 3 studies either in progress or planned: MajesTEC-7 evaluating teclistamab-daratumumab-lenalidomide versus DRd for TI, MajesTEC-2 looking at the safety of combining teclistamab with various combinations of daratumumab, lenalidomide, and bortezomib, and the MASTER-2 trial using an MRD-guided approach after Dara-RVd induction. This trial is of particular interest as MRD- negative patients will be randomized to ASCT or further treatment with Dara-RVd and daratumumab-lenalidomide (DR) maintenance, which may help answer the question of whether ASCT is necessary in the era of highly effective quadruplet induction. Meanwhile, MRD-positive patients will receive ASCT followed by either daratumumab-teclistamab or DR. Of the other BsAbs in development, 2 currently have trials in ND MM: a randomized phase II trial of elranatamab with daratumumab and lenalidomide versus DRd for TI (MagnetisMM-6), and a phase I/II trial evaluating the safety of linvoseltamab in ND MM. Ongoing and upcoming T cell-directed therapeutic regimen in ND MM is summarized in **Tables 3** and **4**.

While highly efficacious, these immunotherapies do pose certain challenges in the newly diagnosed setting. Those targeting BCMA have produced profound hypogammaglobulinemia and high rates of serious infections in the relapsed setting, including several infectious deaths in each study.[46,48,50,51] While this risk may be acceptable in a heavily pretreated population with few available and effective treatment options, and high risk of mortality from MM itself, the level of tolerable risk will be different in a newly diagnosed patient who may be expected to live 10 years or longer. Other toxicities are poorly understood in the long term and require further study, including prolonged cytopenia, transformation to myelodysplastic syndrome and acute myeloid leukemia, and delayed neurotoxicity. Based on early available data, these toxicities do appear to be lesser in earlier lines of therapy.[47,49] Lastly, access may be a barrier to widespread use, especially regarding the current manufacturing limitations of CAR-T and the escalating costs of these therapies when used in

Table 3
Ongoing and upcoming CAR T cell studies in newly diagnosed multiple myeloma

Trial/Identifier	Structure	Phase	Patient Group	No of Patients	Treatment	Primary Endpoint	Status
KarMMA-4 NCT04196491	BCMA CART (Ide-cel)	1	ND MM HR[a]	13	Upto 3 cycles of induction followed by Ide- infusion	DLT, AE	Active, not recruiting
CARTITUDE-5 NCT04923893	BCMA CART (Cilta-cel)	3	ND MM not intended for upfront ASCT	650	RVd × 8 followed by Cilta-cel vs RVd × 8 followed by Rd maintenance	PFS	Recruiting
CARTITUDE-6 NCT05257083	BCMA CART (Cilta-cel)	3	ND MM	750	Dara-RVd followed by Cilta-cel[c] Len maint vs Dara - RVd followed by ASCT[c] Dara-VRd cons[c] Len maint	PFS	Not yet recruiting
NCT04287660	BCMA CART	3 (single arm)	ND MM	20	BiRd followed by BCMA CAR T infusion	ORR	Recruiting
FUMANBA-2 NCT05181501	BCMA CART (CT103 A)	1	ND MM HR	20	Upto 3 cycles of induction (RVd or VCD or PAD) followed by CT103 A infusion	MRD neg, median PFS	Not yet recruiting
FasT CAR T[c] NCT04935580	BCMA-CD-19 CART (GC012 F)	1/2	ND MM TE-HR[b]	20	2 cycles of induction (Bortezomib-based triplet) followed by GC012 F infusion and lenalidomide maintenance	AE, ORR, MRD neg, PFS	Recruiting
BMTCTN1902 NCT05032820	BCMA CART (Ide-cel)	2	ND MM post ASCT with <VGPR	40	Ide-cel followed by lenalidomide maintenance	CR, sCR	Recruiting
NCT05850286	BCMA CART	2 (single arm)	ND MM with P53 abnormalities	20	X-VRd induction followed by CART-ASCT-CART2	CR, ORR, MRD neg	Recruiting

Abbreviations: AE, adverse events; ASCT, autologous stem cell transplantation; BiRd, clarithromycin(biaxin)-lenalidomide-low-dose-dexamethasone; DLT, dose-limiting toxicity; HR, high risk; MM, multiple myeloma; NA, not available; ND, newly diagnosed; sCR, stringent complete response; TE, transplant eligible; VGPR, very good partial response; X, selinexor.
a One or more of - R-ISS 3, t(4;14), del 17p, t(14;16).
b One or more of - R-ISS 2 or 3, t(4;14), del 17p, t(14;16), 1q gain, extramedullary disease, IgD/IgE myeloma, high-risk SMART.
c Preliminary data presented at ASCO 2023.

Table 4
Ongoing and upcoming studies of bispecific antibodies in newly diagnosed multiple myeloma

Trial	Structure	Phase	Patient Group	No of Patients	Treatment	Primary Endpoint	Status	Identifier
MajesTEC-7	BCMA-CD3 BiTE (Teclistamab)	3	ND MM not eligible/intended for upfront ASCT	1060	teclistamab + daratumumab + lenalidomide vs daratumumab + lenalidomide + dexamethasone	MRD neg, PFS	Recruiting	NCT05552222
MagnetisMM-6	BCMA-CD3 BiTE (Elranatamab)	2	ND MM not eligible for ASCT	966	elranatamab + daratumumab + lenalidomide vs daratumumab + lenalidomide + dexamethasone	DLT, PFS, sustained MRD neg	Recruiting	NCT05623020
MajesTEC-2	BCMA-CD3 BiTE (Teclistamab)	Multi-arm phase 1b study	ND MM based on treatment arm. (Arms B,E, F)	140	Arm B- teclistamab + daratumumab + lenalidomide + bortezomib (q21 d) Arm E− teclistamab + daratumumab + lenalidomide Arm F- teclistamab + daratumumab + lenalidomide + bortezomib (q 28 d)	AE, DLT	Not yet recruiting	NCT04722146
MASTER-2	BCMA-CD3 BiTE (Teclistamab)	2	ND MM post Dara-VRD induction if MRD positive	300	Dara-VRD × 6 induction followed by if MRD positive – to randomize to dara-Tec vs dara-R consolidation and maintenance	Sustained MRD neg	Not yet recruiting	NCT05231629
LINKER-MM4	BCMA-CD3 BiTE (Linvoseltamab)	1/2	ND MM	132	Linvoseltamab	AE, DLT	Not yet recruiting	NCT05828511

Abbreviations: AE, adverse events; ASCT, autologous stem cell transplantation; BsAbs, Bi-specific antibodies; DLT, dose-limiting toxicity; MM, multiple myeloma; ND, newly diagnosed.

combination with other novel agents. Nevertheless, if these challenges can be overcome and pending positive results in the aforementioned clinical trials, immunotherapies are poised to revolutionize the treatment of newly diagnosed MM within the next few years.

SUMMARY

Strategies combining novel agents (anti-CD38 monoclonal antibodies, immunomodulators, and proteasome inhibitors) as triplets and quadruplets are the current standard of care frontline treatment for both TI and TE myeloma. These combinations are providing impressive efficacy with manageable toxicity and will continue to be further optimized in the coming years. ASCT continues to be the standard of care for all fit patients until there is evidence of superior outcomes with alternative approaches. While most patients are benefitting from the current treatment paradigm, outcomes for high-risk MM continue to lag behind and there is an urgent need to develop novel approaches for these patients. In the future, potent T-cell-redirecting therapies, including CAR-T and bispecific antibodies, could potentially revolutionize the treatment of ND MM.

CLINICS CARE POINTS

- Triplet induction has been the standard of care until recently for newly diagnosed patients, with RVd being the most preferred and VTD or VCD (CyBorD) as alternatives.
- Addition of daratumumab to triplet induction leads to higher MRD negativity rates and improves PFS, leading to a new standard of care for TE patients.
- Daratumumab with lenalidomide and dexamethasone is the current standard of care for TI patients.
- ASCT should be offered to all fit patients.
- Optimal therapy for high-risk myeloma remains a major clinical challenge and this population represents an urgent unmet need.
- T cell-redirecting therapies, including CAR-T cells and bispecific antibodies, are now being evaluated in the newly diagnosed setting and have the potential to revolutionize the treatment of newly diagnosed MM.

DISCLOSURE

A.J. Devasia has no disclosures; G.S. Lancman -Honoraria from Janssen, Pfizer, Sanofi, Forus, Takeda. Consultancy for Janssen, Takeda; A.K. Stewart -Honoraria from Janssen, Pfizer, Amgen, Sanofi.

REFERENCES

1. Kristinsson SY, Anderson WF, Landgren O. Improved long-term survival in multiple myeloma up to the age of 80 years. Leukemia 2014;28(6):1346–8.
2. Voorhees PM, Kaufman JL, Laubach J, et al. Daratumumab, lenalidomide, bortezomib, and dexamethasone for transplant-eligible newly diagnosed multiple myeloma: the GRIFFIN trial. Blood 2020;136(8):936–45.
3. Moreau P, Attal M, Hulin C, et al. Bortezomib, thalidomide, and dexamethasone with or without daratumumab before and after autologous stem-cell

transplantation for newly diagnosed multiple myeloma (CASSIOPEIA): a randomised, open-label, phase 3 study. Lancet 2019;394(10192):29–38.

4. Facon T, Kumar SK, Plesner T, et al. Daratumumab, lenalidomide, and dexamethasone versus lenalidomide and dexamethasone alone in newly diagnosed multiple myeloma (MAIA): overall survival results from a randomised, open-label, phase 3 trial. Lancet Oncol 2021;22(11):1582–96.

5. Mateos MV, Cavo M, Blade J, et al. Overall survival with daratumumab, bortezomib, melphalan, and prednisone in newly diagnosed multiple myeloma (ALCYONE): a randomised, open-label, phase 3 trial. Lancet 2020;395(10218):132–41.

6. Fonseca R, Usmani SZ, Mehra M, et al. Frontline treatment patterns and attrition rates by subsequent lines of therapy in patients with newly diagnosed multiple myeloma. BMC Cancer 2020;20(1):1087.

7. Yong K, Delforge M, Driessen C, et al. Multiple myeloma: patient outcomes in real-world practice. Br J Haematol 2016;175(2):252–64.

8. Attal M, Lauwers-Cances V, Hulin C, et al. Lenalidomide, Bortezomib, and Dexamethasone with Transplantation for Myeloma. N Engl J Med 2017;376(14):1311–20.

9. Richardson PG, Jacobus SJ, Weller EA, et al. Triplet Therapy, Transplantation, and Maintenance until Progression in Myeloma. N Engl J Med 2022;387(2): 132–47.

10. Gay F, Musto P, Rota-Scalabrini D, et al. Carfilzomib with cyclophosphamide and dexamethasone or lenalidomide and dexamethasone plus autologous transplantation or carfilzomib plus lenalidomide and dexamethasone, followed by maintenance with carfilzomib plus lenalidomide or lenalidomide alone for patients with newly diagnosed multiple myeloma (FORTE): a randomised, open-label, phase 2 trial. Lancet Oncol 2021;22(12):1705–20.

11. Perrot A, Lauwers-Cances V, Cazaubiel T, et al. Early Versus Late Autologous Stem Cell Transplant in Newly Diagnosed Multiple Myeloma: Long-Term Follow-up Analysis of the IFM 2009 Trial. Blood 2020;136(Supplement 1):39.

12. Palumbo A, Bringhen S, Mateos M-V, et al. Geriatric assessment predicts survival and toxicities in elderly myeloma patients: an International Myeloma Working Group report. Blood 2015;125(13):2068–74.

13. Engelhardt M, Domm AS, Dold SM, et al. A concise revised Myeloma Comorbidity Index as a valid prognostic instrument in a large cohort of 801 multiple myeloma patients. Haematologica 2017;102(5):910–21.

14. Durie BGM, Hoering A, Abidi MH, et al. Bortezomib with lenalidomide and dexamethasone versus lenalidomide and dexamethasone alone in patients with newly diagnosed myeloma without intent for immediate autologous stem-cell transplant (SWOG S0777): a randomised, open-label, phase 3 trial. Lancet 2017;389(10068): 519–27.

15. Kumar S, Flinn I, Richardson PG, et al. Randomized, multicenter, phase 2 study (EVOLUTION) of combinations of bortezomib, dexamethasone, cyclophosphamide, and lenalidomide in previously untreated multiple myeloma. Blood 2012;119(19): 4375–82.

16. Sidana S, Kumar S, Fraser R, et al. Impact of Induction Therapy with VRD versus VCD on Outcomes in Patients with Multiple Myeloma in Partial Response or Better Undergoing Upfront Autologous Stem Cell Transplantation. Transplant Cell Ther 2022;28(2):83.e1–9.

17. Cherniawsky HM, Kukreti V, Reece D, et al. The survival impact of maintenance lenalidomide: an analysis of real-world data from the Canadian Myeloma Research Group national database. Haematologica 2021;106(6):1733–6.

18. Moreau P, Hulin C, Macro M, et al. VTD is superior to VCD prior to intensive therapy in multiple myeloma: results of the prospective IFM2013-04 trial. Blood 2016; 127(21):2569–74.

19. Kumar SK, Jacobus SJ, Cohen AD, et al. Carfilzomib or bortezomib in combination with lenalidomide and dexamethasone for patients with newly diagnosed multiple myeloma without intention for immediate autologous stem-cell transplantation (ENDURANCE): a multicentre, open-label, phase 3, randomised, controlled trial. Lancet Oncol 2020;21(10):1317–30.

20. Sweeney NW, Sborov DW, Martínez JAH, et al. Real-world analysis of D-RVd v. RVd at induction for newly diagnosed transplant eligible multiple myeloma patients. J Clin Oncol 2023;41(16_suppl):e20024.

21. Costa LJ, Chhabra S, Medvedova E, et al. Daratumumab, Carfilzomib, Lenalidomide, and Dexamethasone With Minimal Residual Disease Response-Adapted Therapy in Newly Diagnosed Multiple Myeloma. J Clin Oncol 2022;40(25):2901–12.

22. Touzeau C, Perrot A, Hulin C, et al. Daratumumab carfilzomib lenalidomide and dexamethasone as induction therapy in high-risk, transplant-eligible patients with newly diagnosed myeloma: Results of the phase 2 study IFM 2018-04. J Clin Oncol 2022;40(16_suppl):8002.

23. Yimer H, Melear J, Faber E, et al. Daratumumab, cyclophosphamide, bortezomib, and dexamethasone for multiple myeloma: final results of the LYRA study. Leuk Lymphoma 2022;63(10):2383–92.

24. Kastritis E, Palladini G, Minnema MC, et al. Daratumumab-Based Treatment for Immunoglobulin Light-Chain Amyloidosis. N Engl J Med 2021;385(1):46–58.

25. Palladini G, Kastritis E, Maurer MS, et al. Daratumumab plus CyBorD for patients with newly diagnosed AL amyloidosis: safety run-in results of ANDROMEDA. Blood 2020;136(1):71–80.

26. Aurore Perrot VL-C, Touzeau C, Decaux O, et al. Daratumumab Plus Ixazomib, Lenalidomide, and Dexamethasone as Extended Induction and Consolidation Followed by Lenalidomide Maintenance in Standard - Risk Transplant Eligible Newly Diagnosed Multiple Myeloma (NDMM) Patients (IFM 2018-01): A Phase II Study of the Intergroupe Francophone Du Myeloma (IFM). Conference abstract presented at: ASH 2021; December 2021, Atlanta, USA; Session 1.

27. Goldschmidt H, Mai EK, Bertsch U, et al. Addition of isatuximab to lenalidomide, bortezomib, and dexamethasone as induction therapy for newly diagnosed, transplantation-eligible patients with multiple myeloma (GMMG-HD7): part 1 of an open-label, multicentre, randomised, active-controlled, phase 3 trial. Lancet Haematol 2022;9(11):e810–21.

28. Goldschmidt H, Mai EK, Bertsch U, et al. Elotuzumab in Combination with Lenalidomide, Bortezomib, Dexamethasone and Autologous Transplantation for Newly-Diagnosed Multiple Myeloma: Results from the Randomized Phase III GMMG-HD6 Trial. Blood 2021;138:486.

29. Usmani SZ, Hoering A, Ailawadhi S, et al. Bortezomib, lenalidomide, and dexamethasone with or without elotuzumab in patients with untreated, high-risk multiple myeloma (SWOG-1211): primary analysis of a randomised, phase 2 trial. Lancet Haematol 2021;8(1):e45–54.

30. Stuebig T, Kull M, Greil R, et al. Carfilzomib, lenalidomide, and dexamethasone (KRd) versus elotuzumab and KRd in transplant-eligible patients with newly diagnosed multiple myeloma: Post-induction response and MRD results from an open-label randomized phase 3 study. J Clin Oncol 2023;41(16_suppl):8000.

31. Moreau P, Hulin C, Perrot A, et al. Maintenance with daratumumab or observation following treatment with bortezomib, thalidomide, and dexamethasone with or

without daratumumab and autologous stem-cell transplant in patients with newly diagnosed multiple myeloma (CASSIOPEIA): an open-label, randomised, phase 3 trial. Lancet Oncol 2021;22(10):1378–90.

32. Kaiser MF, Hall A, Walker K, et al. Depth of response and minimal residual disease status in ultra high-risk multiple myeloma and plasma cell leukemia treated with daratumumab, bortezomib, lenalidomide, cyclophosphamide and dexamethasone (Dara-CVRd): Results of the UK optimum/MUKnine trial. J Clin Oncol 2021;39(15_suppl):8001.

33. Cavo M, Gay F, Beksac M, et al. Autologous haematopoietic stem-cell transplantation versus bortezomib-melphalan-prednisone, with or without bortezomib-lenalidomide-dexamethasone consolidation therapy, and lenalidomide maintenance for newly diagnosed multiple myeloma (EMN02/HO95): a multicentre, randomised, open-label, phase 3 study. Lancet Haematol 2020;7(6):e456–68.

34. Cavo M, Goldschmidt H, Rosinol L, et al. Double Vs Single Autologous Stem Cell Transplantation for Newly Diagnosed Multiple Myeloma: Long-Term Follow-up (10-Years) Analysis of Randomized Phase 3 Studies. Blood 2018;132:124.

35. Hari P, Pasquini MC, Stadtmauer EA, et al. Long-term follow-up of BMT CTN 0702 (STaMINA) of postautologous hematopoietic cell transplantation (autoHCT) strategies in the upfront treatment of multiple myeloma (MM). J Clin Oncol 2020; 38(15_suppl):8506.

36. De La Torre A, Atenafu EG, Smith AC, et al. Myeloma Patients with Deletion of 17p: Impact of Tandem Transplant and Clone Size. Blood 2021;138(Supplement 1):460.

37. Mateos MV, Dimopoulos MA, Cavo M, et al. Daratumumab Plus Bortezomib, Melphalan, and Prednisone Versus Bortezomib, Melphalan, and Prednisone in Transplant-Ineligible Newly Diagnosed Multiple Myeloma: Frailty Subgroup Analysis of ALCYONE. Clin Lymphoma, Myeloma & Leukemia 2021;21(11):785–98.

38. Palumbo A, Anderson K. Multiple Myeloma. N Engl J Med 2011;364(11):1046–60.

39. Palumbo A, Bringhen S, Ludwig H, et al. Personalized therapy in multiple myeloma according to patient age and vulnerability: a report of the European Myeloma Network (EMN). Blood 2011;118(17):4519–29.

40. Benboubker L, Dimopoulos MA, Dispenzieri A, et al. Lenalidomide and dexamethasone in transplant-ineligible patients with myeloma. N Engl J Med 2014; 371(10):906–17.

41. Durie BGM, Hoering A, Sexton R, et al. Longer term follow-up of the randomized phase III trial SWOG S0777: bortezomib, lenalidomide and dexamethasone vs. lenalidomide and dexamethasone in patients (Pts) with previously untreated multiple myeloma without an intent for immediate autologous stem cell transplant (ASCT). Blood Cancer J 2020;10(5):53.

42. O'Donnell EK, Laubach JP, Yee AJ, et al. Updated Results of a Phase 2 Study of Modified Lenalidomide, Bortezomib, and Dexamethasone (RVd-lite) in Transplant-Ineligible Multiple Myeloma. Blood 2019;134(Supplement_1):3178.

43. Chari A, Romanus D, Palumbo A, et al. Randomized Clinical Trial Representativeness and Outcomes in Real-World Patients: Comparison of 6 Hallmark Randomized Clinical Trials of Relapsed/Refractory Multiple Myeloma. Clin Lymphoma, Myeloma & Leukemia 2020;20(1):8–17.e16.

44. Lancman G, Sastow D, Aslanova M, et al. Effect of intravenous immunoglobulin on infections in multiple myeloma (MM) patients receiving daratumumab. Blood 2020;136:6–7.

45. Facon T, Venner CP, Bahlis NJ, et al. Oral ixazomib, lenalidomide, and dexamethasone for transplant-ineligible patients with newly diagnosed multiple myeloma. Blood 2021;137(26):3616–28.

46. Munshi NC, Anderson LD, Shah N, et al. Idecabtagene Vicleucel in Relapsed and Refractory Multiple Myeloma. N Engl J Med 2021;384(8):705–16.
47. Rodriguez-Otero P, Ailawadhi S, Arnulf B, et al. Ide-cel or Standard Regimens in Relapsed and Refractory Multiple Myeloma. N Engl J Med 2023;388(11): 1002–14.
48. Martin TG, Usmani SZ, Berdeja JG, et al. CARTITUDE-1 final results: Phase 1b/2 study of ciltacabtagene autoleucel in heavily pretreated patients with relapsed/refractory multiple myeloma. J Clin Oncol 2023;41(16_suppl):8009.
49. Yong K, Harrison SJ, Mateos M-V, et al. First phase 3 results from CARTITUDE-4: Cilta-cel versus standard of care (PVd or DPd) in lenalidomide-refractory multiple myeloma. J Clin Oncol 2023;41(17_suppl):LBA106.
50. Moreau P, Garfall AL, van de Donk N, et al. Teclistamab in Relapsed or Refractory Multiple Myeloma. N Engl J Med 2022;387(6):495–505.
51. Lancman G, Parsa K, Rodriguez C, et al. Infections and Severe Hypogammaglobulinemia in Multiple Myeloma Patients Treated with Anti-BCMA Bispecific Antibodies. Blood 2022;140(Supplement 1):10073–4.

Impact of Clonal Heterogeneity in Multiple Myeloma

Carolina Schinke, MD[a], Leo Rasche, MD[b,c], Marc S. Raab, MD[d], Niels Weinhold, PhD[d],*

KEYWORDS

• Myeloma • Clonal heterogeneity • Microenvironment • Evolution • Relapse

KEY POINTS

- Clonal heterogeneity is one of the biggest obstacles to overcome therapy resistance.
- The accumulation of genetic hits seems to occur in a nonrandom fashion, predetermined by initial genetic events.
- The distribution of myeloma within the bone marrow-containing skeletal system can be highly imbalanced with regionally restricted evolution and formation of highly resistant subclones only at specific sites.
- Myeloma evolution is usually driven by a limited number of major subclones that generate the majority of diversity at relapse.

INTRODUCTION

Multiple myeloma (MM) is a malignancy of terminally differentiated plasma cells (PCs) and the most common bone marrow (BM) cancer.[1] Despite impressive therapeutic improvements, the disease remains largely incurable with disease relapses ultimately leading to patient death.[2] Survival rates vary greatly and are significantly affected by the genetic makeup of the disease. Patients with survival rates of less than 5 years usually present with high-risk genetic features at diagnosis.[3] In contrast, other patients often show such features only after treatment.[4] Historically, it has been postulated that high-risk aberrations in these patients develop because of longitudinal evolution and continuous therapeutic pressure on MM cells. Yet, with the advances of novel technologies, particularly single cell analysis, more recent research has shown that

[a] Myeloma Center, University of Arkansas for Medical Sciences, Little Rock, AR, USA; [b] Department of Internal Medicine 2, University Hospital of Würzburg, Würzburg, Germany; [c] Mildred Scheel Early Career Center (MSNZ), University Hospital of Würzburg, Würzburg, Germany; [d] Department of Internal Medicine V, Heidelberg University Clinic Hospital, Heidelberg, Germany
* Corresponding author.
E-mail address: niels.weinhold@med.uni-heidelberg.de

Hematol Oncol Clin N Am 38 (2024) 461–476
https://doi.org/10.1016/j.hoc.2023.12.012   **hemonc.theclinics.com**
0889-8588/24/© 2024 Elsevier Inc. All rights reserved.

aggressive, treatment-resistant MM cells can already preexist as small subclones and expand during treatment when other, more sensitive subclones are being eradicated.[5,6] Expanding, aggressive subclones have a high propensity to acquire additional genetic hits leading to chromosomal instability, high proliferation, and increased treatment resistance.[7–9] Furthermore, it has become increasingly clear that the molecular events occurring during MM progression are not only acquired in a linear fashion but also through branching, nonlinear pathways.[8–11] This phenomenon has been shown to be true not only during MM progression after initial diagnosis but also already at precursor stages, such as monoclonal gammopathy of undetermined significance (MGUS) and or smoldering MM (SMM). Hence, patients who ultimately develop clinical MM usually already harbor a very complex tumor architecture with widespread subclonal heterogeneity. The spatial distribution of MM throughout the BM further complicates the identification of the genetic landscape, making a comprehensive description of the clonal heterogeneity within one patient extremely challenging.[12,13] In this review, we will discuss the molecular basics, extent, and clinical impact of clonal heterogeneity, which is thought to be one of the biggest obstacles to overcome therapy resistance and to achieve cure.

INITIATING AND PROGRESSION EVENTS AND THEIR IMPACT ON OUTCOME

The basic premise underlying the development of MM is that tumor-initiating and successive key genetic events deregulate intrinsic PC pathways leading to clonal expansion over time and thereby generating features of MM, including cytopenias, immunosuppression, and bone lesions. Yet, there is no universal path to malignant PCs. Rather MM is a collection of related disorders with distinct and unique genetic constellations that are manifested as clonal proliferations of PCs.[14,15] The main events that are crucial to initiate the transformation of a normal PC into a myelomatous one can be broadly split into immunoglobulin (Ig) translocations and a hyperdiploid karyotype (HRD, Table 1). Ig translocations are generated by aberrant class switch recombination and place one of the oncogenes cyclin D1 (CCND1), cyclin D3 (CCND3), fibroblast growth factor receptor 3 (FGFR3), multiple myeloma SET domain (MMSET, also known as nuclear receptor binding SET Domain protein 2 (NSD2)), MAF, and MAFB under the strong enhancers of the Ig loci on chromosome 14, leading to their dysregulation. The Ig translocations t(4;14) and t(14;16) are high-risk markers according to the International Myeloma Working Group (IMWG) criteria, whereas translocation t(11;14) is categorized as standard risk. Yet, prognostic implications are often more so driven by the clinical and cellular background in which the genetic lesion occurs and the presence and abundance of secondary genetic events, which tend to further deregulate MM cells. For

---

Table 1
Genetic events at multiple myeloma diagnosis identified by fluorescence in situ hybridization and/or karyotype[10,113]

Primary Genetic Events (% of MM)	Secondary Genetic Events (% of MM)
1. IGH translocations and affected genes	1. Gains
t(4;14); FGFR3 and MMSET (11%–15%)	1q; CKS1B (40%)
t(6;14); CCND3 (1%)	2. Deletions
t(11;14); CCND1 (15%)	1p; CDKN2C and FAM46C (11%)
t(14;16); MAF (3%–5%)	11q; BIRC2 and BIRC3 (7%)
t(14;20); MAFB (1%)	13; RB1 and DIS3 (40%)
2. Hyperdiploidy (approx. 55%)	14q; TRAF3 (38%)
Trisomies of chromosomes	16q; CYLD and WWOX (35%)
3, 5, 7, 9, 11, 15, 19, and 21	17p; TP53 (10%)

example, the *MAF* translocations t(14;16) and t(14;20) are associated with poor prognosis in newly diagnosed MM (NDMM) but not in MGUS.[16,17] However, the standard risk translocation t(11;14) is seen in up to 35% of patients with primary PC leukemia, one of the most aggressive forms of MM with dismal outcomes.[18,19]

HRD as another primary event is associated with multiple trisomies of odd-numbered chromosomes. The mechanism underlying the pathogenesis of HRD MM remains unknown but it has been hypothesized that the gain of multiple whole chromosomes occurs during a single catastrophic mitosis rather than through serial events.[10,20] HRD has been associated with standard risk, although some studies suggest that the prognostic impact is being driven by which chromosomes carry an additional gain. For example, trisomies 3 and 5 have been shown to predict for better survival but not trisomy 21.[21]

It is important to note that initiating events do not lead to the development of clinical MM on their own.[22] Further genetic hits, including secondary translocations, copy number abnormalities, mutations as well as dysregulation of methylation and microRNA expression are required for the development of clinically relevant disease as are alterations in the BM microenvironment (BM-ME, see **Table 1**). In contrast to initiating events, these secondary hits occur in a subclonal fashion, thereby creating various disease branches that evolve over time independently.[10] Hence, genetic complexity develops early in the disease, at the MGUS stage, and increases with disease progression.[23] Although the number and constellations of genetic events required to develop clinical MM remain elusive, MM presents with a higher mutational load and increased genetic events compared with its precursor stages with further increase of such events at subsequent relapses.[18,23] Most, if not all, secondary chromosomal events are associated with adverse prognosis because they lead to overexpression of oncogenes or deletions of tumor suppressor genes, thereby resulting in increased proliferation rates and chromosomal instability. Genetic alterations that are captured by standard cytogenetics used in clinical practice, including fluorescence in situ hybridization (FISH) and karyotyping include chromosome 1p deletion (with loss of the target genes *CDKN2C* and *FAF1* at 1p32, *RPL5* and *EVI* at 1p22, and *FAM46C* at 1p12),[24] deletion of chromosome 17p (with loss of the tumor suppressor gene *TP53*), and gain of 1q (with gain of the oncogene *CKS1B*).[25,26]

More sensitive techniques, such as next-generation sequencing, have identified alterations on a level not captured with standard cytogenetic methods.[8,9,11,27] These studies have uncovered frequently occurring mutations in MM that affect similar pathways leading to PC deregulation and resulting in adverse prognosis. For example, activation by the mitogen-activated protein kinase (MAPK) kinase (MEK)/extracellular signal-regulated kinase (ERK) signaling pathway through mutations in *KRAS*, *NRAS*, *BRAF*, *PTPN11*, *RASA2*, *NF1*, *PRKD2*, or *FGFR3* are seen in up to 50% of patients with NDMM.[11] Other affected mechanisms include the nuclear factor-κB (NF-κB) signaling pathway (through mutations in *TRAF2*, *TRAF3*, *CYLD*, *NFKB2*, or *NFKBIA*) and the G1/S cell cycle transition (*CCND1*, *RB1*, *CDKN2C*, or *CDKN1B*) in 14% and 5% of NDMM, respectively. Importantly, these studies have further highlighted the oncologic dependencies between primary and secondary events, underscoring that the genomic landscape in MM is predetermined by the primary events on which further genetic alterations are built.[11] These dependencies include the association of the primary translocation t(4;14) with mutations in *FGFR3*, *DIS3*, and *PRKD2*, whereas translocation t(11;14) is associated with mutations in *CCND1* and *IRF4* and translocation t(14;16) is associated with mutations in *MAF*, *BRAF*, *DIS3*, and *ATM*.[9,11] HRD as a primary event has been associated with mutations in *FAM46C* and rearrangements of the *MYC* oncogene. Hence, although genomic heterogeneity is very complex, the accumulation of genetic hits seems to occur in a nonrandom fashion, predetermined by initial genetic events. Understanding these dependencies could shed light on potential evolutionary patterns and lead to better therapeutic approaches.

Finally, single cell technologies have further advanced the field and are able to dissect clonal and subclonal populations with high resolution.[6,28–33] In line with their prognostic impact, the translocations t(4;14), and t(14;16) are associated with a higher degree of intratumoral heterogeneity (based on the number of subclones) compared with translocation t(11;14), whereas HRD presented with an intermediate level of intratumoral heterogeneity. Notably, secondary hits, such as gain(1q), had significantly higher levels of intratumoral heterogeneity. Furthermore, a recent study elegantly reconstructed distinct evolutionary patterns and confirmed an initial linear growth pattern in early disease stages after which the MM cells evolve in a branching pattern leading to rapid expansion, increased heterogeneity, and disease progression.[34]

SPATIAL CLONAL HETEROGENEITY

MM has long been assumed to be a cancer evolving via Darwinian selective sweeps, with more advanced subclones replacing less-fit subclones. Based on this assumption, a rapid and homogenous dissemination of clones throughout the BM has been anticipated. However, the distribution of the disease can be highly imbalanced with regionally restricted evolution and formation of highly resistant subclones only at specific BM sites.[12,13,32] Therefore, samples derived from the random BM site might not be representative of the whole disease process, which can pose a major challenge for adequate prognosis and even treatment. This imbalanced disease distribution can be visualized using whole body imaging techniques, such as MRI or PET, which highlight that up to 80% of patients with NDMM harbor focal lesions (FLs) at baseline.[35] As FLs are hotspots of MM evolution superimposed on diffuse interstitial growth patterns, their presence and increased number has been shown to correlate with adverse prognostic risk.[36–38] Recent studies analyzing the genomic background of multiple regions within the same patients have highlighted that advanced clones growing within FLs contain strong and more numerous driver events compared with subclones that dominate at the iliac crest. The number of site-specific events (in terms of mutations and copy number alterations) correlates positively with the size of the FL. Importantly, the IMWG recognized FLs on whole body imaging as a diagnostic criteria for MM in 2014, thereby acknowledging that this clinical picture represents already advanced disease in need of treatment, even when other criteria, such as random BM infiltration of MM cells and cytopenias, are not met.[39] The assessment of FLs by functional imaging is hence a crucial part in the diagnosis and follow-up of patients with MM.[37,38,40]

Intriguingly, the spatial clonal heterogeneity observed in MM differs greatly from other BM cancers, such as acute myeloid leukemia or acute lymphoblastic leukemia, where disease heterogeneity is low and site-restricted evolution is generally not observed.[27,41] Spatial heterogeneity poses major challenges to identifying subclonal heterogeneity and high-risk clones because the detection of those in FLs would require separate biopsies. Although peripheral blood assays to detect and analyze the spatial heterogeneity in MM have been applied, their specificity and sensitivity remain unclear and they are currently not in clinical use.[42,43] Functional imaging is another potential solution. Indeed, using the size of lesions as a surrogate marker for spatial heterogeneity, Rasche and colleagues recently identified the presence of at least 3 large FLs as a feature of high-risk MM.[38] Yet, functional imaging lacks sensitivity to assess deep responses within FLs after therapy. Although the vast majority of FLs tend to resolve quickly on PET imaging after therapy, minimal residual disease within FLs is not well captured and remaining cells can regrow quickly despite seemingly deep remissions on random BM biopsies taken from the iliac crest.[44–46]

CLONAL HETEROGENEITY AND THE BONE MARROW MICROENVIRONMENT

Clonal heterogeneity and evolution are not only the result of tumor-intrinsic events but are also influenced by extrinsic mechanisms. Particularly, the BM-ME plays a crucial role in MM growth and progression and has long been a subject of intense research.[47,48] Increasing evidence supports the ability of MM cells to shape their own advantageous BM-ME, thereby creating a supportive niche to survive, proliferate, and evade therapies, whereas in other instances, the BM-ME can impose constraints on MM growth through resource limitations, immune predation, and adverse growth conditions.[49] Consequently, the BM-ME plays a key role in clonal selection and evolution and has wide implications on prognosis and therapy.[50–52] With the advance of novel technologies, particularly single-cell techniques, recent studies have tried to thoroughly dissect these complex interactions between MM cells and the BM-ME.[48] Alterations in the BM-ME are already present at precursor stages, including MGUS, and are characterized by distinct immune transcriptomes and phenotypes.[53–55] For example, PC dyscrasias harbor increased proportions of natural killer cells, regulatory T cells, and CD16+ and CD14+ monocyte populations compared with healthy subjects. Furthermore, the increased expression of major histocompatibility complex type II genes on monocytes and loss of granzyme K+ expression in memory T cells leads to impaired T-cell function, particularly cytotoxicity and immune surveillance facilitating the progression to clinical MM.

Intriguingly, distinct immune cell alterations and constellations seem to be associated with certain genetic alterations, thereby directly supporting the hypothesis of immune-mediated clonal selection. In relapsed/refractory MM (RRMM) gain(1q) was recently associated with depletion of CD4+/CD8+ naïve and CD4+ memory cells and an enrichment of CD14+/CD16+ monocytes, effector T-cell populations (CD8+ memory and cytotoxic cells) as well as gamma/delta T cells with an increase of inflammatory markers in the BM.[33] In a different patient population t(11;14) was associated with separate T-cell clusters compared with other genetic subgroups with upregulation of lysine methyltransferase genes *KMT2A* and *KMT2C* in CD8+ T cells.[31] These results underscore that distinct and unique immune phenotypes can provide signals that favor the growth of certain subclones with specific genetic alterations, ultimately leading to the expansion of more aggressive and resistant populations. It has also been shown that the microenvironment in FLs, where clonal evolution and heterogeneity is highest, differs from random BM, including proportional differences for macrophages and the T cell repertoire.[56] Additionally, the changes in the BM-ME leading to altered bone metabolism are highly active in FLs.[32] Secretion of sclerotin, Dickkopf-1 (DKK1), receptor activator of nuclear factor kappa-B ligand (RANKL), and interleukin-6 (IL-6) by MM and surrounding cells leads to activation of osteoclasts and inhibition of osteoblasts resulting in increased bone resorption with ultimately lysis and fracture of the bone. Moreover, it has been shown that the interaction between MM cells and osteoblasts, or osteoblast-like cells, is crucial for MM dormancy, a phenomenon where MM cells go into a quiescent state, are shielded from systemic therapy and can grow back leading to relapse after many years.[57] Coculture of MM cells with osteoblasts switches on dormant genes in MM cells and can transition them into a quiescent state for a prolonged period.

CLONAL HETEROGENEITY AND TREATMENT RESISTANCE

A critical mechanism for tumor progression is the competition between individual subclones for the same BM niche, combined with the process of adaptation and natural selection.[58,59] Therapy exerts a selective pressure on MM cells, facilitating the death or expansion of distinct tumor subclones. As a result, subclonal complexity diminishes initially after the start of therapy, with only fitter and resistant subclones surviving.[23] These surviving subclones continue to acquire further genetic hits and continue to evolve in branching patterns eventually leading to a rapid increase of clonal heterogeneity and relapse.[60]

Intriguingly, patients with high-risk genetic features at diagnosis have similar complete response rates after autologous stem cell transplantation (ASCT) compared with patients without these features. However, they tend to relapse quickly, within 1 to 2 years after ASCT, usually during maintenance, leading to significantly shorter progression free survival (PFS) and overall survival (OS). The mechanisms leading to this rapid regrowth of high-risk subclones are complex and are thought to be due to a combination of (1) high proliferation rate, (2) intrinsic resistance mechanisms, and (3) activation of antiapoptotic pathways. A high-proliferation rate has long been known to be associated with high-risk cytogenetics[61,62] and most recently was confirmed to be an independent prognostic risk factor.[63] Conversely, MM with the standard risk translocation (t11;14) or HRD tends to have a low-proliferation index.[34,61] MM cells are usually sensitive to alkylating agents, such as melphalan but few remaining tumor cells after treatment can then grow back rapidly. Because these subclones tend to expand during maintenance therapy, it is clear that they are also equipped with or have acquired resistance mechanisms to immunomodulatory drugs (IMiDs) and/or proteasome inhibitors (PIs). Consequently, it has been shown that adverse risk genetic events are associated with intrinsic treatment resistance. For example, high MAF expression as seen in translocations t(14;16) and (14;20) mediates innate resistance to PIs[64,65] while some Ig translocations have been associated with IMiD resistance through dysregulation of the Cereblon and Ikaros/Aiolos/IRF4 axis.[66,67] Yet for the most part, disease heterogeneity and its impact on treatment resistance on a molecular level remain elusive. Data from recent single-cell studies indicate that downstream pathways of adverse genetic events converge on a molecular level and lead to the activation of similar mechanisms resulting in treatment resistance. Converging adaptation mechanisms to treatment was also described at the subclonal level, with the majority of therapy-induced changes in gene expression being shared across distinct resistant subclones.[68] Importantly, antiapoptotic pathways are highly activated in RRMM. This includes the activation of the MEK/ERK and NF-κB pathway in up to 65% of relapsed patients with MM, followed by dysregulation in the MYC pathway and cell cycle/DNA damage checkpoints.[29,69]

A longitudinal analysis of FLs in patients with MM from diagnosis to relapse has emphasized that site-restricted subclones within FLs respond differently to treatment and apart from local disease progression can also disseminate to other medullary or extramedullary sites and/or lead to clonal sweeps, where the whole BM is repopulated by one specific subclone.[13,70] It is hence unsurprising that relapse subclones often tend to have a close phylogenetic relationship to baseline FLs. Relapse patterns can vary depending on the number of FLs at baseline and response to therapy. For example, in patients with less than 3 FLs at baseline, who achieve deep treatment responses, expansion of a single resistant cell usually occurs.[71] Relapse driven by 2 to 3 coexisting expanding (and competing) subclones is particularly observed when responses are not deep and 3 or more FLs are seen at baseline. Finally, in deep-responding patients with multiple baseline FLs, distinct subclones can drive relapse at different anatomic locations leading to a pattern of "alternating spatial clonal dominance" (**Fig. 1**).[71] Hence, MM evolution is most often driven by a limited number of major subclones that generate the majority of diversity at relapse.

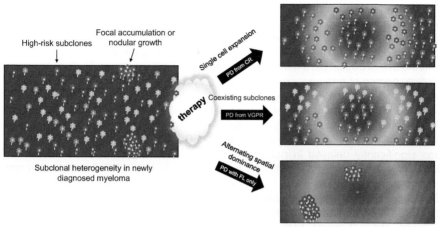

Fig. 1. The spatio-temporal evolution of myeloma. Newly diagnosed patients with myeloma typically show a complex tumor architecture with widespread subclonal heterogeneity. High-risk subclones can be site-specific and grow within FLs. During treatment, there are 3 main evolutionary patterns, which are associated with the depth of response. They include (1) relapse driven by single expanding tumor cells, (2) coexisting expanding subclones, and (3) expansion of distinct subclones at different sites. The anatomic location of subclones is the main difference between the second and the third patterns.

Importantly, treatment resistance is not only driven by tumor cell intrinsic mechanisms. The BM-ME contributes to drug resistance by secreting factors that protect MM cells and enhance cell survival, thereby fostering clonal selection and evolution.[72,73] As MM subclones compete for their niche, they eventually create a network of supporting cells, including mesenchymal stromal cells, fibroblasts, endothelial cells, and hematopoietic cells, which help to shield them from therapy. Intercellular communication and dynamic interactions between MM cells and the surrounding BM-ME in a reciprocal prosurvival loop are essential for therapy resistance and can be distinguished into soluble factors-mediated drug resistance (eg, IL-6 and vascular endothelial growth factor [VEGF]),[74,75] and cell adhesion-mediated drug resistance. The latter occurs via interactions with BM stromal cells and or extracellular matrix components through integrins, CD138 (syndecan-1), CD44, vascular adhesion molecule-1 (VCAM1), and intercellular adhesion molecule-1 (ICAM1).[76–78] In a recent single-cell study, subclone-specific interactions of MM cells with the BM-ME were observed in patients with differential treatment response at the subclonal level, highlighting a complex reciprocal network of MM and the BM-ME.[68] These results suggest that in order to treat and cure MM, it will be necessary to also target the BM-ME.

OVERCOMING CLONAL HETEROGENEITY

Therapeutic approaches have been intensified during the last decades in order to deepen response.[2] The use of novel and prolonged multidrug combination approaches consisting of PIs, IMiDs, CD38 targeting monoclonal antibodies, high-dose chemotherapy, and ASCT followed by continuous maintenance have significantly improved PFS and OS. Maintenance ensures that constant therapeutic pressure is exerted on slowly growing subclones that might not have been significantly affected by high-dose chemotherapy.[59] However, regardless of the intensity and length of the regimen, a complete eradication of all subclones is usually not possible with standard treatment options.

To break this pattern of perpetuating tumor evolution, novel treatment strategies are being investigated. One concept is to treat MM early, at precursor stages, before genetic complexity becomes extreme and insurmountable.[79] Since not every precursor condition progresses to MM, this concept is not justifiable for all of patients.[80,81] Yet, with the use of clinical parameters, such as level of free light chains (FLC), monoclonal protein, degree of immunoparesis, abnormal cytogenetics, and BM PC infiltration, a subset of patients with high-risk SMM can be identified (**Table 2**).[82–85] Treating these patients before symptomatic MM develops has been an intense focus in recent clinical trials. Two phase 3 clinical trials randomized high-risk patients with SMM to receive either lenalidomide or placebo (QuiRedex,[86] ECOG E3A06[87]). Progression to MM was significantly delayed in patients receiving lenalidomide but the effect on OS was less clear. A significantly longer OS for patients in the lenalidomide arm was only observed in the QuiRedex trial. However, most patients enrolled into this study did not have routine imaging at baseline, raising the possibility that patients with multiple FLs, and hence, clinical MM were overseen and treated as high-risk SMM. Although phase 2 clinical trials using other treatment regimen have been conducted,[88–91] equally showing delay to MM progression, it needs to be emphasized that only approximately 75% of the enrolled patients with SMM would have progressed to MM within 5 years without treatment, suggesting that up to 25% of patients have unnecessarily been exposed to toxic side effects.[79] These and other limitations, including poor overlap between populations defined as high-risk in different studies, have hampered the translation of universal early treatment in high-risk patients with SMM into standard clinical practice.[79,92] Of note, on a molecular level, most genetic changes necessary to give rise to MM are already present in high-risk SMM.[59] More intriguingly, the gene expression signatures predicting for high-risk disease in MM also correlate with a higher risk of transformation from precursor stages to symptomatic MM,[93] indicating that some aggressive intrinsic features, or even aggressive subclones, already exist at very early disease stages and early treatment on its own might not be sufficient to overcome malignant transformation in all patients.

In MM, treatment concepts have focused on more personalized approaches. For example, the use of gene expression profiling has shown to be one of the best tools

Table 2
Risk models for progression of smoldering multiple myeloma to clinical multiple myeloma[82,85]

Model	Risk Factors	Risk Groups	Outcomes
PETHEMA	1. ≥95% aberrant BM PCs by flow cytometry 2. Immunoparesis	0: low risk 1: intermediate risk 2: high risk	PFS at 5 y 0%–4% 1%–36% 2%–72%
Mayo 2018	1. BM PCs ≥20% 2. M Protein >2 g/dL 3. sFLC ratio ≤0.125 or ≥8	0: low risk 1: intermediate risk 2/3: high risk	Median TTP 0: 110 min 1: 68 min 2/3: 29 min
IMWG 2020**	1. sFLC ratio (0–5 pts) 2. M Protein (0–4 pts) 3. BM PC % (0–6 pts) 4. FISH abnormalities (0–2 pts)	0–4 pts: low risk 5–8 pts: low/intermediate risk 9–12 pts: intermediate risk >12 pts: high risk	Risk of progression at 2 y Low risk: 3.8% Low/intermediate risk: 26% Intermediate risk: 51% High risk: 72.5%

**, International Myeloma Working Group

to identify high-risk disease.[94–96] Accordingly, patients with MM have been treated with different approaches based on their risk profile.[97] Similarly, whole exome or targeted sequencing can improve prognostic models, such as the International Staging System (ISS) or the revised ISS (R-ISS) and are able to better capture clonal diversity as compared with standard cytogenetics.[98,99] Yet, as mentioned previously, there is currently no technology to capture all clonal heterogeneity within the MM BM.

In recent studies, progression events, particularly activation of the MEK/ERK pathway, have been targeted.[100–102] The use of BRAF-inhibitors and MEK-inhibitors has shown therapeutic success; however, because mutations in this pathway are typically not present in all cells and/or subclones with resistance-driving RAS mutations were selected, a long-term disease control was usually not possible.[102,103]

Targeting somatic events that are shared by all tumor cells, such as initiating events, is currently under investigation. For example, translocation t(11;14) is associated with high bcl-2 expression, leading to downstream antiapoptotic effects.[104] The use of Venetoclax, an oral bcl-2 inhibitor, has shown impressive therapeutic results in patients carrying this translocation, even in those with adverse secondary genetic events.[105,106] Similarly, inhibitors of the histone lysine methyl transferase MMSET, which is highly expressed in patients with translocation t(4;14), are now in clinical trials.[107] MMSET is the principal methyl transferase of histone H3K36, thereby regulating transcriptional activation and DNA repair.[107–109] Blocking this oncogenic pathway could lead to improved outcomes.

Finally, novel immunotherapies, such as bispecific antibodies and chimeric antigen receptor (CAR)-T cell therapy, have shown impressive results in patients with highly advanced disease, suggesting that these therapies have the potential to overcome clonal heterogeneity.[110] However, loss of surface protein targets, assumed to be essential for PCs, have been identified as a mechanism of resistance in RRMM, demonstrating that pronounced clonal heterogeneity and further evolution at this disease stage provides the tumor the ability to survive even under such a strong selective pressure.[111,112]

Considered together, with the therapeutic landscape rapidly expanding and the presence of better prognostic tools in MM, personalized medicine will be inevitable. Adjustment of therapy based on identified clonal heterogeneity and therapeutic response will hopefully lead to improved outcomes and reduced toxicities in the near future.

SUMMARY

The knowledge that intraclonal heterogeneity and differences in the spatial distribution of subclones are important features of MM biology has changed our way to address the disease. MM is considered to be a composite mixture of subclones with continuous branching evolution and fierce competition for medullary and eventually also extramedullary space. It is hence of primary importance to consider the impact that evolutionary biology and clonal heterogeneity have on the presentation, prognosis, and treatment of MM and also the emergence of treatment resistance. By doing so, we will be able to effectively use all of the tools to ultimately cure MM with best efficacy and least toxicity.

CLINICS CARE POINTS

- The spatial distribution of subclones can be highly heterogeneous in myeloma. Hence, samples derived from a random BM site are often not representative.

- There is currently no technology to capture all clonal heterogeneity within patients with myeloma.
- The prognostic impact of initiating events is driven by the clinical and cellular background in which they occur as well as by secondary genetic events.
- The size of FLs is a surrogate marker for spatial heterogeneity and is associated with poor outcome in myeloma.
- Targeting progression events, such as mutations in the MEK/ERK pathway, usually does not result in long-term disease control.
- Events that are shared by all tumor cells, for example, tumor initiating events and pathways associated with them, are promising therapy targets, which are currently under investigation.

FUNDING

Carolina Schinke was supported by the NIGMS/NIH P20 GM109005 grant. Leo Rasche was funded by the Deutsche Krebshilfe via the MSNZ program Würzburg, and the Interdisciplinary Center for Clinical Research Würzburg (IZKF). Marc S. Raab and Niels Weinhold were supported by the Dietmar-Hopp Foundation.

DISCLOSURE

The authors have nothing to disclose.

REFERENCES

1. Palumbo A, Anderson K. Multiple Myeloma. N Engl J Med 2011;1046–60. https://doi.org/10.1056/nejmra1011442.
2. Rajkumar SV. Multiple myeloma: 2022 update on diagnosis, risk stratification, and management. Am J Hematol 2022;97(8):1086–107.
3. Sonneveld P, Avet-Loiseau H, Lonial S, et al. Treatment of multiple myeloma with high-risk cytogenetics: a consensus of the International Myeloma Working Group. Blood 2016;127(24):2955–62.
4. Lonial S. Relapsed Multiple Myeloma. Hematology Am Soc Hematol Educ Program 2010;2010(1):303–9.
5. Lannes R, Samur M, Perrot A, et al. In Multiple Myeloma, High-Risk Secondary Genetic Events Observed at Relapse Are Present From Diagnosis in Tiny, Undetectable Subclonal Populations. J Clin Oncol 2023;41(9):1695–702.
6. Cohen YC, Zada M, Wang S-Y, et al. Identification of resistance pathways and therapeutic targets in relapsed multiple myeloma patients through single-cell sequencing. Nat Med 2021;27(3):491–503.
7. Walker BA, Mavrommatis K, Wardell CP, et al. A high-risk, Double-Hit, group of newly diagnosed myeloma identified by genomic analysis. Leukemia 2019; 33(1):159–70.
8. Bolli N, Avet-Loiseau H, Wedge DC, et al. Heterogeneity of genomic evolution and mutational profiles in multiple myeloma. Nat Commun 2014;5:2997.
9. Lohr JG, Stojanov P, Carter SL, et al. Widespread genetic heterogeneity in multiple myeloma: implications for targeted therapy. Cancer Cell 2014;25(1): 91–101.
10. Morgan GJ, Walker BA, Davies FE. The genetic architecture of multiple myeloma. Nat Rev Cancer 2012;12(5):335–48.

11. Walker BA, Mavrommatis K, Wardell CP, et al. Identification of novel mutational drivers reveals oncogene dependencies in multiple myeloma. Blood 2018; 132(6):587–97.

12. Rasche L, Chavan SS, Stephens OW, et al. Spatial genomic heterogeneity in multiple myeloma revealed by multi-region sequencing. Nat Commun 2017; 8(1):268.

13. Rasche L, Schinke C, Maura F, et al. The spatio-temporal evolution of multiple myeloma from baseline to relapse-refractory states. Nat Commun 2022. https://doi.org/10.1038/s41467-022-32145-y.

14. Manier S, Salem KZ, Park J, et al. Genomic complexity of multiple myeloma and its clinical implications. Nat Rev Clin Oncol 2017;14(2):100–13.

15. Maura F, Bolli N, Angelopoulos N, et al. Genomic landscape and chronological reconstruction of driver events in multiple myeloma. Nat Commun 2019;10(1): 3835.

16. Boyd KD, Ross FM, Chiecchio L, et al. A novel prognostic model in myeloma based on co-segregating adverse FISH lesions and the ISS: analysis of patients treated in the MRC Myeloma IX trial. Leukemia 2012;26(2):349–55.

17. Ross FM, Chiecchio L, Dagrada G, et al. The t(14;20) is a poor prognostic factor in myeloma but is associated with long-term stable disease in monoclonal gammopathies of undetermined significance. Haematologica 2010;95(7):1221–5.

18. Schinke C, Boyle EM, Ashby C, et al. Genomic analysis of primary plasma cell leukemia reveals complex structural alterations and high-risk mutational patterns. Blood Cancer J 2020;10(6):70.

19. Tuazon SA, Holmberg LA, Nadeem O, et al. A clinical perspective on plasma cell leukemia; current status and future directions. Blood Cancer J 2021; 11(2):23.

20. Wiedmeier-Nutor JE, Bergsagel PL. Review of Multiple Myeloma Genetics including Effects on Prognosis, Response to Treatment, and Diagnostic Workup. Life 2022;12(6). https://doi.org/10.3390/life12060812.

21. Chretien M-L, Corre J, Lauwers-Cances V, et al. Understanding the role of hyperdiploidy in myeloma prognosis: which trisomies really matter? Blood 2015; 126(25):2713–9.

22. Bolli N, Maura F, Minvielle S, et al. Genomic patterns of progression in smoldering multiple myeloma. Nat Commun 2018;9(1):3363.

23. Walker BA, Wardell CP, Melchor L, et al. Intraclonal heterogeneity is a critical early event in the development of myeloma and precedes the development of clinical symptoms. Leukemia 2014;28(2):384–90.

24. Hanamura I. Multiple myeloma with high-risk cytogenetics and its treatment approach. Int J Hematol 2022;115(6):762–77.

25. Schmidt TM, Fonseca R, Usmani SZ. Chromosome 1q21 abnormalities in multiple myeloma. Blood Cancer J 2021;11(4):83.

26. Shaughnessy J. Amplification and overexpression of CKS1B at chromosome band 1q21 is associated with reduced levels of p27 Kip1 and an aggressive clinical course in multiple myeloma. Hematology 2005;10(sup1):117–26.

27. Chapman MA, Lawrence MS, Keats JJ, et al. Initial genome sequencing and analysis of multiple myeloma. Nature 2011;471(7339):467–72.

28. Jang JS, Li Y, Mitra AK, et al. Molecular signatures of multiple myeloma progression through single cell RNA-Seq. Blood Cancer J 2019;9(1):2.

29. Ledergor G, Weiner A, Zada M, et al. Single cell dissection of plasma cell heterogeneity in symptomatic and asymptomatic myeloma. Nat Med 2018;24(12): 1867–76.

30. de Jong MME, Kellermayer Z, Papazian N, et al. The multiple myeloma microenvironment is defined by an inflammatory stromal cell landscape. Nat Immunol 2021;22(6):769–80.

31. Liu R, Gao Q, Foltz SM, et al. Co-evolution of tumor and immune cells during progression of multiple myeloma. Nat Commun 2021;12(1):2559.

32. Merz M, Merz AMA, Wang J, et al. Deciphering spatial genomic heterogeneity at a single cell resolution in multiple myeloma. Nat Commun 2022;13(1):807.

33. Tirier SM, Mallm J-P, Steiger S, et al. Subclone-specific microenvironmental impact and drug response in refractory multiple myeloma revealed by single-cell transcriptomics. Nat Commun 2021;12(1):1–16.

34. Dang M, Wang R, Lee HC, et al. Single cell clonotypic and transcriptional evolution of multiple myeloma precursor disease. Cancer Cell 2023;41(6): 1032–47.e4.

35. Zamagni E, Tacchetti P, Cavo M. Imaging in multiple myeloma: How? When? Blood 2019;133(7):644–51.

36. Bartel TB, Haessler J, Brown TLY, et al. F18-fluorodeoxyglucose positron emission tomography in the context of other imaging techniques and prognostic factors in multiple myeloma. Blood 2009;114(10):2068–76.

37. Walker R, Barlogie B, Haessler J, et al. Magnetic resonance imaging in multiple myeloma: diagnostic and clinical implications. J Clin Oncol 2007;25(9):1121–8.

38. Rasche L, Angtuaco EJ, Alpe TL, et al. The presence of large focal lesions is a strong independent prognostic factor in multiple myeloma. Blood 2018;132(1): 59–66.

39. Rajkumar SV, Dimopoulos MA, Palumbo A, et al. International Myeloma Working Group updated criteria for the diagnosis of multiple myeloma. Lancet Oncol 2014;15(12):e538–48.

40. Zamagni E, Patriarca F, Nanni C, et al. Prognostic relevance of 18-F FDG PET/CT in newly diagnosed multiple myeloma patients treated with up-front autologous transplantation. Blood 2011;118(23):5989–95.

41. Ley TJ, Mardis ER, Ding L, et al. DNA sequencing of a cytogenetically normal acute myeloid leukaemia genome. Nature 2008;456(7218):66–72.

42. Waldschmidt JM, Yee AJ, Vijaykumar T, et al. Cell-free DNA for the detection of emerging treatment failure in relapsed/refractory multiple myeloma. Leukemia 2022;36(4):1078–87.

43. Deshpande S, Tytarenko RG, Wang Y, et al. Monitoring treatment response and disease progression in myeloma with circulating cell-free DNA. Eur J Haematol 2021;106(2):230–40.

44. Rasche L, Alapat D, Kumar M, et al. Combination of flow cytometry and functional imaging for monitoring of residual disease in myeloma. Leukemia 2019; 33(7):1713–22.

45. Kaddoura M, Dingli D, Buadi FK, et al. Prognostic impact of posttransplant FDG PET/CT scan in multiple myeloma. Blood Adv 2021;5(13):2753–9.

46. Moreau P, Attal M, Caillot D, et al. Prospective Evaluation of Magnetic Resonance Imaging and [18F]Fluorodeoxyglucose Positron Emission Tomography-Computed Tomography at Diagnosis and Before Maintenance Therapy in Symptomatic Patients With Multiple Myeloma Included in the IFM/DFCI 2009 Trial: Results of the IMAJEM Study. J Clin Oncol 2017;35(25):2911–8.

47. García-Ortiz A, Rodríguez-García Y, Encinas J, et al. The Role of Tumor Microenvironment in Multiple Myeloma Development and Progression. Cancers 2021;13(2). https://doi.org/10.3390/cancers13020217.

48. Schinke C, Weinhold N. The Immune Microenvironment in Multiple Myeloma Progression at a Single-cell Level. Hemasphere 2023;7(6):e894.

49. McGranahan N, Swanton C. Clonal Heterogeneity and Tumor Evolution: Past, Present, and the Future. Cell 2017;168(4):613–28.

50. Schinke C, Qu P, Mehdi SJ, et al. The Pattern of Mesenchymal Stem Cell Expression Is an Independent Marker of Outcome in Multiple Myeloma. Clin Cancer Res 2018;24(12):2913–9.

51. Adams HC 3rd, Stevenaert F, Krejcik J, et al. High-parameter mass cytometry evaluation of relapsed/refractory multiple myeloma patients treated with daratumumab demonstrates immune modulation as a novel mechanism of action. Cytometry 2019;95(3):279–89.

52. Chung DJ, Pronschinske KB, Shyer JA, et al. T-cell Exhaustion in Multiple Myeloma Relapse after Autotransplant: Optimal Timing of Immunotherapy. Cancer Immunol Res 2016;4(1):61–71.

53. Zavidij O, Haradhvala NJ, Mouhieddine TH, et al. Single-cell RNA sequencing reveals compromised immune microenvironment in precursor stages of multiple myeloma. Nat Cancer 2020;1(5):493–506.

54. Schinke C, Poos AM, Bauer M, et al. Characterizing the role of the immune microenvironment in multiple myeloma progression at a single-cell level. Blood Adv 2022;6(22):5873–83.

55. Bailur JK, McCachren SS, Doxie DB, et al. Early alterations in stem-like/resident T cells, innate and myeloid cells in the bone marrow in preneoplastic gammopathy. JCI Insight 2019;5(11). https://doi.org/10.1172/jci.insight.127807.

56. John L, Poos A, Brobeil A, et al. Resolving the spatial architecture of myeloma and its microenvironment at the single-cell level. Nat Commun 2023;14(1):5011.

57. Khoo WH, Ledergor G, Weiner A, et al. A niche-dependent myeloid transcriptome signature defines dormant myeloma cells. Blood 2019;134(1):30–43.

58. Greaves M, Maley CC. Clonal evolution in cancer. Nature 2012;481(7381): 306–13.

59. Brioli A, Melchor L, Cavo M, et al. The impact of intra-clonal heterogeneity on the treatment of multiple myeloma. Br J Haematol 2014;165(4):441–54.

60. Keats JJ, Chesi M, Egan JB, et al. Clonal competition with alternating dominance in multiple myeloma. Blood 2012;120(5):1067–76.

61. Fonseca R, Barlogie B, Bataille R, et al. Genetics and cytogenetics of multiple myeloma: a workshop report. Cancer Res 2004;64(4):1546–58.

62. Hanamura I. Gain/Amplification of Chromosome Arm 1q21 in Multiple Myeloma. Cancers 2021;13(2). https://doi.org/10.3390/cancers13020256.

63. Mellors PW, Binder M, Ketterling RP, et al. Metaphase cytogenetics and plasma cell proliferation index for risk stratification in newly diagnosed multiple myeloma. Blood Adv 2020;4(10):2236–44.

64. Qiang Y-W, Ye S, Chen Y, et al. MAF protein mediates innate resistance to proteasome inhibition therapy in multiple myeloma. Blood, The Journal of the American Society of Hematology 2016;128(25):2919–30.

65. Qiang Y-W, Ye S, Huang Y, et al. MAFb protein confers intrinsic resistance to proteasome inhibitors in multiple myeloma. BMC Cancer 2018;18(1):724.

66. Bird SA, Pawlyn C. IMiD Resistance in Multiple Myeloma: Current Understanding of the Underpinning Biology and Clinical Impact. Blood 2023. https://doi.org/10.1182/blood.2023019637.

67. Barwick BG, Neri P, Bahlis NJ, et al. Multiple myeloma immunoglobulin lambda translocations portend poor prognosis. Nat Commun 2019;10(1):1911.

68. Poos AM, Prokoph N, Przybilla MJ, et al. Resolving therapy resistance mechanisms in multiple myeloma by multi-omics subclone analysis. Blood 2023. https://doi.org/10.1182/blood.2023019758.

69. Vo JN, Wu Y-M, Mishler J, et al. The genetic heterogeneity and drug resistance mechanisms of relapsed refractory multiple myeloma. Nat Commun 2022;13(1):3750.

70. Melchor L, Jones JR, Lenive O, et al. Spatiotemporal Analysis of Intraclonal Heterogeneity in Multiple Myeloma: Unravelling the Impact of Treatment and the Propagating Capacity of Subclones Using Whole Exome Sequencing. Blood 2015;126(23):371.

71. Landau HJ, Yellapantula V, Diamond BT, et al. Accelerated single cell seeding in relapsed multiple myeloma. Nat Commun 2020;11(1):3617.

72. Ria R, Vacca A. Bone Marrow Stromal Cells-Induced Drug Resistance in Multiple Myeloma. Int J Mol Sci 2020;21(2). https://doi.org/10.3390/ijms21020613.

73. Di Marzo L, Desantis V, Solimando AG, et al. Microenvironment drug resistance in multiple myeloma: emerging new players. Oncotarget 2016;7(37):60698–711.

74. Chauhan D, Kharbanda S, Ogata A, et al. Interleukin-6 inhibits Fas-induced apoptosis and stress-activated protein kinase activation in multiple myeloma cells. Blood 1997;89(1):227–34.

75. Hideshima T, Mitsiades C, Tonon G, et al. Understanding multiple myeloma pathogenesis in the bone marrow to identify new therapeutic targets. Nat Rev Cancer 2007;7(8):585–98.

76. Katz B-Z. Adhesion molecules—The lifelines of multiple myeloma cells. Semin Cancer Biol 2010;20(3):186–95.

77. Hazlehurst LA, Damiano JS, Buyuksal I, et al. Adhesion to fibronectin via beta1 integrins regulates p27kip1 levels and contributes to cell adhesion mediated drug resistance (CAM-DR). Oncogene 2000;19(38):4319–27.

78. Neri P, Ren L, Azab AK, et al. Integrin β7-mediated regulation of multiple myeloma cell adhesion, migration, and invasion. Blood 2011;117(23):6202–13.

79. Vaxman I, Gertz MA. How I approach smoldering multiple myeloma. Blood 2022;140(8):828–38.

80. Zingone A, Kuehl WM. Pathogenesis of monoclonal gammopathy of undetermined significance and progression to multiple myeloma. Semin Hematol 2011;48(1):4–12.

81. Visram A, Cook J, Warsame R. Smoldering multiple myeloma: evolving diagnostic criteria and treatment strategies. Hematology Am Soc Hematol Educ Program 2021;2021(1):673–81.

82. Pérez-Persona E, Vidriales M-B, Mateo G, et al. New criteria to identify risk of progression in monoclonal gammopathy of uncertain significance and smoldering multiple myeloma based on multiparameter flow cytometry analysis of bone marrow plasma cells. Blood. The Journal of the American Society of Hematology 2007;110(7):2586–92.

83. Dispenzieri A, Kyle RA, Katzmann JA, et al. Immunoglobulin free light chain ratio is an independent risk factor for progression of smoldering (asymptomatic) multiple myeloma. Blood 2008;111(2):785–9.

84. Lakshman A, Rajkumar SV, Buadi FK, et al. Risk stratification of smoldering multiple myeloma incorporating revised IMWG diagnostic criteria. Blood Cancer J 2018;8(6):59.

85. Mateos M-V, Kumar S, Dimopoulos MA, et al. International Myeloma Working Group risk stratification model for smoldering multiple myeloma (SMM). Blood Cancer J 2020. https://doi.org/10.1038/s41408-020-00366-3.

86. Mateos M-V, Hernández M-T, Giraldo P, et al. Lenalidomide plus dexamethasone versus observation in patients with high-risk smouldering multiple myeloma (QuiRedex): long-term follow-up of a randomised, controlled, phase 3 trial. Lancet Oncol 2016;17(8):1127–36.

87. Lonial S, Jacobus S, Fonseca R, et al. Randomized Trial of Lenalidomide Versus Observation in Smoldering Multiple Myeloma. J Clin Oncol 2020;38(11):1126–37.

88. Landgren CO, Chari A, Cohen YC, et al. Daratumumab monotherapy for patients with intermediate-risk or high-risk smoldering multiple myeloma: a randomized, open-label, multicenter, phase 2 study (CENTAURUS). Leukemia 2020;34(7):1840–52.

89. Kumar SK, Abdallah A-O, Badros AZ, et al. Aggressive smoldering curative approach evaluating novel therapies (ASCENT): A phase 2 trial of induction, consolidation and maintenance in subjects with high risk smoldering multiple myeloma (SMM): Initial analysis of safety data. Blood 2020;136(Supplement 1):35–6.

90. Mateos M-V, Martinez Lopez J, Rodríguez-Otero P, et al. Curative Strategy (GEM-CESAR) for High-Risk Smoldering Myeloma (SMM): Carfilzomib, Lenalidomide and Dexamethasone (KRd) As Induction Followed By HDT-ASCT, Consolidation with Krd and Maintenance with Rd. Blood 2021;138:1829.

91. Kazandjian D, Hill E, Dew A, et al. Carfilzomib, Lenalidomide, and Dexamethasone Followed by Lenalidomide Maintenance for Prevention of Symptomatic Multiple Myeloma in Patients With High-risk Smoldering Myeloma: A Phase 2 Nonrandomized Controlled Trial. JAMA Oncol 2021;7(11):1678–85.

92. Cherry BM, Korde N, Kwok M, et al. Modeling progression risk for smoldering multiple myeloma: results from a prospective clinical study. Leuk Lymphoma 2013;54(10):2215–8.

93. Dhodapkar MV, Sexton R, Waheed S, et al. Clinical, genomic, and imaging predictors of myeloma progression from asymptomatic monoclonal gammopathies (SWOG S0120). Blood 2014;123(1):78–85.

94. Zhan F, Huang Y, Colla S, et al. The molecular classification of multiple myeloma. Blood 2006;108(6):2020–8.

95. Kuiper R, Zweegman S, van Duin M, et al. Prognostic and predictive performance of R-ISS with SKY92 in older patients with multiple myeloma: the HOVON-87/NMSG-18 trial. Blood Adv 2020;4(24):6298–309.

96. Broyl A, Hose D, Lokhorst H, et al. Gene expression profiling for molecular classification of multiple myeloma in newly diagnosed patients. Blood 2010;116(14):2543–53.

97. Usmani SZ, Crowley J, Hoering A, et al. Improvement in long-term outcomes with successive Total Therapy trials for multiple myeloma: are patients now being cured? Leukemia 2013;27(1):226–32.

98. Yellapantula V, Hultcrantz M, Rustad EH, et al. Comprehensive detection of recurring genomic abnormalities: a targeted sequencing approach for multiple myeloma. Blood Cancer J 2019;9(12):101.

99. Bolli N, Genuardi E, Ziccheddu B, et al. Next-Generation Sequencing for Clinical Management of Multiple Myeloma: Ready for Prime Time? Front Oncol 2020;10:189.

100. Heuck CJ, Jethava Y, Khan R, et al. Inhibiting MEK in MAPK pathway-activated myeloma. Leukemia 2016;30(4):976–80.

101. Čepulytė R, Žučenka A, Pečeliūnas V. Combination of Dabrafenib and Trameti-nib for the Treatment of Relapsed and Refractory Multiple Myeloma Harboring BRAF V600E Mutation. Case Rep Hematol 2020;2020:8894031.

102. Giesen N, Chatterjee M, Scheid C, et al. A phase 2 clinical trial of combined BRAF/MEK inhibition for BRAFV600E-mutated multiple myeloma. Blood 2023; 141(14):1685–90.

103. Subbiah V, Kreitman RJ, Wainberg ZA, et al. Dabrafenib plus trametinib in BRAFV600E-mutated rare cancers: the phase 2 ROAR trial. Nat Med 2023; 29(5):1103–12.

104. Paner A, Patel P, Dhakal B. The evolving role of translocation t(11;14) in the biology, prognosis, and management of multiple myeloma. Blood Rev 2020; 41(100643):100643.

105. Kumar S, Kaufman JL, Gasparetto C, et al. Efficacy of venetoclax as targeted therapy for relapsed/refractory t(11;14) multiple myeloma. Blood 2017; 130(22):2401–9.

106. Kumar SK, Harrison SJ, Cavo M, et al. Venetoclax or placebo in combination with bortezomib and dexamethasone in patients with relapsed or refractory mul-tiple myeloma (BELLINI): a randomised, double-blind, multicentre, phase 3 trial. Lancet Oncol 2020;21(12):1630–42.

107. Rogawski DS, Grembecka J, Cierpicki T. H3K36 methyltransferases as cancer drug targets: rationale and perspectives for inhibitor development. Future Med Chem 2016;8(13):1589–607.

108. Martinez-Garcia E, Popovic R, Min D-J, et al. The MMSET histone methyl trans-ferase switches global histone methylation and alters gene expression in t(4;14) multiple myeloma cells. Blood 2011;117(1):211–20.

109. Popovic R, Martinez-Garcia E, Giannopoulou EG, et al. Histone methyltransfer-ase MMSET/NSD2 alters EZH2 binding and reprograms the myeloma epige-nome through global and focal changes in H3K36 and H3K27 methylation. PLoS Genet 2014;10(9):e1004566.

110. Rasche L, Wäsch R, Munder M, et al. Novel immunotherapies in multiple myeloma - chances and challenges. Haematologica 2021;106(10):2555–65.

111. Da Vià MC, Dietrich O, Truger M, et al. Homozygous BCMA gene deletion in response to anti-BCMA CAR T cells in a patient with multiple myeloma. Nat Med 2021;27(4):616–9.

112. Samur MK, Fulciniti M, Aktas Samur A, et al. Biallelic loss of BCMA as a resis-tance mechanism to CAR T cell therapy in a patient with multiple myeloma. Nat Commun 2021;12(1):868.

113. Bianchi G, Ghobrial IM. Biological and Clinical Implications of Clonal Heteroge-neity and Clonal Evolution in Multiple Myeloma. Curr Cancer Ther Rev 2014; 10(2):70–9.

Measurable Residual Disease and Decision-Making in Multiple Myeloma

Benjamin A. Derman, MD[a,*], Rafael Fonseca, MD[b]

KEYWORDS

- Multiple myeloma • MRD • Minimal residual disease • Measurable residual disease

KEY POINTS

- Measurable (minimal) residual disease (MRD) is one of the most powerful prognostic factors for progression-free survival and overall survival in multiple myeloma (MM).
- There are several ways to assess for MRD in MM; bone marrow methods such as next-generation sequencing and next-generation flow cytometry can achieve sensitivity up to 10^{-6}.
- Each increase in MRD sensitivity threshold is associated with improved prognostication, and sustained MRD negativity carries greater significance than a single instance of MRD negativity.
- Peripheral blood techniques (ie, mass spectrometry) to assess for MRD are quickly moving from research only to clinical use.
- MRD-adapted clinical decision-making is controversial, but there is mounting evidence that MRD-guided de-escalation of therapy is feasible and may not compromise clinical outcomes.

INTRODUCTION

Measurable (or minimal) residual disease (MRD) in multiple myeloma (MM) refers to low levels of myeloma cells detectable using advanced diagnostics. MRD testing is evolving, initially limited to bone marrow-based assays and now expanding to sophisticated peripheral blood techniques such as mass spectrometry (MS) and circulating tumor DNA (ctDNA). MRD status has been established as a powerful prognostic tool, but two key functions remain controversial: the role of MRD as surrogate regulatory endpoint and its role for decision-making in MM, where some have stated that it may not be ready for "primetime." Much like the transition of prestige dramas to on-demand platforms, the

[a] Section of Hematology/Oncology, University of Chicago, 5841 South Maryland Avenue, Chicago, IL 60637, USA; [b] Division of Hematology and Medical Oncology, Mayo Clinic in Arizona, 13400 East Shea Boulevard, MCCRB 3-001, Phoenix, AZ 85259, USA
* Corresponding author. 5841 South Maryland Avenue, M/C 2115, Chicago, IL 60637.
E-mail address: bderman@bsd.uchicago.edu

Hematol Oncol Clin N Am 38 (2024) 477–495
https://doi.org/10.1016/j.hoc.2023.12.009
0889-8588/24/© 2023 Elsevier Inc. All rights reserved.

hemonc.theclinics.com

authors eschew the notion of MRD in primetime in favor of its utility as a "streaming" service to optimize the care in real-time for patients living with MM.

A PRIMER ON MEASURABLE RESIDUAL DISEASE IN MYELOMA

Imagine a diver is preparing to dive into a pool whose depth increases along its length (**Fig. 1**); the deepest end of the pool is just beyond their skills to reach and remains inaccessible to them. They have been tasked with finding a small coin that may have been cast somewhere into the pool, but they are not certain that it has been. It is possible that the coin will be found at the shallow end of the pool and will not require much effort to detect. More challenging would be if the coin is found in the lower depths of the pool but still within their capacity to obtain. However, it is still possible that the coin could be in the deepest end of the pool which cannot be reached, or it may not be in the pool at all; how could they know?

As an analogy to MRD in myeloma, the pool is analogous to the "compartment" of the patient being analyzed, the diver is the MRD assay, the pool depth is the sensitivity of the assay, and the coin is the residual disease. The bone marrow can be assessed using multiparametric flow cytometry (MFC) and next-generation sequencing (NGS). The extramedullary compartments can be explored using PET or MRI. The peripheral blood compartment remains the least explored, though MFC, NGS, circulating tumor cells, cell-free DNA, and MS are all under investigation.

Flow Cytometry

Transitioning from first-generation MFC—which carried a sensitivity of 10^{-4} (ability to identify one plasma cell in 10,000 cells)—to second-generation eight-color MFC (MRD

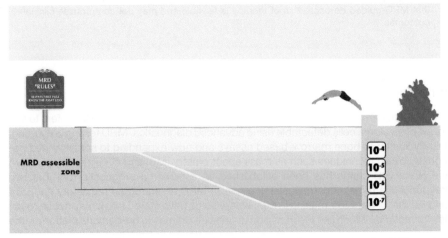

Fig. 1. Measurable residual disease (MRD) depth and uncertainty. Assessing for MRD can be likened to a diver jumping into a pool. The deepest end of the pool is just beyond their skills to reach and remains inaccessible. They have been tasked with finding a small coin (ie, MRD) that may have been cast somewhere into the pool, but they are not certain that it has been. It is possible that the coin will be found at the shallow end of the pool (ie, less sensitive MRD techniques) and will not require much effort to find. More challenging would be if the coin is found in the lower depths of the pool but still within their capacity to obtain (MRD 10^{-5}–10^{-6}). However, it is still possible that the coin could be in the deepest end of the pool which cannot be reached (10^{-7} or beyond), or it may not be in the pool at all (truly no disease present).

sensitivity of 10^{-5}) carried with it an improvement in prognostication of PFS and OS.[1] Patients who were MRD negative at a level of 10^{-4} but MRD positive at a level of 10^{-5} had inferior outcomes to patients who were MRD negative at 10^{-5}. With this method, Lahuerta performed a pooled analysis of 609 patients to show that MFC MRD negativity was much better in discriminating prolonged PFS and OS than CR achievement. Indeed, the entire survival benefit of CR could be attributed to MRD negativity.[2]

The EuroFlow Consortium later devised what has become known as "next generation flow" using a two-tube 8-color MFC method with a limit of detection (LoD) of 2×10^{-6} (20 aberrant plasma cells per 10 million events) and a limit of quantitation (LoQ) of 5×10^{-6} (50 aberrant plasma cells per 10 million events).[3]

MFC requires assessment within 24 to 48 hours, and no baseline diagnostic sample is needed. With second-generation MFC, there is considerable heterogeneity in marker expression and analytical strategies between laboratories, leading to inconsistent clinical interpretation of results.[4] NGF is standardized but requires a substantial number of cells (10 million events) to achieve 10^{-6} sensitivity, requires experienced laboratories, and carries a higher risk of false negatives from hemodiluted samples. The addition of anti-CD38 monoclonal antibodies daratumumab and isatuximab to the treatment armamentarium may also make interpretation of results even more difficult.[5]

Next-Generation Sequencing

NGS MRD testing for MM identifies and quantifies rearranged immunoglobulin heavy chain (IgH) variable, diversity, and joining (VDJ) and diversity and joining (DJ) rearrangements and kappa and lambda rearrangements.[5] An initial high tumor burden sample is needed to identify clonotypic sequences (clone identification [ID]) for tracking on subsequent assessments. Close to 95% of patients will have an identifiable clone ID at the time of diagnosis.[6,7] MRD by NGS can be performed using the FDA-cleared clonoSEQ assay (Adaptive Biotechnologies), though other similar assays exist as well. With the maximum input of 20 μg of DNA (which equates to approximately 2–3 million cellular equivalents), clonoSEQ has the highest sensitivity of the assays with an LoD of 6.8×10^{-7} and an LoQ of 1.76×10^{-6}.

MRD negativity by NGS has been shown on a number of occasions to be associated with longer PFS and OS, regardless of International Staging System (ISS) staging, cytogenetic risk, or treatment.[8–11] Although NGS offers a standardized way to achieve 10^{-6} sensitivity with fewer cells than next generation flow (NGF), it requires a baseline high tumor burden sample and offers no way to determine if samples are hemodiluted.

Imaging

PET can detect extramedullary disease in MM and is especially useful in non/oligo-secretory MM. Patients who were MRD negative by MFC (10^{-4}) and without evidence of hypermetabolic lesions on PET imaging had superior PFS to patients who were either MRD MFC positive or PET positive.[12] The FORTE trial found pre-maintenance PET to be prognostic and complementary to MFC (10^{-5}).[13] On the other hand, the CASSIOPET study found that only 12 of 114 (11%) patients with MRD less than 10^{-5} (MFC) had a positive PET following consolidation therapy.[14] In a retrospective analysis of patients with paired bone marrow MRD by NGS (10^{-5} to 10^{-6}) and PET assessments at day 100 post-ASCT, only 23 of 102 (23%) of patients with MRD positivity had a positive PET.[15] Moreover, only 2 of 34 (6%) patients with MRD negativity were PET positive, suggesting the role of PET in the age of high-sensitivity MRD testing is less clear. PET scans carry the advantage of being able to identify hypermetabolic areas of active disease, though they are expensive and expose patients to radiation.

Whole body diffusion-weighted imaging, MRI, may be more sensitive in detecting disease,[16–18] though this remains a nascent field.

Peripheral Blood Techniques

Perhaps the "holy grail" in MRD detection for myeloma is a method to assess for MRD in the peripheral blood without the need for costly imaging or the discomfort of bone marrow biopsies. This might also help to circumvent current limitations with bone marrow assays that are believed to lead to false-negative results: patchy myeloma disease leading to inconsistent results, hemodilution of aspirate samples, and extramedullary disease that is undetectable by bone marrow assessment.

Next-Generation Flow Cytometry in the Peripheral Blood

The presence of circulating tumor cells by NGF in the peripheral blood at MM diagnosis is associated with inferior outcomes.[19–22] As a peripheral blood MRD test, NGF was able to detect circulating tumor plasma cells in 26% of cases in one study, though every single one of these cases had NGF MRD positivity in the bone marrow.[23] Moreover, 40% of samples were NGF MRD negative in the peripheral blood but MRD positive in the bone marrow, suggesting significantly lower sensitivity for NGF in the peripheral blood compared with the bone marrow.[23] To overcome this, Notarfranchi and colleagues devised a novel technique called BloodFlow" in which a 50-mL peripheral blood sample underwent immunomagnetic enrichment for plasma cells and the reduced volume was then analyzed using NGF.[24] BloodFlow detected MRD in 9% of analyzed on-treatment samples with the lowest MRD level at 6×10^{-8}, including in two bone marrow NGF-negative cases; notably, 41 of 60 (68%) bone marrow NGF-positive cases were still BloodFlow negative.[24]

Next-Generation Sequencing in the Peripheral Blood

The same interest lies in NGS assessment of the peripheral blood. Vij and colleagues found that peripheral blood myeloma clone levels were 2 logs (100-fold) lower than paired bone marrow samples.[25] When paired bone marrow and peripheral blood samples were compared using the clonoSEQ assay for patients in follow-up, there was no correlation between MRD in the peripheral blood and the bone marrow; only 1 of 11 (9%) of cases were peripheral blood MRD positive but bone marrow MRD negative, whereas 18 of 26 (69%) were bone marrow MRD positive but peripheral blood MRD negative.[26]

Other techniques to detect ctDNA have been evaluated as well. A bespoke tumor-informed NGS assay has been used to measure up to 16 patient-specific somatic mutations and then track them in patient's plasma.[27] Patients who were ctDNA negative had longer PFS than ctDNA-positive patients.[27] It remains to be seen how such technology compares with more sensitive MRD techniques.

In their totality, NGF and NGS performed on peripheral blood are less sensitive compared with bone marrow methods. Although a peripheral blood MRD-positive result might circumvent the need for bone marrow assessment, a negative result does not.

Mass Spectrometry in the Peripheral Blood

The sensitivity of serum protein electrophoresis (monoclonal protein of 0.1 g/dL) and immunofixation (monoclonal protein 0.05 g/dL) can be improved by MS. The premise relies on the fact that plasma cells achieve their uniqueness through somatic recombination and hypermutation, which leads to unique heavy and light chain genes. Each plasma cell produces a unique immunoglobulin with a specific amino acid sequence and mass, and MS is able to identify and quantify this M-protein.[31]

In the "top-down" (intact immunoglobin light chain) approach, the intact protein is introduced into the mass spectrometer and analyzed directly. There are two methods that use the top-down approach: matrix-assisted laser desorption–ionization (MALDI) time of flight MS and liquid chromatography MS (LC-MS). With MALDI, samples are ionized into the gas phase and measured for their mass-to-charge (m/z) ratio based on their time of flight through the flight tube. MALDI is performed after immunoglobulins are purified from serum and then heavy chains and light chains are dissociated from each other by reducing disulfide bonds. The MASS-FIX assay uses camelid-derived nanobodies, linked to agarose beads, which are directed against the respective heavy (IgG, IgA, and IgM) and light (kappa and lambda) chains. The beads are then washed and the bound proteins are eluted to make five immunoglobulin isolations, which are the analyzed using MALDI MS.[32,33] The MASS-FIX assay has been implemented into routine practice at the Mayo Clinic.[34] The EXENT assay (The Binding Site Group) is similar; five immunoglobulin isolations are performed with polyclonal sheep nanobodies against IgG, IgA, IgM, kappa, and lambda, and which are covalently linked to paramagnetic beads. These intact proteins are ionized and then analyzed in the mass spectrometer.[35,36] MALDI analyzes samples quickly (10 seconds) and it can be done in an automated fashion using the EXENT system; the limit of quantification with EXENT is as low as 0.015 g/dL, providing a significantly more sensitive assay than immunofixation.[33–38]

A comparison of MALDI in the peripheral blood and 10-color MFC (10^{-5}) in the bone marrow found a concordance of 62%, with the discordance split between MALDI positive only and MFC positive only.[39] Comparison of EXENT (MALDI) and NGF showed only 15% disagreement, with 10% NGF positive only and 5% EXENT positive only.[40] Paired bone marrow and peripheral blood samples found that MALDI and NGS (10^{-5} to 10^{-6}) had 17% disagreement, nearly all of which (90%) was attributed to MALDI-positive and NGS-negative cases.[41]

LC-MS is another top-down approach that first separates proteins by their size and charge using LC before being passed through a mass spectrometer, which measures their mass and charge. Although this process is more time-consuming (20 minutes) than MALDI alone, the added discriminatory capacity decreases the limit of quantification to 0.005 g/dL, which is substantially lower than that of MALDI or immunofixation (**Table 1**).[36] LC-MS in the peripheral blood and NGS (10^{-5} to 10^{-6}) in the bone marrow were shown to have 63% agreement; all discordant cases (37%) were LC-MS positive and NGS negative.[41] The Spanish PETHEMA group analyzed paired peripheral blood EXENT and LC-MS with bone marrow NGF. NGF and EXENT were found to be complementary. LC-MS was able to detect disease in 58% of EXENT-negative samples; this increased discordance with NGF to 35%, largely favoring MS positive only cases.[42] Concordance between LC-MS and NGS seems to increase with time from treatment initiation, likely reflecting dissipation of recycled immunoglobulins over time.[43]

In the bottom-up (clonotypic peptide) approach, the protein of interest is first digested into smaller peptides before analysis, typically with trypsin. The peptides are then separated by LC and analyzed by MS. The clonotypic peptides are identified by comparing their m/z ratios and fragmentation patterns to those of known peptides, often with the assistance of a bioinformatics algorithm. This clonotypic peptide identification can be accomplished when the M-protein concentration is at least 0.2 g/dL, and it can be acquired from serum or gel electrophoreses. Subsequent follow-up samples are analyzed using targeted MS for the clonotypic peptides of interest; whereas MALDI and LC-MS methods require the monoclonal protein to be detectable above

Table 1
Mass spectrometry methods for minimal (measurable) residual disease detection in multiple myeloma

Mass Spectrometry Method	Alternative Names	Limit of Detection	Advantages	Disadvantages
MALDI-TOF	MASS-FIX EXENT	0.015 g/dL	• Quick (10 s) • Can be automated	• Not as sensitive as other MS assays
Liquid chromatography	miRAMM	0.005 g/dL	• Higher sensitivity than MALDI	• Time-consuming (20 min per sample) • M-spike lags significantly behind tumor lysis
Clonotypic peptide	EasyM M-InSight	0.00001–0.00005 g/dL	• Highest sensitivity • No interference from polyclonal background	• Expensive • Time-consuming • M-spike lags significantly behind tumor lysis

the polyclonal background, the clonotypic peptide approach is not interfered with by the polyclonal background or therapeutic monoclonal antibodies.

EasyM (RapidNovor) and M-InSight (Sebia) are clonotypic peptide assays, where the limit of quantification is 0.00001 to 0.00005 g/dL.[44–46] EasyM can detect MRD in the peripheral blood and also monitor M-protein kinetics to predict relapse in MM; it detected MRD in 62 of 72 (86%) of MFC (10^{-4})-negative cases in one study[44] and in 79% of NGS (10^{-5})-negative cases in another.[47] NGS at 10^{-6} still detected MRD when EasyM could not. M-InSight was studied in 926 serial samples from 41 patients treated on the IFM-2009 clinical trial.[48] M-InSight detected MRD in 864 of 926 (93%) samples compared with only 195 (21%) by serum protein electrophoresis (SPEP).[48] M-InSight was negative for MRD in only 3 of 66 (4.5%) NGS-positive cases, and M-Insight was positive for MRD in 14 of 15 (93%) NGS-negative cases.[48]

Could LC-MS and clonotypic peptide analysis be *too* sensitive as MRD assays?! The half-life of IgG antibodies in the serum (21–25 days) is prolonged due to the neonatal Fc receptor (FcRn), which rescues IgG antibodies from lysosomal degradation and recycles them back into circulation. The IgG–FcRn interaction is saturable; thus, when serum IgG levels are low, more IgG is salvaged and recycled.[49] This phenomenon makes assessment of disease response challenging in IgG myelomas using serum immunofixation owing to a time lag between tumor lysis and monoclonal protein decrease. This is even more pronounced by the most sensitive MS techniques.[50] This is less of a concern for IgA isotype M-proteins or light chain only disease, where the half-lives are significantly shorter.[50] Given the exquisite sensitivities of these assays, it may be more sensible to track the kinetics of such proteins over time to determine concerning profiles for relapse rather than setting cutoffs at a particular concentration. Identifying when FcRn recycling of monoclonal IgG is no longer occurring will be key to understanding the optimal timepoint for assessing MRD with MS.

MEASURABLE RESIDUAL DISEASE AS A PROGNOSTIC TOOL

Historically, achievement of a complete response (CR)—the absence of a monoclonal protein in the peripheral blood and urine with less than 5% plasmacytosis in the bone marrow—has been an important prognostic marker.[51–53] The advent of stringent CR (sCR) unfortunately did not led to meaningful discrimination in outcomes.[54–56] Critical analyses of the International Myeloma Working Group (IMWG) response criteria show no discernible differences in PFS and OS between those with the various response categories if MRD was detected.[56] Said differently, MRD status provides superior prognostication of PFS and OS compared with IMWG response criteria.[57,58]

Measurable Residual Disease Negativity Is Prognostic, Regardless of Assay or Sensitivity Threshold

Despite differences in assays and depth, Munshi and colleagues showed in a meta-analysis that MRD negativity was associated with superior PFS and OS, even among patients in a CR.[57] An updated meta-analysis of 44 studies involving 8098 patients confirmed this finding, but went further to show that MRD negativity was associated with improved PFS and OS regardless of the disease setting, assay, sensitivity threshold, cytogenetic risk, and timing of assessment.[58]

Chimeric antigen receptor (CAR) T-cell therapy presents a unique opportunity to understand the role of MRD in disease monitoring; owing to delayed clearance of paraprotein, patients continue to have detectable paraprotein in their blood long after the CAR T-cells have destroyed the source of these paraproteins. In a retrospective analysis of patients treated with CAR T-cell therapy for relapsed/refractory MM, 78% were MRD negative 1 month after infusion, but the rate of sustained MRD negativity was only 40%.[59] The KarMMa study involving idecabtagene vicleucel found that MRD negativity 1 month after therapy was associated with improved PFS (median 11.5 vs 2 months, $P<.001$), though PFS was significantly longer (median 30 months) for patients with sustained MRD negativity at 12 months.[60] Of the 56 patients who achieved MRD negativity with ciltacabtagene autoleucel in CARTITUDE-1, 26 (46%) had sustained MRD negativity at 12 months and 18 (32%) had sustained MRD negativity with at least a CR at 24 months.[61,62] These data drive home the point that although early MRD negativity post-CAR T is favorable, it is sustained MRD negativity that must be achieved in order to achieve durable outcomes.

Sustained Measurable Residual Disease Negativity Is More Important than a Single Instance

Patients who reach MRD negativity may still experience progression. For example, patients with MRD negativity after 1 year of maintenance lenalidomide in the IFM-2009 trial had a 3-year PFS of approximately 75%.[11] This has led to an understanding of the importance of *sustained* MRD negativity, defined by the IMWG as two consecutive MRD-negative results separated by at least 1 year.

The randomized phase II FORTE study compared three different treatment strategies in newly diagnosed MM and found that PFS was similar regardless of the treatment strategy if sustained MRD negativity by MFC (10^{-5}) was achieved.[63] In a pooled analysis of the MAIA and ALCYONE studies of newly diagnosed MM without transplant intent, sustained MRD negativity for $\geq$ 12 months was associated with superior PFS compared with less than 12 months.[64] The same was shown in a pooled analysis of the POLLUX and CASTOR trials in relapsed/refractory MM.[65]

Although sustained MRD negativity seems to be a key biomarker for deep and durable responses, we also know that MRD resurgence (ie, conversion from MRD negative to positive) portends a poor prognosis. A large analysis of patients treated at the University of Arkansas found that 73% of patients with MRD resurgence experienced disease relapse, and MRD resurgence preceded relapse by a median of 1 year.[66] This has also been shown in other prospective settings.[67,68] It will be important to better understand the implications of a single MRD negative determination; is it better to have reached MRD negativity at least once even if it is followed by MRD resurgence? As for the impact of sustained MRD negativity, it can become circular logic to state that many years of MRD negativity will lead to better outcomes; what is the shortest duration of sustained MRD negativity where it may still be a relevant biomarker?

Depth of Measurable Residual Disease Testing Matters

Improvements in MRD technologies have led to the enhanced ability to detect disease, which have also led to improvements in prognostication. When different MRD cutoffs were used (10^{-4}, 10^{-5}, and 10^{-6}) in the IFM-2009 trial, each log-fold improvement in sensitivity was accompanied by improved discrimination of PFS.[11] A meta-analysis of MRD in MM by Munshi and colleagues also showed decreasing hazard ratios for each MRD threshold,[58] suggesting the superiority of higher sensitivity analysis.

The type of assay used is less important if the sensitivity threshold is the same. A comparative analysis from the FORTE trial found that MFC/NGF and NGS demonstrated a high degree of concordance when using the same cutoffs (10^{-5} and 10^{-6}) and each showed similar PFS hazard ratios.[69]

Although an MRD sensitivity threshold of 10^{-6} is optimal, it can be aspirational at times due to hemodilution of specimens. This may be unavoidable in cases of low bone marrow cellularity (ie, after intensive therapy). However, prioritizing MRD assessments during bone marrow aspiration, when MRD negativity is the primary goal, is essential; it should always be the "first pull."[70]

Moving beyond 10^{-6} sensitivity presents additional challenges, largely due to the constraints of current technologies. Efforts to increase sensitivity to 10^{-7} are currently underway by using CD138 enrichment of larger aspirate samples followed by NGS MRD assessment; preliminary findings suggest that it can detect disease where the conventional 10^{-6} NGS assay cannot and this might carry prognostic significance.[71]

MS performed on peripheral blood samples has been shown to be a prognostic biomarker as well. MALDI status was demonstrated to be associated with PFS in several studies, including the GEM2012MENOS65, GEM2014MAIN, and STAMINA trials and a Mayo Clinic retrospective study.[40,42,72,73] LC-MS status was also associated with PFS based on analyses from the GEM2014MAIN and KRd/autologous stem cell transplant (ASCT) trials.[41,42]

MEASURABLE RESIDUAL DISEASE RESULT INTERPRETATION

The proliferation of MRD testing in MM makes result interpretation a critical skill. The key elements of interpretation include the assay type, the number of cells input into the assay, the LoD and/or quantitation (which depends on the input), and the trend of MRD results over time (**Fig. 2**). An assay such as NGS with a sensitivity threshold of 10^{-6} will only provide such discrimination if 20 µg DNA ($\sim$2–3 million cellular equivalents) are input. A hemodilute or hypocellular sample will not be sufficient to make a determination at 10^{-6}. In some cases, particularly with NGS, MRD may be detected below the LoD. This can occur in the setting of a less unique clonal sequence that may be shared with other nonmalignant plasma cells, which is typically not of concern. However, there may also be situations where MRD is detected at less than 1 cell/million for unique clonal sequences; it is unknown whether this represents true residual disease.

MEASURABLE RESIDUAL DISEASE AS A SURROGATE ENDPOINT

It should follow that if MRD negativity is associated with PFS and OS, then it would serve as an ideal surrogate endpoint for clinical trials. This would carry the advantage of allowing more rapid readouts of important randomized studies.

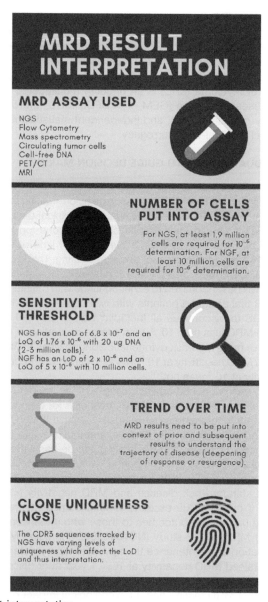

Fig. 2. MRD result interpretation.

Much of the consternation regarding MRD as a surrogate endpoint relates to the concepts of patient-level and trial-level surrogacy.[74] Patient-level surrogacy refers to whether the surrogate endpoint has prognostic value for an individual.[75] In the case of MRD in myeloma, patient-level surrogacy has been established as evidenced by the meta-analysis showing the association between MRD negativity and longer PFS and OS.[58]

However, it has been argued that for MRD to be accepted as a valid surrogate endpoint for OS, trial-level surrogacy must be established. Trial-level surrogacy refers to whether an intervention that improves the surrogate also improves survival. To prove trial-level surrogacy in MM, it must be shown that interventions that improve

MRD also improve OS in a consistent way across different trials. This requires many trials with a long follow-up period. One aggregate data analysis showed that for newly diagnosed transplant-eligible MM, the R^2 for the correlation between treatment effects on MRD and PFS was 0.74, surpassing the typically defined 0.7 threshold for a stastically acceptable correlation.[76,77] The i²TEAMM (International Independent Team for Endpoint Approval of Myeloma MRD) is an ongoing multifaceted initiative involving several myeloma research groups (GEM, IFM/DFCI, MRC, EMN/HOVON, GMMG, BMT-CTN), industry representatives, and independent statisticians to help generate data for patient-level and trial-level surrogacy.

MEASURABLE RESIDUAL DISEASE TO GUIDE DECISION-MAKING

Although prognostication and surrogacy are important elements in the evolution of MRD in MM, most significant is whether MRD can guide decision-making in MM. The FDA has issued guidance that when MRD is being evaluated for clinical decision-making in the trial setting, the MRD threshold used should be at least one log less sensitive than the assay's lower LoD.[79] In other words, if the technical limit of the assay is 10^{-6}, then a threshold of 10^{-5} should be used for decision-making. This is being implemented in the randomized SWOG S1803; after 2 years of post-ASCT maintenance, patients with MRD less than 10^{-5} will be randomized to either continue with maintenance or stop therapy.[80] The MASTER trial assigned patients with two consecutive MRD less than 10^{-5} assessments by NGS to discontinue all therapy.[6] Half of enrolled patients remained off therapy and with MRD less than 10^{-5}, with a large proportion of relapses occurring in patients with two or more high-risk cytogenetic abnormalities.[78] An updated analysis found that sustained MRD negativity at 10^{-6} was associated with improved PFS but sustained MRD negativity at 10^{-5} was not.[78]

Although the FDA has cautioned against using 10^{-6} as the detection threshold for guiding decision-making, using less sensitive thresholds for de-escalation potentially exposes patients to an increased risk of relapse. A phase II study of MRD-adapted elotuzumab, carfilzomib, lenalidomide, and dexamethasone (Elo-KRd) showed that MRD by NGS 10^{-6} could be used to effectively guide de-escalation of carfilzomib.[43] The randomized phase III ATLAS trial comparing carfilzomib, lenalidomide, and dexamethasone (KRd) versus lenalidomide for post-ASCT maintenance allowed patients receiving KRd with standard-risk disease and MRD negativity ($<10^{-6}$, or $< 10^{-5}$ if not available) after 6 cycles to de-escalate to lenalidomide; patients who received all 36 cycles of KRd had similar outcomes to those who underwent early de-escalation.[82] The ongoing MRD2STOP study (NCT04108624) is using MRD by NGS 10^{-6} to guide discontinuation of maintenance therapy; preliminary data showed that 84% of patients had sustained MRD negativity at 10^{-6} 1 year after discontinuation.[71]

What is the patient perspective? A study of 68 patients and their perspectives on MRD in MM found that MRD testing had a psychological impact on patients.[83] Interestingly, 10 of 19 (53%) patients with MRD-positive results felt the result had a negative psychological impact on them, though 100% were glad to have known the result.[83] Only 79% of patients with MRD-positive results felt that their medical team explained the significance of the result. This stresses the need for clinicians to preemptively explain to patients the reason for and implications of performing MRD testing before moving forward.

"HOT TAKES" AND BURNING QUESTIONS

We posit that it is irrelevant whether MRD is ready for primetime in MM (though it is!). More importantly, we believe that MRD is ready for on-demand streaming to help guide decision-making in MM. It is imperative that we use our best available tools to mitigate physical, psychological, financial, and time toxicities in the setting of excellent disease control and to potentially press harder in the face of recalcitrant MRD-positive disease.

MRD negativity's association with outcomes is not simply a reflection of favorable disease biology. This would (falsely) suggest that patients with excellent conventional responses such as CR or sCR but MRD positivity do not have favorable "substrate." Furthermore, patients who achieve MRD negativity are not guaranteed to sustain it. However, the evolving evidence suggests that the optimal goal is for patients to *safely* achieve MRD negativity.

Although some might state that more evidence may be needed to convincingly show that MRD status can inform practice, it is important to note that MM clinicians routinely make decisions based on biomarkers (serum protein electrophoresis, immunofixation, and serum free light chains) that have not been rigorously validated. An MM clinician survey using common clinical scenarios in MM to see how MRD status might impact decision-making found that 60% would change at least one decision based on an MRD result.[84] A retrospective study involving 400 patients with newly diagnosed MM found that 67 (17%) underwent a clinical decision based on an MRD result and PFS was prolonged in patients for whom a treatment change was made.[85]

Deeper testing will likely always be possible, but a relevant threshold eventually must be chosen; at this time, we believe that MRD 10^{-6} is that threshold. Let us explore some scenarios in which MRD can be used to guide decision-making (**Table 2**). Patients with sustained MRD negativity during maintenance therapy, especially those with standard-risk disease, face the unenviable prospect of indefinite therapy and must deal with both the short-term effects of maintenance therapy in addition to longer term issues such as second cancers. Continuing maintenance indefinitely may lead to a pyrrhic victory, where the patient has won the battle (eradicated myeloma) but lost the war (succumbed to a second hematologic malignancy). There is no clearer imperative than to use sustained MRD negativity to trigger discontinuation of maintenance therapy. De-escalation measures need not necessarily end in full treatment discontinuation and should be drug agnostic. Patients on multi-agent maintenance therapy with MRD negativity might also benefit from de-escalation of their regimen to decrease toxicity and time spent in clinic. For instance, patients

Table 2
Potential minimal (measurable) residual disease-adapted strategies in multiple myeloma

Scenario	Information Learned	Potential Intervention
Sustained MRD negativity	Deep/durable responders	Single-agent maintenance: discontinue Multi-agent maintenance: de-escalate
MRD(+) to MRD(−)	Benefit conferred by intervention (ie, ASCT, maintenance)	De-escalation of intensive therapy
MRD(+) to MRD(+)	Signifies persistent disease	Careful monitoring for disease progression Early intervention before progression
MRD(−) to MRD(+)	Harbinger of progression	Early intervention before progression

receiving a proteasome inhibitor (PI) as part of maintenance therapy could decrease the frequency or discontinue the PI if MRD negativity is achieved.

Patients with MRD positivity present a different challenge, because it is unclear what is the timepoint at which a best response is expected to be achieved. MRD positivity following induction therapy is common; even with quadruplet therapy in the MASTER trial (Dara-KRd), the post-induction MRD negativity rates were 38% (10^{-5}) and 24% (10^{-6}).[6] This makes post-induction MRD status less attractive as a timepoint for decision-making, suggesting that the standard 4 to 6 cycles of induction therapy is a historical precedent and not substantiated by prospective clinical trials. MRD status post ASCT or following eight cycles may be more suitable; indeed, 65% achieved MRD less than 10^{-5} post-ASCT (48% at 10^{-6}) in the MASTER trial and the rate of MRD negativity has been shown to increase over time in transplant-deferred settings.[43,86]

Single-agent maintenance therapy can convert patients from an MRD-positive to MRD-negative state at a rate of 12% to 45% in the first year and 2.5% to 26% in the second year.[11,67–69,87–90] Dual maintenance therapy may be able to convert even more patients to MRD negativity and sustain it.[63,82] Thus, it is critical to characterize the kinetics of MRD for the individual patient over time rather than evaluating response at a single timepoint. Establishing MRD status at various points along the patient journey—following extended induction, ASCT, and during maintenance therapy—can provide key data points for the clinician and the patient to make the decisions that are most appropriate. Clinicians may be dissuaded from assessing MRD when asking themselves, "How will this change management?" without realizing that the trend of MRD over time carries more weight than a single moment in time. If a patient undergoes MRD testing that shows 10 cells per million, the meaning of such a result is far different if the result a year before was undetectable versus 100 cells per million. In one case, MRD resurgence has occurred and is a harbinger of disease relapse; in the other, deepening of response has occurred!

MRD resurgence from a negative state presents a unique challenge, as prevailing evidence suggests this predicts disease relapse within a short period of time.[66,67] Should these patients wait for the inevitable—progression of their disease—to occur? Or would they be benefitted from alternative therapy to attempt to re-induce MRD negativity? Chasing MRD positivity as a "myeloma thought crime" may not lead to improved outcomes and instead just introduce additional toxicities. The availability of immunotherapies such as T-cell engagers and CAR T-cell therapy hold great promise to potentially induce MRD negativity, but with tradeoffs due to toxicity. If MRD negativity at the deepest thresholds can be regularly attained and sustained with these approaches, their risk and expense might well be justified.

The introduction of peripheral blood MRD assays affords the ability to expand the frequency of testing given its convenience. As these assays become validated, it is conceivable that patients could be screened for MRD with a peripheral blood test and then undergo reflexive bone marrow MRD assessment only if found to be undetectable for disease by the former.

There is no doubt that the applications of MRD in MM will only continue to grow, and the role of MRD in decision-making will be further elucidated with time by ongoing pivotal studies. However, questions remain. Is 10^{-6} deep enough of a threshold? If not, can deeper thresholds be reliably achieved? Will MRD negativity ever serve as a valid surrogate endpoint for OS? Do attempts at driving MRD-positive disease toward MRD negativity change long-term outcomes or just increase toxicity? Will peripheral blood tests complement or supplant bone marrow evaluation? The next "season" of MRD in MM will hopefully help to answer these questions and more.

CLINICS CARE POINTS

- Measurable (minimal) residual disease (MRD) is one of the most powerful prognostic factors for progression-free survival and overall survival.

- There are several ways to assess for MRD; bone marrow methods such as next-generation sequencing and next-generation flow cytometry can achieve sensitivity thresholds of 10^{-6}.

- Each increase in MRD sensitivity threshold is associated with improved prognostication, and sustained MRD negativity carries greater significance than a single instance of MRD negativity.

- Peripheral blood techniques, chiefly mass spectrometry, to assess for MRD are quickly moving from research only to clinical use.

- MRD-adapted clinical decision-making is controversial, but there is mounting evidence that MRD-guided de-escalation of therapy is feasible and may not compromise clinical outcomes.

DISCLOSURE

B.A. Derman declares consultancy for COTA Inc, GLG Consulting, Guidepoint, Janssen, and PRECISIONheor; honoraria from the American Physician Institute, Multiple Myeloma Research Foundation, and Plexus Communications; independent clinical trial reviewer for BMS. R. Fonseca declares consultancy for AbbVie, Adaptive Biotechnologies, AMGEN, AZeneca, Bayer, Binding Site, BMS (Celgene), Millenium Takeda, Jansen, Juno, Kite, Merck, Pfizer, Pharmacyclics, Regeneron, Sanofi; scientific advisory boards for Adaptive Biotechnologies, Caris Life Sciences, Oncotracker; board of directors for Antegene, AZBio; and patents for FISH in myeloma.

REFERENCES

1. Paiva B, Cedena MT, Puig N, et al. Minimal residual disease monitoring and immune profiling in multiple myeloma in elderly patients. Blood 2016;127(25): 3165–74.

2. Lahuerta JJ, Paiva B, Vidriales MB, et al. Depth of Response in Multiple Myeloma: A Pooled Analysis of Three PETHEMA/GFM Clinical Trials. J Clin Oncol 2017; 35(25):2900–10.

3. Flores-Montero J, Sanoja-Flores L, Paiva B, et al. Next Generation Flow for highly sensitive and standardized detection of minimal residual disease in multiple myeloma. Leukemia 2017;31(10):2094–103.

4. Kumar S, Paiva B, Anderson KC, et al. International Myeloma Working Group consensus criteria for response and minimal residual disease assessment in multiple myeloma. Lancet Oncol 2016;17(8):e328–46.

5. Yanamandra U, Kumar SK. Minimal residual disease analysis in myeloma – when, why and where. Leuk Lymphoma 2017;1–13. https://doi.org/10.1080/10428194. 2017.1386304.

6. Costa LJ, Chhabra S, Medvedova E, et al. Daratumumab, Carfilzomib, Lenalidomide, and Dexamethasone With Minimal Residual Disease Response-Adapted Therapy in Newly Diagnosed Multiple Myeloma. J Clin Orthod 2021. https://doi. org/10.1200/JCO.21.01935. JCO.21.01935.

7. Adaptive Biotechnologies Corporation. clonoSEQ Assay Technical Information. Available at: https://www.clonoseq.com/sites/default/files/clonoSEQ_TechnicalInformation Summary_21Sept2018.pdf. Accessed February 10, 2020.

8. Attal M, Lauwers-Cances V, Hulin C, et al. Lenalidomide, Bortezomib, and Dexamethasone with Transplantation for Myeloma. N Engl J Med 2017;376(14): 1311–20.

9. Martinez-Lopez J, Lahuerta JJ, Pepin F, et al. Prognostic value of deep sequencing method for minimal residual disease detection in multiple myeloma. Blood 2014;123(20):3073–9.

10. Avet-Loiseau H, Lauwers-Cances V, Corre J, et al. Minimal Residual Disease in Multiple Myeloma: Final Analysis of the IFM2009 Trial. Blood 2017;130(Suppl 1):435.

11. Perrot A, Lauwers-Cances V, Corre J, et al. Minimal residual disease negativity using deep sequencing is a major prognostic factor in multiple myeloma. Blood 2018;132(23):2456–64.

12. Moreau P, Attal M, Caillot D, et al. Prospective Evaluation of Magnetic Resonance Imaging and [18F]Fluorodeoxyglucose Positron Emission Tomography-Computed Tomography at Diagnosis and Before Maintenance Therapy in Symptomatic Patients With Multiple Myeloma Included in the IFM/DFCI 2009 Trial: Results of the IMAJEM Study. J Clin Oncol 2017;35(25):2911–8.

13. Zamagni E, Oliva S, Gay F, et al. Impact of minimal residual disease standardised assessment by FDG-PET/CT in transplant-eligible patients with newly diagnosed multiple myeloma enrolled in the imaging sub-study of the FORTE trial. eClinicalMedicine 2023;60. https://doi.org/10.1016/j.eclinm.2023.102017.

14. Kraeber-Bodéré F, Zweegman S, Perrot A, et al. Prognostic value of positron emission tomography/computed tomography in transplant-eligible newly diagnosed multiple myeloma patients from CASSIOPEIA: the CASSIOPET study. Haematologica 2023;108(2):621–6.

15. Fonseca R, Arribas M, Wiedmeier-Nutor JE, et al. Integrated analysis of next generation sequencing minimal residual disease (MRD) and PET scan in transplant eligible myeloma patients. Blood Cancer J 2023;13(1):1–9.

16. Rasche L, Angtuaco E, McDonald JE, et al. Low expression of hexokinase-2 is associated with false-negative FDG-positron emission tomography in multiple myeloma. Blood 2017;130(1):30–4.

17. Sachpekidis C, Mosebach J, Freitag MT, et al. Application of (18)F-FDG PET and diffusion weighted imaging (DWI) in multiple myeloma: comparison of functional imaging modalities. Am J Nucl Med Mol Imaging 2015;5(5):479–92.

18. Kaiser MF, Porta N, Sharma B, et al. Prospective comparison of whole body MRI and FDG PET/CT for detection of multiple myeloma and correlation with markers of disease burden: Results of the iTIMM trial. J Clin Orthod 2021;39(15_suppl): 8012.

19. Sanoja-Flores L, Flores-Montero J, Garcés JJ, et al. Next generation flow for minimally-invasive blood characterization of MGUS and multiple myeloma at diagnosis based on circulating tumor plasma cells (CTPC). Blood Cancer J 2018;8(12):117.

20. Garcés JJ, Cedena MT, Puig N, et al. Circulating Tumor Cells for the Staging of Patients With Newly Diagnosed Transplant-Eligible Multiple Myeloma. J Clin Oncol 2022;40(27):3151–61.

21. Jelinek T, Bezdekova R, Zihala D, et al. More Than 2% of Circulating Tumor Plasma Cells Defines Plasma Cell Leukemia–Like Multiple Myeloma. J Clin Orthod 2023;41(7):1383–92.

22. Bertamini L, Oliva S, Rota-Scalabrini D, et al. High Levels of Circulating Tumor Plasma Cells as a Key Hallmark of Aggressive Disease in Transplant-Eligible

Patients With Newly Diagnosed Multiple Myeloma. J Clin Oncol 2022;40(27): 3120–31.

23. Sanoja-Flores L, Flores-Montero J, Puig N, et al. Blood monitoring of circulating tumor plasma cells by next generation flow in multiple myeloma after therapy. Blood 2019;134(24):2218–22.

24. Notarfranchi L, Zherniakova A, Lasa M, et al. Ultra-Sensitive Assessment of Measurable Residual Disease (MRD) in Peripheral Blood (PB) of Multiple Myeloma (MM) Patients Using Bloodflow. Blood 2022;140(Supplement 1): 2095–7.

25. Vij R, Mazumder A, Klinger M, et al. Deep sequencing reveals myeloma cells in peripheral blood in majority of multiple myeloma patients. Clin Lymphoma Myeloma Leuk 2014;14(2):131–9.e1.

26. Mazzotti C, Buisson L, Maheo S, et al. Myeloma MRD by deep sequencing from circulating tumor DNA does not correlate with results obtained in the bone marrow. Blood Advances 2018;2(21):2811–3.

27. Dhakal B, Sharma S, Balcioglu M, et al. Assessment of Molecular Residual Disease Using Circulating Tumor DNA to Identify Multiple Myeloma Patients at High Risk of Relapse. Front Oncol 2022;12:786451.

31. Thoren KL. Mass spectrometry methods for detecting monoclonal immunoglobulins in multiple myeloma minimal residual disease. Semin Hematol 2018; 55(1):41–3.

32. Kohlhagen MC, Barnidge DR, Mills JR, et al. Screening Method for M-Proteins in Serum Using Nanobody Enrichment Coupled to MALDI-TOF Mass Spectrometry. Clin Chem 2016;62(10):1345–52.

33. Mills JR, Kohlhagen MC, Dasari S, et al. Comprehensive Assessment of M-Proteins Using Nanobody Enrichment Coupled to MALDI-TOF Mass Spectrometry. Clin Chem 2016;62(10):1334–44.

34. Kohlhagen M, Dasari S, Willrich M, et al. Automation and validation of a MALDI-TOF MS (Mass-Fix) replacement of immunofixation electrophoresis in the clinical lab. Clin Chem Lab Med 2020;59(1):155–63.

35. Barnidge DR, Dasari S, Botz CM, et al. Using Mass Spectrometry to Monitor Monoclonal Immunoglobulins in Patients with a Monoclonal Gammopathy. J Proteome Res 2014;13(3):1419–27.

36. Zajec M, Langerhorst P, VanDuijn MM, et al. Mass Spoctrometry for Identification, Monitoring, and Minimal Residual Disease Detection of M-Proteins. Clin Chem 2020;66(3):421–33.

37. Li K, Barnidge D, Krevvata M, et al. Comparison of the Analytical Performance of EXENT®, a Mass Spectrometry-Based Assessment of M-Protein, to SPEP and NGS-Based MRD in Multiple Myeloma Patient Samples. Blood 2022; 140(Supplement 1):12446–7.

38. Barnidge DR, Krick TP, Griffin TJ, et al. Using matrix-assisted laser desorption/ionization time-of-flight mass spectrometry to detect monoclonal immunoglobulin light chains in serum and urine. Rapid Commun Mass Spectrom 2015;29(21): 2057–60.

39. Eveillard M, Rustad E, Roshal M, et al. Comparison of MALDI-TOF mass spectrometry analysis of peripheral blood and bone marrow-based flow cytometry for tracking measurable residual disease in patients with multiple myeloma. Br J Haematol 2020;189(5):904–7.

40. Puig N, Agulló C, Contreras Sanfeliciano T, et al. Clinical Impact of Next Generation Flow in Bone Marrow Vs Qip-Mass Spectrometry in Peripheral Blood to Assess Minimal Residual Disease in Newly Diagnosed Multiple Myeloma Patients

Receiving Maintenance As Part of the GEM2014MAIN Trial. Blood 2022; 140(Supplement 1):2098–100.

41. Derman BA, Stefka AT, Jiang K, et al. Measurable residual disease assessed by mass spectrometry in peripheral blood in multiple myeloma in a phase II trial of carfilzomib, lenalidomide, dexamethasone and autologous stem cell transplantation. Blood Cancer J 2021;11(2):1–4.

42. Puig N, Contreras Sanfeliciano T, Paiva B, et al. Assessment of Treatment Response By Ife, Next Generation Flow Cytometry and Mass Spectrometry Coupled with Liquid Chromatography in the GEM2012MENOS65 Clinical Trial. Blood 2021;138(Supplement 1):544.

43. Derman BA, Kansagra A, Zonder J, et al. Elotuzumab and Weekly Carfilzomib, Lenalidomide, and Dexamethasone in Patients With Newly Diagnosed Multiple Myeloma Without Transplant Intent: A Phase 2 Measurable Residual Disease–Adapted Study. JAMA Oncol 2022;8(9):1278–86.

44. Liyasova M, McDonald Z, Taylor P, et al. A Personalized Mass Spectrometry-Based Assay to Monitor M-Protein in Patients with Multiple Myeloma (EasyM). Clin Cancer Res 2021;27(18):5028–37.

45. McDonald Z, Taylor P, Liyasova M, et al. Mass Spectrometry Provides a Highly Sensitive Noninvasive Means of Sequencing and Tracking M-Protein in the Blood of Multiple Myeloma Patients. J Proteome Res 2021;20(8):4176–85.

46. Bonifay V, Vimard V, Noori S, et al. P10 AN ULTRA-SENSITIVE METHOD FOR SEQUENCING AND MONITORING OF M-PROTEIN IN PERIPHERAL BLOOD (M-INSIGHT). HemaSphere 2023;7(S2):15.

47. Slade MJ, Khalid A, Fiala MA, et al. Clonotypic Mass Spectrometry with Easym Assay for Detection of Measurable Residual Disease in Multiple Myeloma. Blood 2022;140(Supplement 1):4376–7.

48. Noori S, Wijnands C, Langerhorst P, et al. Dynamic monitoring of myeloma minimal residual disease with targeted mass spectrometry. Blood Cancer J 2023; 13(1):1–3.

49. Kendrick F, Harding S, Chappell MJ, et al. Immunoglobulin G (IgG) and neonatal Fc-receptor (FcRn) dynamics in IgG multiple myeloma**Felicity Kendrick is a member of the Midlands Integrative Bio- sciences Training Partnership funded by the Biotechnology and Bi-ological Sciences Research Council (BBSRC). IFAC-PapersOnLine 2015;48(20):106–11.

50. Kendrick F, Evans ND, Arnulf B, et al. Analysis of a Compartmental Model of Endogenous Immunoglobulin G Metabolism with Application to Multiple Myeloma. Front Physiol 2017;8:149.

51. van de Velde HJK, Liu X, Chen G, et al. Complete response correlates with long-term survival and progression-free survival in high-dose therapy in multiple myeloma. Haematologica 2007;92(10):1399–406.

52. Gay F, Larocca A, Wijermans P, et al. Complete response correlates with long-term progression-free and overall survival in elderly myeloma treated with novel agents: analysis of 1175 patients. Blood 2011;117(11):3025–31.

53. Lahuerta JJ, Mateos MV, Martínez-López J, et al. Influence of pre- and post-transplantation responses on outcome of patients with multiple myeloma: sequential improvement of response and achievement of complete response are associated with longer survival. J Clin Oncol 2008;26(35):5775–82.

54. Martínez-López J, Paiva B, López-Anglada L, et al. Critical analysis of the stringent complete response in multiple myeloma: contribution of sFLC and bone marrow clonality. Blood 2015;126(7):858–62.

55. Cedena MT, Martin-Clavero E, Wong S, et al. The clinical significance of stringent complete response in multiple myeloma is surpassed by minimal residual disease measurements. PLoS One 2020;15(8):e0237155.

56. Jiménez Ubieto A, Paiva B, Puig N, et al. Validation of the IMWG standard response criteria in the PETHEMA/GEM2012MENOS65 study: are these times of change? Blood 2021. https://doi.org/10.1182/blood.2021012319. blood.2021012319.

57. Munshi NC, Avet-Loiseau H, Rawstron AC, et al. Association of Minimal Residual Disease With Superior Survival Outcomes in Patients With Multiple Myeloma: A Meta-analysis. JAMA Oncol 2017;3(1):28.

58. Munshi NC, Avet-Loiseau H, Anderson KC, et al. A large meta-analysis establishes the role of MRD negativity in long-term survival outcomes in patients with multiple myeloma. Blood Advances 2020;4(23):5988–99.

59. Bansal R, Baksh M, Larsen JT, et al. Prognostic value of early bone marrow MRD status in CAR-T therapy for myeloma. Blood Cancer J 2023;13(1):1–5.

60. Paiva B, Manrique I, Rytlewski J, et al. Time-dependent prognostic value of serological and measurable residual disease assessments after idecabtagene vicleucel. Blood Cancer Discovery 2023. https://doi.org/10.1158/2643-3230.BCD-23-0044. BCD-23-0044.

61. Martin T, Usmani SZ, Berdeja JG, et al. Ciltacabtagene Autoleucel, an Anti–B-cell Maturation Antigen Chimeric Antigen Receptor T-Cell Therapy, for Relapsed/Refractory Multiple Myeloma: CARTITUDE-1 2-Year Follow-Up. JCO 2022. https://doi.org/10.1200/JCO.22.00842. JCO.22.00842.

62. Lin Y, Martin TG, Usmani SZ, et al. CARTITUDE-1 final results: Phase 1b/2 study of ciltacabtagene autoleucel in heavily pretreated patients with relapsed/refractory multiple myeloma. J Clin Orthod 2023;41(16_suppl):8009.

63. Gay F, Musto P, Rota-Scalabrini D, et al. Carfilzomib with cyclophosphamide and dexamethasone or lenalidomide and dexamethasone plus autologous transplantation or carfilzomib plus lenalidomide and dexamethasone, followed by maintenance with carfilzomib plus lenalidomide or lenalidomide alone for patients with newly diagnosed multiple myeloma (FORTE): a randomised, open-label, phase 2 trial. Lancet Oncol 2021;22(12):1705–20.

64. San-Miguel J, Avet-Loiseau H, Paiva B, et al. Sustained minimal residual disease negativity in newly diagnosed multiple myeloma and the impact of daratumumab in MAIA and ALCYONE. Blood 2022;139(4):492–501.

65. Avet-Loiseau H, San-Miguel J, Casneuf T, et al. Evaluation of Sustained Minimal Residual Disease Negativity With Daratumumab-Combination Regimens in Relapsed and/or Refractory Multiple Myeloma: Analysis of POLLUX and CASTOR. J Clin Oncol 2021;39(10):1139–49.

66. Mohan M, Kendrick S, Szabo A, et al. Clinical implications of loss of bone marrow minimal residual disease negativity in multiple myeloma. Blood Advances 2022; 6(3):808–17.

67. Diamond B, Korde N, Lesokhin AM, et al. Dynamics of minimal residual disease in patients with multiple myeloma on continuous lenalidomide maintenance: a single-arm, single-centre, phase 2 trial. The Lancet Haematology 2021;8(6): e422–32.

68. Paiva B, Manrique I, Dimopoulos MA, et al. MRD dynamics during maintenance for improved prognostication of 1280 patients with myeloma in the TOURMALINE-MM3 and -MM4 trials. Blood 2023;141(6):579–91.

69. Oliva S, Genuardi E, Paris L, et al. Prospective evaluation of minimal residual disease in the phase II FORTE trial: a head-to-head comparison between

multiparameter flow cytometry and next-generation sequencing. eClinicalMedicine 2023;60.

70. Costa LJ, Derman BA, Bal S, et al. International harmonization in performing and reporting minimal residual disease assessment in multiple myeloma trials. Leukemia 2021;35(1):18–30.

71. Derman BA, Major A, Major S, et al. Prospective Trial Using Multimodal Measurable Residual Disease Negativity to Guide Discontinuation of Maintenance Therapy in Multiple Myeloma (MRD2STOP). Blood 2022;140(Supplement 1):2108–9.

72. Dispenzieri A, Krishnan A, Arendt B, et al. Mass-Fix better predicts for PFS and OS than standard methods among multiple myeloma patients participating on the STAMINA trial (BMT CTN 0702/07LT). Blood Cancer J 2022;12(2):1–8.

73. Claveau JS, Murray DL, Dispenzieri A, et al. Value of bone marrow examination in determining response to therapy in patients with multiple myeloma in the context of mass spectrometry-based M-protein assessment. Leukemia 2023;37(1):1–4.

74. Buyse M, Molenberghs G, Burzykowski T, et al. The validation of surrogate endpoints in meta-analyses of randomized experiments. Biostatistics 2000;1(1): 49–67.

75. Etekal T, Koehn K, Sborov DW, et al. Time-to-event surrogate end-points in multiple myeloma randomised trials from 2005 to 2019: A surrogacy analysis. Br J Haematol 2023;200(5):587–94.

76. Xie W, Halabi S, Tierney JF, et al. A Systematic Review and Recommendation for Reporting of Surrogate Endpoint Evaluation Using Meta-analyses. JNCI Cancer Spectr 2019;3(1):kz002.

77. Paiva B, Zherniakova A, Nuñez-Córdoba JM, et al. Impact of treatment effect on MRD and PFS: an aggregate analysis from randomized clinical trials in multiple myeloma. Blood Adv 2023;1, bloodadvances.202301082.

78. Costa LJ, Chhabra S, Medvedova E, et al. Minimal residual disease response-adapted therapy in newly diagnosed multiple myeloma (MASTER): final report of the multicentre, single-arm, phase 2 trial. Lancet Haematol 2023;10(11): e890–901.

79. Research C for DE and. Hematologic Malignancies: Regulatory Considerations for Use of Minimal Residual Disease in Development of Drug and Biological Products for Treatment. U.S. Food and Drug Administration. Published January 24, 2020. Available at: https://www.fda.gov/regulatory-information/search-fda-guidance-documents/hematologic-malignancies-regulatory-considerations-use-minimal-residual-disease-development-drug-and. Accessed June 30, 2023.

80. Dhakal B, Usmani S. Daratumumab and Lenalidomide Maintenance Guided by Minimal Residual Disease in Multiple Myeloma. The Hematologist 2021;18(6). https://doi.org/10.1182/hem.V18.6.202166.

82. Dytfeld D, Wróbel T, Jamroziak K, et al. Carfilzomib, lenalidomide, and dexamethasone or lenalidomide alone as maintenance therapy after autologous stem-cell transplantation in patients with multiple myeloma (ATLAS): interim analysis of a randomised, open-label, phase 3 trial. Lancet Oncol 2023;24(2):139–50.

83. Correia N, Dowling E, Popat R, et al. Functional and psychological impact of minimal residual disease assessment on patients with multiple myeloma. Br J Haematol 2023. https://doi.org/10.1111/bjh.18948.

84. Derman BA, Jakubowiak AJ, Thompson MA. Clinician survey regarding measurable residual disease-guided decision-making in multiple myeloma. Blood Cancer J 2022;12(7):108.

85. Martinez-Lopez J, Alonso R, Wong SW, et al. Making clinical decisions based on measurable residual disease improves the outcome in multiple myeloma. J Hematol Oncol 2021;14(1):126.
86. Derman BA, Major A, Rosenblatt J, et al. A Phase 2 Study of Extended Daratumumab, Carfilzomib, Lenalidomide, and Dexamethasone in Newly Diagnosed Multiple Myeloma. Blood 2021;138(Supplement 1):2759.
87. de Tute RM, Pawlyn C, Cairns DA, et al. Minimal Residual Disease After Autologous Stem-Cell Transplant for Patients With Myeloma: Prognostic Significance and the Impact of Lenalidomide Maintenance and Molecular Risk. J Clin Orthod 2022;40(25):2889–900.
88. Alonso R, Cedena MT, Wong S, et al. Prolonged lenalidomide maintenance therapy improves the depth of response in multiple myeloma. Blood Advances 2020; 4(10):2163–71.
89. Hahn TE, Wallace PK, Fraser R, et al. Minimal Residual Disease (MRD) Assessment before and after Autologous Hematopoietic Cell Transplantation (AutoHCT) and Maintenance for Multiple Myeloma (MM): Results of the Prognostic Immunophenotyping for Myeloma Response (PRIMeR) Study. Biol Blood Marrow Transplant 2019;25(3):S4–6.
90. Paiva B, Puig N, Cedena MT, et al. Measurable Residual Disease by Next-Generation Flow Cytometry in Multiple Myeloma. J Clin Orthod 2019. https://doi.org/10.1200/JCO.19.01231. JCO.19.01231.

Approach to High-Risk Multiple Myeloma

Xiaoyi Chen, MD, PhD, Gaurav Varma, MD, Faith Davies, MD,
Gareth Morgan, MB BCh, PhD*

KEYWORDS

- High-risk • Aggressive • Myeloma • Biology • Genetics • Treatment • Guidance

KEY POINTS

- Aggressive clinical behavior in myeloma, high-risk multiple myeloma (HRMM), has proven difficult to treat with only a limited impact of the treatments developed in the last 2 decades.
- Only a limited number of genetic groups make up the majority of cases with HRMM. The size of the HRMM group increases with each relapse, making it a significant clinical problem.
- Risk-stratified treatment and focused clinical trials for HRMM are now possible, with single-arm phase II designs being typical
- Eradicating detectable disease using sensitive testing strategies is a key to improving long-term outcome for HRMM. One way of achieving this is to integrate immunotherapeutic agents into clinical treatment combinations.
- A concerted effort to understand the biology underlying aggressive clinical behavior and the systematic use of this knowledge to design and evaluate therapeutic strategies are likely to improve outcomes of HRMM over the next decade.

INTRODUCTION

Clinical experience of treating multiple myeloma (MM) with different strategies has led to the fundamental understanding that a subgroup of cases is associated with adverse outcomes.[1,2] The comparison of the impact of treatment on this group of high-risk MM (HRMM) compared to cases with standard risk features has shown a less significant impact of treatment, forcing a consideration of how to specifically treat and improve the outcome of this group of cases which has a distinct clinical course and biology.[3]

Center Blood Cancer, Perlmutter Cancer Center, New York University, NYCLangone, Room# 496, Medical Science Building 4th Floor, 540 1st Avenue, New York, NY 10016, USA
* Corresponding author.
E-mail address: Gareth.morgan@NYULangone.org

Hematol Oncol Clin N Am 38 (2024) 497–510
https://doi.org/10.1016/j.hoc.2023.12.008
0889-8588/24/© 2023 Elsevier Inc. All rights reserved.

hemonc.theclinics.com

THE CLINICAL PROBLEM ASSOCIATED WITH HIGH-RISK MYELOMA

The analysis of cases with early relapse after autologous stem cell transplant, the presence of extra-medullary disease, plasma cell leukemia, large focal lesions in the bone marrow and either primary refractoriness to treatment or short response duration with relapse occurring within 12 to 18 months identified a group of cases, HRMM, characterized by adverse cytogenetic features and poor survival .[2,4–6] The group of HRMM is a significant clinical problem with up to 20% to 30% of cases of newly diagnosed multiple melanomas (NDMMs) falling into this group.[7–9] The size of the group increases at each relapse, with cases often relapsing with high-risk clinical or cytogenetic features.[10] Overall HRMM constitutes a large unmet clinical need for which a solution is required. In order to address this unmet need and to improve communication, recent clinical work has focused on the generation of consensus definitions of the HR group.[8,9,11] Further, to address the clinical problem of HRMM, it is important to move toward a risk-stratified trial approach, as the therapy for this group is likely to require different approaches to cases with standard-risk biology. As the therapeutic tool box has expanded over time, optimizing therapy for HRMM using a risk-stratified trial approach has become a clinical reality.

CONCEPTUALLY WHAT IS HIGH-RISK MYELOMA, AND HOW SHOULD IT BE ADDRESSED THERAPEUTICALLY?

In order to treat HRMM effectively, it is crucial to understand how it develops and the drivers of the clinical stages leading to it. The progression of monoclonal gammopathy of unknown significance (MGUS) through smoldering multiple myeloma (SMM) to MM and HRMM occurs via a process that involves the co-evolution of the plasma cell clone with its bone marrow microenvironment.[12,13] Acquired genetic features in the clonal plasma cells are the main drivers of progression, but it is recognized that there is a complex interplay between these drivers and the exhaustion of effective immune editing that acts to control disease progression. Even at the earliest precursor stage, genomic analysis demonstrates significant subclonal heterogeneity, which provides an essential substrate for Darwinian-based disease evolution. Phylogenetic reconstruction of the clone has shown that there are up to 5 to 6 major myeloma subclones and branching evolutionary changes are typical.[14,15] To deal with this disease complexity, therapeutic strategies need to be built based on the induction of deep responses with treatment and addressing the multiple levels of sensitivity and resistance to therapy seen in such diverse subclonal populations of cells.

CYTOGENETIC MARKERS OF HIGH-RISK DISEASE

The use of metaphase cytogenetics and then the widespread application of interphase fluorescence in situ hybridization (FISH) led to the identification of a range of molecular markers associated with HRMM. Classifications of MM divide it into at least 6 subgroups, each with a distinct biology and outcome based on the cytogenetic abnormalities they carry and the expression of a D group cyclin.[16] The cytogenetic groups identified include hyperdiploidy, where there are 3 copies of the odd-numbered chromosomes and the translocation subtypes t(11;14), t(4;14), t(14;16), or t(14;20).[17,18] These recurrent translocations involve structural variants at the immunoglobulin gene enhancers, where an oncogene is placed under the influence of a strong enhancer, leading to its deregulated expression and the initiation of the disease. HR is an acquired abnormality that can occur in any of the etiologic subgroups of MM;

it is more frequent with some of the subgroups but predominantly falls into a limited number of etiologic groups including predominantly the t(4;14), t(14;16).[12,19]

PROGNOSTIC SCORING SYSTEMS
International Staging System

Many different prognostic scores and markers have been proposed to capture MM heterogeneity and stratify NDMM patients, for example, International Staging System (ISS), Revised ISS (R-ISS) and Second Revision ISS (R2-ISS).[8,9,11] These prognostic scores have been built by integrating cytogenetic features into the ISS. However, despite some improvements, there remains considerable patient-to-patient variability within individual risk groups. To date, these scores have rarely influenced clinical or personalized therapeutic decisions and merely define the relative risk of either progression or death for a group of patients with similar features (ie, high, moderate, low risk). A comparison of the different risk groups identified using the different risk stratification tools shows that they identify a variable proportion of HRMM. All of them are characterized by a failure to identify the entirety of the HRMM group, with a variable proportion falling into the low-/intermediate-risk groups. Given what is known about genetic mutations and their frequency, it is clear that no single marker other than chromothripsis can enhance current prognostic systems because of either their frequency or penetrance.[20,21]

Proliferative Multiple Myeloma

Gene expression-based scores such as the GEP70 can effectively identify a group of 12% to 15% of cases with HRMM.[22] These scores are effective and correlate with adverse outcome but do not define its biology. Despite widespread evaluation and having been shown to be effective, the widespread application of such scores has not proven to be taken up in the clinical environment. The proliferative MM (PR) group is of significant size and is an important acquired feature.

Double-Hit Multiple Myeloma

The first recognition of a double-hit group of HRMM recognized that the cosegregation of the adverse translocations and adverse copy number abnormalities (CNAs) increased the adverse prognostic risk.[23] A subsequent comprehensive analysis of whole-exome mutation data showed that 2 major groups contributed to HRMM including biallelic inactivation of P53 and ISS III with gain/amp 1q.[24] While only identifying 8% of all cases, the associated outcome was extremely poor. The value of the double-hit concept was shown again recently on the myeloma XI trial set, where it proved to be a simple and reliable way to identify HRMM.[25,26] Patients who lacked any of the adverse genetic markers and were less than 65 years of age had an extremely good outcome and could be considered as low risk. A key group to disentangle is the residual intermediate-risk group cases.

An all molecular classifier of Multiple Myeloma IRMMa

Using clustering and hierarchical dirichlet processes approaches applied to a large clinical series with whole-exome sequencing, an all-genomic approach to the classification of MM has been developed. A key feature of this approach has been to move away from a single gene classifier to an approach identifying broad groups of cases such as those with complex genetics that could be used to effectively assign risk. Advances in machine learning that take into account tumor-specific treatment and response data have been used to explore the same data set and identified a prognostic approach named IRMMa, which outperforms other scores and can predict response to a specific therapy such as transplant (Maura and colleagues, JCO in press). Approaches such as this are likely to be more generally applied as data sets accrue overtime.

Imaging

Functional imaging, such as positron emission tomography-computed tomography (PET-CT) or diffusion weighted MRI allow the identification of patients with BM abnormalities such as focal lesions.[27–29] These features have been incorporated into the definitions of MM, moving some cases out of the smoldering group to MM (more than a single FL) and defining cases with HR behavior (more than 3 FL).[30–32]

BIOLOGIC, GENETIC, AND EPIGENETIC FEATURES OF HIGH RISK

MM is initiated by either a chromosomal translocation or hyperdiploidy with an excess of t(4;14), t(14;16), and t(MYC) in HRMM.[12,33] The progression of the MGUS stage to HRMM is based on the acquisition of mutations in disease driver genes that result in the biologic features of an increased proliferation rate, resistance to apoptosis, and focal and bone marrow-independent growth. These mutations include single nucleotide variants (SNV), structural variants, and CNAs.[34] As these variants are largely acquired independently and some give rise to a survival benefit, progression is associated with multiple subclones within the single initiated clone. The diversity within the clone increases as it progresses, and it behaves as a complex biological system that is difficult to fully eradicate with treatment.[10] An important component of HRMM is the development of bone marrow independent growth that allows subclones to escape the bone marrow into the organs and peripheral blood. At least in part, mutations in the RAS/MAPK and NFkB pathways allow this by providing constitutive signaling through these pathways and as such constitute good therapeutic targets.[35,36] A further key biological feature of HRMM is bi-allelic inactivation of P53 and G1S cell cycle deregulation.[37,38] Clinical series suggest that most HR cases fall within the group defined by a t(4;14), t(14;16), gain 1q, del 17p or the proliferative group defined by the UAMS classifier.[18] It is, therefore, important to fully understand the biology and vulnerabilities imposed by these specific subsets if HRMM is to be treated effectively.

t(4;14), NSD2 and Epigenetic Change

The t(4;14) (p16;q32) occurs in approximately 10% to 15% of MM patients and results in a histone methyltransferase NSD2 and a tyrosine kinase FGFR3 being upregulated, with NSD2 being thought the be the key driver gene.[33,39] Cases with this translocation are associated with clinically aggressive disease in 40% of cases. Importantly, NSD2 is a member of a family of epigenetically active SET oncogenes that are upregulated in several aggressive cancers including pediatric ALL and ovarian cancer.[40,41] NSD2 encodes a histone methyl transferase that deposits the H3K36me2 marks on actively transcribed genes, with high levels of expression only being seen in the t(4;14) subtype of MM.[42] Currently it is thought that NSD2 expression results in the epigenetic reprogramming of the MM cells by altering the balance of H3K36 and H3K27 methylation leading to altered adhesion, enhanced growth, increased cell survival, and genetic instability.

Several gene variants suggest an epigenetic basis for HRMM.[43,44] Mutations are seen in several genes but have little relevance to HR. NSD2 is epigenetically active and has been discussed in detail. High expression of EZH2 is associated with poor prognosis as is expression of PHF19, focusing attention on the role played by the

PRC2 complex.[45,46] The expression of *PHF19* increases with increasing disease stage and during the progression from the premalignant stages MGUS to MM, with the highest *PHF19* expression being seen in PCL. Overall, data from different cell-context and experimental studies strongly implicates PHF19 in the regulation of genes important in cell cycle regulation and the genetic stability of cancer cells, making it highly relevant to the biology of HR MM.[47,48]

t(14;16) and maf

The t(14;16) is present in less than 5% of NDMM and is associated with HRMM in some 50% of cases.[49] The t(14;16) deregulates maf, an oncogenic transcription factor, and is associated with a hyper-APOBEC mutational signature.[50,51]

t(MYC)

Most cell MM lines carry an *MYC* abnormality, and translocations to the MYC locus at 8q24 are common in clinical samples.[52,53] Although primary Ig translocations to MYC are relatively rare, as the disease progresses, secondary translocations to *MYC* using alternate superenhancers become more common (up to 40% of hyperdiploid MM) and seem to be associated with adverse outcomes.[54–56]

Mutational Drivers and APOBEC

Taking mutations as a whole, there are 7 main mutational signatures in MM, including 2 age-related signatures, SBS1 and SBS5.[57–59] SBS9 reflects adenine-induced DNA deaminase (AID) activity in the germinal center.[51] Two APOBEC signatures are associated with the t(14;16) (IGH;MAF) subgroup and with poor prognosis.[60] The 2 remaining signatures SBS8 and SBS18 are of unknown function or potentially associated with oxygen radical exposure or homologous recombination.[61] The prevalence of each signature varies among patients in absolute and relative contribution. All patients have evidence of AID and/or APOBEC activity, consistent with an important role for inflammatory states and germinal center mutational processes in the evolution to HRMM.[62] It has been suggested that the presence of an APOBEC signature is associated with genetic complexity and proliferation and is a signature associated with progression of SMM to MM and with HRMM.[50]

Structural Variation

An important role for simple and complex structural variants (SVs) and CNAs in the progression to HRMM has been noted.[63] Whole-genome sequencing has identified a role for 3 complex structural events: chromothripsis, chromoplexy, and templated insertion chains (TIC) in MM, of which chromothripsis plays a key role in HRMM.[20] Chromosomal translocations to *MYC* at 8q24 are also key features of HRMM.[54]

Copy Number Change on Chromosome 1

Chr1 is a key driver of aggressive clinical behavior, with gain(1q) being seen in 40% of cases, and amplification (>3 copies) seen in 10% of cases.[64–66] The chr1 centromere is prone to arm-length chromosomal rearrangements. Consistent with a driver role for chr1q, fewer events are seen in smoldering MM compared with NDMM, and analysis of paired presentation-relapse samples shows that 13% to 19% of patients acquire a gain(1q) at relapse.[67] Complicating prognostic assessment, gain(1q) is not evenly distributed through the molecular subgroups of MM with an association with the t(4;14), t(14;16), del(13), and del(17p), and the expression of CCND2. Change in expression of genes on chr1 is frequent, with up to 30% of the genes making up the GEP70 being on the long and short arms of chr1.[22] Previous studies have identified several regions associated with changes in gene expression, including 1p32, the site of *CDKN2C/FAF1*; 1p12, the site of *TENT5C;* and 1p22.1, the site of *RPL5/EVI5*.[68–70] At 1q12 to 21, potential drivers include *CKS1B, PDZK1, BCL9, ANP32 E, ILF2, ADAR, MDM2,* and *MCL1*.[23,71–75] The region of copy number gain at 1q21.1-1q25.2 can be separated into at least 6 distinct hotspots rather than being a single homogeneous region as has been implied previously. Multiple potential novel driver genes have been identified at 1q21.1, including *SLAMF7, MCL1, SETDB1, S100A4, NOTCH2NL,* and *BGLAP*.[76] It is likely that that multiple transcriptional units located at more than 1 region of chr1 provide a strong selective advantage that is crucial to MM pathogenesis rather than there being a single candidate gene that drives progression. In terms of the definition of HRMM, co-occurrence of 1q+ with another HR molecular abnormality or ISSIII is crucial.

Deletion of the Short Arm of Chromosome 17

Deletion of the short arm of chromosome 17 (17p-) because of P53 inactivation is a recurrent feature of HRMM.[77] It has become clear that the size of the subclone carrying the abnormality is important for the definition of HRMM, with a cut point of 50% or higher being key to defining a very poor outcome.[78,79] A further important feature is bi-allelic inactivation of P53, with loss of copy number on 1 allele and mutation of the other allele being critical.[38,80]

THE HIGH-RISK MICROENVIRONMENT

Although much of the focus of disease progression in HRMM has focused been on genetic drivers in the clonal plasma cells, it is now clear that the clone evolves in the context of the bone marrow microenvironment. In normal plasma cell development, plasmablasts exit the GC and home to the BM plasma-cell niche, where they gain survival signals from the niche.[81,82] The availability of specialized niches likely restricts growth of the MM clone in its early stages, and the clonal plasma cells expand the niche, increasing its capacity to support their expansion. An intricate network of endothelial, perivascular, mesenchymal stem cells (MSCs), osteoclasts, and immune cells constitute the niche.[83] Survival signals include cell extrinsic signals from cytokines including interleukin-6 (IL6) and BCMA/APRIL/BLyS, integrins such as LFA4 and VLA4 together with chemokines such as CXCL12.[84–86] Acquired mutations in the clone, such as those in the NFkB, RAS/MAPK pathway, and structural variants to MYC provide likely independence from these niches as the clone moves toward plasma cell leukemia. Flow cytometry, RNA expression analysis and single-cell RNA-seq have identified multiple changes in the immune microenvironment associated with disease progression.[87,88] In MGUS, there is little evidence of immune dysregulation, with normal numbers of innate and adaptive immune populations. In SMM, although is more heterogeneity in these immune populations, the overall content of the microenvironment is still largely preserved. At the MM stage, however, there is considerable variation, with clusters of cases being defined by the loss of CD4 T central memory and effector populations and B-cell subsets.[87] Analyses of the microenvironment in the context of therapy have suggested the microenvironment exerts important effects on treatment response, especially for immune therapies with monocytes, NK-cells, T-cells and B-cell depletion appearing to be important.[89]

THERAPEUTIC CONSIDERATIONS

A key approach for the treatment of HRMM is to induce deep MRD-negative responses. Despite the recognition of the mutational signatures driven by melphalan that could drive progression/relapse, high-dose melphalan and autologous stem cell transplantation remain a mainstay of therapy. Inducing deep remissions before transplant is important; therefore, 4-drug combinations given to maximum response that incorporate anti-CD38 monoclonal antibody are currently central to optimized treatment strategies.[90–92] The application of bi-specific antibodies and Car-T therapies that are associated with high response rates in RRMM open the way for their inclusion into induction regimens to increase the number and depth of responses. Based on current outcomes in RRMM, even with these agents the used in combination, it is likely that cases will still relapse. These agents impact the recovery of B-cell numbers after treatment and the chances of infection but these can be readily managed in the clinic.

To date, few risk-stratified trials have been carried out in MM. The most important series of cases having been entered into the total therapy (TT) trials showed failure to enhance outcomes significantly in GEP-defined HR cases. They also showed the importance of ASCT for t(14;16) cases with a lack of improvement being seen for the IMiDS and proteosome inhibitors.[49] The Forte study showed that the use of carfilzomib consolidation maintenance can improve the outcomes of patients with HRMM.[93] The SWOG study of Elotuzumab-VRD was completed but did not show good outcomes and highlighted the inadequacy of this combination alone.[94] The OPTIMUM study examined enhanced induction, autologous stem cell transplantation, and maintenance in a group of cases defined by gene expression analysis and showed an excellent outcome and the feasibility of risk stratification across populations.[95] Several single-arm HR trials are underway currently including the German concept study and studies utilizing bispecific antibodies. It is likely that single-arm phase II studies will continue to be explored to identify a common control arm against which new combinations can be examined in future randomized studies. These trials will also have a focus on translational science to identify biomarkers and the biology of HR.

MECHANISMS OF RELAPSE

The percentage of cases with HR features increases at each relapse. Despite unprecedented improvements in outcome and depth of response, more than half of all patients with NDMM relapse within 5 years. Key mechanisms of relapse involve copy number changes and biallelic inactivation of key tumor suppressor genes.[96,97] Mutational diversity generated within focal lesions favors relapse and is associated with HRMM. Resistance to specific drugs such as IMiDs is often driven by mutations within the ubiquitin proteosome targeting machinery that they use to target Ikaros and Aiolos for degradation.[98] With the use of anti-BCMA and anti-GPRC5D bispecific antibodies, a major mechanism of resistance is by means of deletion and mutation of these targets.[99,100] What would be predicted is that if this is correct, swapping therapy from one target to the other would be effective as a way of treating relapse.

CONSENSUS DEFINITIONS

At a recent consensus meeting to clarify the definitions of HRMM, the features associated with true aggressive clinical behavior were discussed to bring clarity to the area. The importance of age as an adverse prognostic factor was recognized as was the importance of frailty in the older age groups and the penetrance of the cytogenetic risk factors. Double-hit events, where an adverse translocation and an adverse prognosis CNA, such as 1q+, 17p- or 1p, occur together was accepted as being an important group of HR cases. The t(4;14) alone was therefore omitted from the HR definition. In contrast, cases with t(14;16) were retained within the HR group because of their association with a defined biology, hyper-APOBEC, and poor outcomes. The presence of del 17p-was considered HR only when present at a clonal fraction of more than

20%, and there was a recognition that more than 60% of clonal cell involvement was a marker of true HR behavior. Biallelic inactivation of P53, the likely gene involved on 17p, by mutation and loss of copy was also considered HR. Cases with 1q gain alone may not be considered HR, but in the presence of ISSIII, the combination defines an HR group and may be incorporated into definitions. Similarly, 1p-in the presence of ISSIII can be considered HR. Several features were acknowledged as constituting relevant markers for the future including chromothripsis and an APOBEC signature. The importance of building diagnostic mutation approaches/panels able to identify adverse translocations, mutations, signatures, and CNA to enhance the ease and reproducibility of the genetic features of HR was noted. These panels should be able to detect all of the recurrent translocations typical of MM including those impacting *MYC*.

SUMMARY

A focus on HRMM can enhance progress toward improving outcomes these cases that have a consistently poor prognosis. Going forward, it is essential to carry out specific trials of HRMM, because it has a specific biology that needs to be effectively managed and is different to standard-risk disease. Carrying out translational research using biologic material derived from the trials can help make progress in the search for a biologic-based therapy for HRMM. There is progress in understanding and defining HR myeloma and by focusing clinical trials on these poor outcome cases, outcomes can be sequentially improved over time.

CLINICS CARE POINTS

- The use of IMS guidance for the definition of HR is recommended for use in future clinical trials.
- A rapid move to the uniform application of molecular diagnostic panels to identify HR features including chromothripsis and hyper-APOBEC signatures is recommended.
- The application of functional imaging strategies to identify extramedullary disease and focal lesions is critical.
- Therapy should include combinations of different agents with different modalities of action to overcome the diversity associated with HRMM.
- Going forward, the use of high-dose alkylating agents such as melphalan should be avoided, because they have been shown to contribute to the pattern of mutations seen at relapse.
- Maintenance should not induce mutations and should be given long term.
- Infection prophylaxis is crucial, because of the B-cell depletion associated with effective therapy.
- Monitoring response with functional imaging is crucial to ensure resolution of focal lesions and marrow uptake following treatment.
- The use of sensitive markers of MRD applied sequentially over time to monitor the depth of response is crucial, with the achievement of MRD negativity being a key therapeutic goal.

FUNDING

The work was funded by the Myeloma Solutions Fund.

DISCLOSURES

X. Chen, G. Varma declare no related conflict of interests.

REFERENCES

1. Majithia N, Rajkumar SV, Lacy MQ, et al. Early relapse following initial therapy for multiple myeloma predicts poor outcomes in the era of novel agents. Leukemia 2016;30:2208–13.
2. Bygrave C, Pawlyn C, Davies F, et al. Early relapse after high-dose melphalan autologous stem cell transplant predicts inferior survival and is associated with high disease burden and genetically high-risk disease in multiple myeloma. Br J Haematol 2021;193:551–5.
3. Sonneveld P, Avet-Loiseau H, Lonial S, et al. Treatment of multiple myeloma with high-risk cytogenetics: a consensus of the International Myeloma Working Group. Blood 2016;127:2955–62.
4. Jagosky MH, Usmani SZ. Extramedullary disease in multiple myeloma. Curr Hematol Malig Rep 2020;15:62–71.
5. Bansal R, Rakshit S, Kumar S. Extramedullary disease in multiple myeloma. Blood Cancer J 2021;11:161.
6. Schinke C, Boyle EM, Ashby C, et al. Genomic analysis of primary plasma cell leukemia reveals complex structural alterations and high-risk mutational patterns. Blood Cancer J 2020;10:70.
7. Chng WJ, Dispenzieri A, Chim CS, et al. IMWG consensus on risk stratification in multiple myeloma. Leukemia 2014;28:269–77.
8. Greipp PR, San Miguel J, Durie BG, et al. International staging system for multiple myeloma. J Clin Oncol 2005;23:3412–20.
9. Palumbo A, Avet-Loiseau H, Oliva S, et al. Revised international staging system for multiple myeloma: a report from International Myeloma Working Group. J Clin Oncol 2015;33:2863–9.
10. Boyle EM, Rosenthal A, Wang Y, et al. High-risk transcriptional profiles in multiple myeloma are an acquired feature that can occur in any subtype and more frequently with each subsequent relapse. Br J Haematol 2021;195:283–6.
11. D'Agostino M, Cairns DA, Lahuerta JJ, et al. Second Revision of the International Staging System (R2-ISS) for overall survival in multiple myeloma: a European Myeloma Network (EMN) report within the HARMONY Project. J Clin Oncol 2022;40:3406–18.
12. Pawlyn C, Morgan GJ. Evolutionary biology of high-risk multiple myeloma. Nat Rev Cancer 2017;17:543–56.
13. Maura F, Rustad EH, Boyle EM, et al. Reconstructing the evolutionary history of multiple myeloma. Best Pract Res Clin Haematol 2020;33:101145.
14. Melchor L, Brioli A, Wardell CP, et al. Single-cell genetic analysis reveals the composition of initiating clones and phylogenetic patterns of branching and parallel evolution in myeloma. Leukemia 2014;28:1705–15.
15. Walker BA, Wardell CP, Melchor L, et al. Intraclonal heterogeneity is a critical early event in the development of myeloma and precedes the development of clinical symptoms. Leukemia 2014;28:384–90.
16. Landgren O, Morgan GJ. Biologic frontiers in multiple myeloma: from biomarker identification to clinical practice. Clin Cancer Res 2014;20:804–13.
17. Bergsagel PL, Kuehl WM, Zhan F, et al. Cyclin D dysregulation: an early and unifying pathogenic event in multiple myeloma. Blood 2005;106:296–303.
18. Zhan F, Huang Y, Colla S, et al. The molecular classification of multiple myeloma. Blood 2006;108:2020–8.
19. Joseph NS, Gentili S, Kaufman JL, et al. High-risk multiple myeloma: definition and management. Clin Lymphoma Myeloma Leuk 2017;17S:S80–7.

20. Maura F, Boyle EM, Rustad EH, et al. Chromothripsis as a pathogenic driver of multiple myeloma. Semin Cell Dev Biol 2022;123:115–23.

21. Maura F, Bolli N, Angelopoulos N, et al. Genomic landscape and chronological reconstruction of driver events in multiple myeloma. Nat Commun 2019;10:3835.

22. Shaughnessy JD Jr, Zhan F, Burington BE, et al. A validated gene expression model of high-risk multiple myeloma is defined by deregulated expression of genes mapping to chromosome 1. Blood 2007;109:2276–84.

23. Walker BA, Leone PE, Chiecchio L, et al. A compendium of myeloma-associated chromosomal copy number abnormalities and their prognostic value. Blood 2010;116:e56–65.

24. Walker BA, Mavrommatis K, Wardell CP, et al. A high-risk, double-hit, group of newly diagnosed myeloma identified by genomic analysis. Leukemia 2019;33: 159–70.

25. Panopoulou A, Cairns DA, Holroyd A, et al. Optimizing the value of lenalidomide maintenance by extended genetic profiling: an analysis of 556 patients in the Myeloma XI trial. Blood 2023;141:1666–74.

26. Panopoulou A, Easdale S, Ethell M, et al. Impact of ultra high-risk genetics on real-world outcomes of transplant-eligible multiple myeloma patients. Hemasphere 2023;7:e831.

27. Messiou C, Giles S, Collins DJ, et al. Assessing response of myeloma bone disease with diffusion-weighted MRI. Br J Radiol 2012;85:e1198–203.

28. Giles SL, Messiou C, Collins DJ, et al. Whole-body diffusion-weighted MR imaging for assessment of treatment response in myeloma. Radiology 2014;271: 785–94.

29. Rasche L, Alapat D, Kumar M, et al. Combination of flow cytometry and functional imaging for monitoring of residual disease in myeloma. Leukemia 2019; 33:1713–22.

30. Dimopoulos M, Terpos E, Comenzo RL, et al. International myeloma working group consensus statement and guidelines regarding the current role of imaging techniques in the diagnosis and monitoring of multiple myeloma. Leukemia 2009;23:1545–56.

31. Rasche L, Angtuaco EJ, Alpe TL, et al. The presence of large focal lesions is a strong independent prognostic factor in multiple myeloma. Blood 2018;132: 59–66.

32. McDonald JE, Kessler MM, Gardner MW, et al. Assessment of total lesion glycolysis by (18)F FDG PET/CT significantly improves prognostic value of GEP and ISS in myeloma. Clin Cancer Res 2017;23:1981–7.

33. Morgan GJ, Walker BA, Davies FE. The genetic architecture of multiple myeloma. Nat Rev Cancer 2012;12:335–48.

34. Hoang PH, Dobbins SE, Cornish AJ, et al. Whole-genome sequencing of multiple myeloma reveals oncogenic pathways are targeted somatically through multiple mechanisms. Leukemia 2018;32:2459–70.

35. Stein CK, Pawlyn C, Chavan S, et al. The varied distribution and impact of RAS codon and other key DNA alterations across the translocation cyclin D subgroups in multiple myeloma. Oncotarget 2017;8:27854–67.

36. Heuck CJ, Jethava Y, Khan R, et al. Inhibiting MEK in MAPK pathway-activated myeloma. Leukemia 2016;30:976–80.

37. Hose D, Reme T, Hielscher T, et al. Proliferation is a central independent prognostic factor and target for personalized and risk-adapted treatment in multiple myeloma. Haematologica 2011;96:87–95.

38. Thanendrarajan S, Tian E, Qu P, et al. The level of deletion 17p and bi-allelic inactivation of TP53 has a significant impact on clinical outcome in multiple myeloma. Haematologica 2017;102:e364–7.
39. Dring AM, Davies FE, Fenton JA, et al. A global expression-based analysis of the consequences of the t(4;14) translocation in myeloma. Clin Cancer Res 2004;10:5692–701.
40. Woo JS, Alberti MO, Tirado CA. Childhood B-acute lymphoblastic leukemia: a genetic update. Exp Hematol Oncol 2014;3:16.
41. Topchu I, Pangeni RP, Bychkov I, et al. The role of NSD1, NSD2, and NSD3 histone methyltransferases in solid tumors. Cell Mol Life Sci 2022;79:285.
42. Popovic R, Martinez-Garcia E, Giannopoulou EG, et al. Histone methyltransferase MMSET/NSD2 alters EZH2 binding and reprograms the myeloma epigenome through global and focal changes in H3K36 and H3K27 methylation. PLoS Genet 2014;10:e1004566.
43. Walker BA, Wardell CP, Chiecchio L, et al. Aberrant global methylation patterns affect the molecular pathogenesis and prognosis of multiple myeloma. Blood 2011;117:553–62.
44. Pawlyn C, Kaiser MF, Heuck C, et al. The spectrum and clinical impact of epigenetic modifier mutations in myeloma. Clin Cancer Res 2016;22:5783–94.
45. Pawlyn C, Kaiser MF, Davies FE, et al. Current and potential epigenetic targets in multiple myeloma. Epigenomics 2014;6:215–28.
46. Pawlyn C, Bright MD, Buros AF, et al. Overexpression of EZH2 in multiple myeloma is associated with poor prognosis and dysregulation of cell cycle control. Blood Cancer J 2017;7:e549.
47. Ghamlouch H, Boyle EM, Blaney P, et al. Insights into high-risk multiple myeloma from an analysis of the role of PHF19 in cancer. J Exp Clin Cancer Res 2021; 40:380.
48. Mason MJ, Schinke C, Eng CLP, et al. Multiple myeloma DREAM Challenge reveals epigenetic regulator PHF19 as marker of aggressive disease. Leukemia 2020;34:1866–74.
49. Qiang YW, Ye S, Huang Y, et al. MAFb protein confers intrinsic resistance to proteasome inhibitors in multiple myeloma. BMC Cancer 2018;18:724.
50. Walker BA, Wardell CP, Murison A, et al. APOBEC family mutational signatures are associated with poor prognosis translocations in multiple myeloma. Nat Commun 2015;6:6997.
51. Maura F, Rustad EH, Yellapantula V, et al. Role of AID in the temporal pattern of acquisition of driver mutations in multiple myeloma. Leukemia 2020;34:1476–80.
52. Shou Y, Martelli ML, Gabrea A, et al. Diverse karyotypic abnormalities of the c-myc locus associated with c-myc dysregulation and tumor progression in multiple myeloma. Proc Natl Acad Sci U S A 2000;97:228–33.
53. Avet-Loiseau H, Gerson F, Magrangeas F, et al. Rearrangements of the c-myc oncogene are present in 15% of primary human multiple myeloma tumors. Blood 2001;98:3082–6.
54. Walker BA, Wardell CP, Brioli A, et al. Translocations at 8q24 juxtapose MYC with genes that harbor superenhancers resulting in overexpression and poor prognosis in myeloma patients. Blood Cancer J 2014;4:e191.
55. Affer M, Chesi M, Chen WG, et al. Promiscuous MYC locus rearrangements hijack enhancers but mostly super-enhancers to dysregulate MYC expression in multiple myeloma. Leukemia 2014;28:1725–35.
56. Misund K, Keane N, Stein CK, et al. MYC dysregulation in the progression of multiple myeloma. Leukemia 2020;34:322–6.

57. Maura F, Petljak M, Lionetti M, et al. Biological and prognostic impact of APOBEC-induced mutations in the spectrum of plasma cell dyscrasias and multiple myeloma cell lines. Leukemia 2018;32:1044–8.

58. Alexandrov LB, Nik-Zainal S, Wedge DC, et al. Signatures of mutational processes in human cancer. Nature 2013;500:415–21.

59. Bolli N, Avet-Loiseau H, Wedge DC, et al. Heterogeneity of genomic evolution and mutational profiles in multiple myeloma. Nat Commun 2014;5:2997.

60. Hoang PH, Cornish AJ, Dobbins SE, et al. Mutational processes contributing to the development of multiple myeloma. Blood Cancer J 2019;9:60.

61. Rustad EH, Yellapantula V, Leongamornlert D, et al. Timing the initiation of multiple myeloma. Nat Commun 2020;11:1917.

62. Cowan G, Weston-Bell NJ, Bryant D, et al. Massive parallel IGHV gene sequencing reveals a germinal center pathway in origins of human multiple myeloma. Oncotarget 2015;6:13229–40.

63. Rustad EH, Yellapantula VD, Glodzik D, et al. Revealing the impact of structural variants in multiple myeloma. Blood Cancer Discov 2020;1:258–73.

64. Morgan GJ. Jumping translocations and high-risk myeloma. Blood 2014;123:2442–3.

65. Sawyer JR, Tian E, Heuck CJ, et al. Jumping translocations of 1q12 in multiple myeloma: a novel mechanism for deletion of 17p in cytogenetically defined high-risk disease. Blood 2014;123:2504–12.

66. Hanamura I, Stewart JP, Huang Y, et al. Frequent gain of chromosome band 1q21 in plasma-cell dyscrasias detected by fluorescence in situ hybridization: incidence increases from MGUS to relapsed myeloma and is related to prognosis and disease progression following tandem stem-cell transplantation. Blood 2006;108:1724–32.

67. Sawyer JR, Tian E, Walker BA, et al. An acquired high-risk chromosome instability phenotype in multiple myeloma: jumping 1q syndrome. Blood Cancer J 2019;9:62.

68. Hebraud B, Leleu X, Lauwers-Cances V, et al. Deletion of the 1p32 region is a major independent prognostic factor in young patients with myeloma: the IFM experience on 1195 patients. Leukemia 2014;28:675–9.

69. Hofman IJF, van Duin M, De Bruyne E, et al. RPL5 on 1p22.1 is recurrently deleted in multiple myeloma and its expression is linked to bortezomib response. Leukemia 2017;31:1706–14.

70. Boyd KD, Ross FM, Walker BA, et al. Mapping of chromosome 1p deletions in myeloma identifies FAM46C at 1p12 and CDKN2C at 1p32.3 as being genes in regions associated with adverse survival. Clin Cancer Res 2011;17:7776–84.

71. Inoue J, Otsuki T, Hirasawa A, et al. Overexpression of PDZK1 within the 1q12-q22 amplicon is likely to be associated with drug-resistance phenotype in multiple myeloma. Am J Pathol 2004;165:71–81.

72. Mani M, Carrasco DE, Zhang Y, et al. BCL9 promotes tumor progression by conferring enhanced proliferative, metastatic, and angiogenic properties to cancer cells. Cancer Res 2009;69:7577–86.

73. Marchesini M, Ogoti Y, Fiorini E, et al. ILF2 Is a regulator of RNA splicing and DNA damage response in 1q21-amplified multiple myeloma. Cancer Cell 2017;32:88–100 e6.

74. Teoh PJ, An O, Chung TH, et al. Aberrant hyperediting of the myeloma transcriptome by ADAR1 confers oncogenicity and is a marker of poor prognosis. Blood 2018;132:1304–17.

75. Samo AA, Li J, Zhou M, et al. MCL1 gene co-expression module stratifies multiple myeloma and predicts response to proteasome inhibitor-based therapy. Genes Chromosomes Cancer 2018;57:420–9.
76. Boyle EM, Blaney P, Stoeckle JH, et al. Multiomic Mapping of Acquired Chromosome 1 Copy-Number and Structural Variants to Identify Therapeutic Vulnerabilities in Multiple Myeloma. Clin Cancer Res 2023;29(19):3901–13.
77. Owen RG, Davis SA, Randerson J, et al. p53 gene mutations in multiple myeloma. Mol Pathol 1997;50:18–20.
78. Shah V, Johnson DC, Sherborne AL, et al. Subclonal TP53 copy number is associated with prognosis in multiple myeloma. Blood 2018;132:2465–9.
79. Thakurta A, Ortiz M, Blecua P, et al. High subclonal fraction of 17p deletion is associated with poor prognosis in multiple myeloma. Blood 2019;133:1217–21.
80. Martello M, Poletti A, Borsi E, et al. Clonal and subclonal TP53 molecular impairment is associated with prognosis and progression in multiple myeloma. Blood Cancer J 2022;12:15.
81. Kunkel EJ, Butcher EC. Plasma-cell homing. Nat Rev Immunol 2003;3:822--9.
82. Cyster JG. Homing of antibody secreting cells. Immunol Rev 2003;194:48–60.
83. Danziger SA, McConnell M, Gockley J, et al. Bone marrow microenvironments that contribute to patient outcomes in newly diagnosed multiple myeloma: A cohort study of patients in the Total Therapy clinical trials. PLoS Med 2020;17: e1003323.
84. Neri P, Ren L, Azab AK, et al. Integrin beta7-mediated regulation of multiple myeloma cell adhesion, migration, and invasion. Blood 2011;117:6202–13.
85. Gupta VA, Matulis SM, Conage-Pough JE, et al. Bone marrow microenvironment-derived signals induce Mcl-1 dependence in multiple myeloma. Blood 2017;129: 1969–79.
86. de Jong MME, Kellermayer Z, Papazian N, et al. The multiple myeloma microenvironment is defined by an inflammatory stromal cell landscape. Nat Immunol 2021;22:769–80.
87. Schinke C, Poos AM, Bauer M, et al. Characterizing the role of the immune microenvironment in multiple myeloma progression at a single-cell level. Blood Adv 2022;6:5873–83.
88. Zavidij O, Haradhvala NJ, Mouhieddine TH, et al. Single-cell RNA sequencing reveals compromised immune microenvironment in precursor stages of multiple myeloma. Nat Cancer 2020;1.493–506.
89. Friedrich MJ, Neri P, Kehl N, et al. The pre-existing T cell landscape determines the response to bispecific T cell engagers in multiple myeloma patients. Cancer Cell 2023;41:711–725 e6.
90. Moreau P, Attal M, Hulin C, et al. Bortezomib, thalidomide, and dexamethasone with or without daratumumab before and after autologous stem-cell transplantation for newly diagnosed multiple myeloma (CASSIOPEIA): a randomised, open-label, phase 3 study. Lancet 2019;394:29–38.
91. Voorhees PM, Kaufman JL, Laubach J, et al. Daratumumab, lenalidomide, bortezomib, and dexamethasone for transplant-eligible newly diagnosed multiple myeloma: the GRIFFIN trial. Blood 2020;136:936–45.
92. Costa LJ, Chhabra S, Medvedova E, et al. Daratumumab, carfilzomib, lenalidomide, and dexamethasone with minimal residual disease response-adapted therapy in newly diagnosed multiple myeloma. J Clin Oncol 2022;40:2901–12.
93. Gay F, Musto P, Rota-Scalabrini D, et al. Carfilzomib with cyclophosphamide and dexamethasone or lenalidomide and dexamethasone plus autologous transplantation or carfilzomib plus lenalidomide and dexamethasone, followed

by maintenance with carfilzomib plus lenalidomide or lenalidomide alone for patients with newly diagnosed multiple myeloma (FORTE): a randomised, open-label, phase 2 trial. Lancet Oncol 2021;22:1705–20.

94. Usmani SZ, Hoering A, Ailawadhi S, et al. Bortezomib, lenalidomide, and dexamethasone with or without elotuzumab in patients with untreated, high-risk multiple myeloma (SWOG-1211): primary analysis of a randomised, phase 2 trial. Lancet Haematol 2021;8:e45–54.

95. Brown S, Sherratt D, Hinsley S, et al. MUKnine OPTIMUM protocol: a screening study to identify high-risk patients with multiple myeloma suitable for novel treatment approaches combined with a phase II study evaluating optimised combination of biological therapy in newly diagnosed high-risk multiple myeloma and plasma cell leukaemia. BMJ Open 2021;11:e046225.

96. Croft J, Ellis S, Sherborne AL, et al. Copy number evolution and its relationship with patient outcome-an analysis of 178 matched presentation-relapse tumor pairs from the Myeloma XI trial. Leukemia 2021;35:2043–53.

97. Chavan SS, He J, Tytarenko R, et al. Bi-allelic inactivation is more prevalent at relapse in multiple myeloma, identifying RB1 as an independent prognostic marker. Blood Cancer J 2017;7:e535.

98. Bird S, Pawlyn C. IMiD resistance in multiple myeloma: current understanding of the underpinning biology and clinical impact. Blood 2023;142:131–40.

99. Da Via MC, Dietrich O, Truger M, et al. Homozygous BCMA gene deletion in response to anti-BCMA CAR T cells in a patient with multiple myeloma. Nat Med 2021;27:616–9.

100. Swamydas M, Murphy EV, Ignatz-Hoover JJ, et al. Deciphering mechanisms of immune escape to inform immunotherapeutic strategies in multiple myeloma. J Hematol Oncol 2022;15:17.

New Therapies on the Horizon for Relapsed Refractory Multiple Myeloma

Nadine Abdallah, MD, Shaji K. Kumar, MD*

KEYWORDS

• Venetoclax • Iberdomide • Mezigdomide • Modakafusp alfa

KEY POINTS

• Patients with relapsed/refractory multiple myeloma (RRMM) have poor outcomes, highlighting the need for new therapies.
• Several novel agents have shown promising signs of efficacy and tolerability in patients with RRMM.
• Venetoclax is a B-cell lymphoma 2 (Bcl-2) inhibitor that is associated with a favorable risk-to-benefit ratio only in patients with t(11;14) or high Bcl-2 expression.
• Iberdomide and mezigdomide are higher potency cereblon E3 ligase modulators, which have demonstrated clinical activity in patients with RRMM including those with triple-class refractory disease.
• Modakafusp alfa (TAK-573), an immunocytokine that delivers attenuated interferon molecules to CD38+ cells, has demonstrated single agent activity in RRMM in the phase 1 setting.

INTRODUCTION

During the past 2 decades, considerable advances have been made in the treatment strategies for multiple myeloma (MM) with the introduction of proteasome inhibitors (PIs), immunomodulatory drugs (IMiDs), and more recently, CD38-targeting antibodies. The availability of highly effective combinations with less toxicity compared with earlier treatment regimens has been associated with significant improvement in survival.[1,2] However, MM remains an incurable disease,[3] and the majority of patients will experience relapses and will need additional treatments. As triplet and quadruplet regimens incorporating PIs, IMiDs, and/or anti-CD38 monoclonal antibodies are increasingly being used in the front-line and early relapse settings, the management of relapses in patients with earlier exposure to these drug classes has become a growing challenge. The LocoMMotion study examined the real-world treatment decisions and outcomes of

Division of Hematology, Mayo Clinic, 200 First Street Southwest, Rochester, MN 55905, USA
* Corresponding author.
E-mail address: kumar.shaji@mayo.edu

Hematol Oncol Clin N Am 38 (2024) 511–532
https://doi.org/10.1016/j.hoc.2023.12.013
0889-8588/24/© 2023 Elsevier Inc. All rights reserved.

patients with relapsed/refractory MM (RRMM) who had been exposed to 3 different classes of drugs. This study, which included patients across greater than 70 medical sites in the United States and Europe, revealed wide heterogeneity in the treatment choices for this subset of patients due to the absence of established standard treatments in this context. Clinical responses were limited, observed in less than one-third of patients, with less than 1% achieving a complete response. Moreover, these responses were short-lived, with a median duration of response lasting 7.4 months. The outcomes in this group of patients were poor, with a median progression-free survival (PFS) of 4.6 months and a median overall survival (OS) of 12.4 months.[4] Similarly, the MAMMOTH study retrospectively evaluated the outcomes for patients in the United States who were refractory to PIs, IMiDs, and anti-CD38 antibodies, showing limited and progressively decreasing responses with successive lines of treatment. Despite salvage therapies, the median OS was only 9.2 and 5.6 months in triple-refractory and penta-refractory patients, respectively.[5] The results of these studies underscore the urgent need for new drugs classes, which are both effective and well tolerated, to address the limitations of currently available strategies in the RR setting. An array of novel therapies have been introduced to the treatment landscape of RRMM in recent years; these include the nuclear export inhibitor selinexor,[6] the antibody–drug conjugate belantamab mafodotin,[7] the anti-CD38 monoclonal antibody isatuximab,[8] and approaches that harness the immune system: T-cell engaging bispecific antibodies[9–11] and chimeric antigen receptor (CAR) T-cell therapies.[12,13] Among these, bispecifics and CAR T-cell therapies are the most promising, with high rates of deep and durable remissions reported in clinical trials.[9–11] Nonetheless, relapses are still common, and some patients may not meet the eligibility or have access to these therapies. Thus, there is an ongoing need for novel drug classes in the RR setting especially for patients who have been heavily pretreated. A wide range of drugs with diverse mechanisms of action and targets are currently under evaluation at various preclinical and clinical stages. In this review, we will focus on novel therapies that have successful transitioned from the laboratory to clinical trial setting and have shown promising signs of efficacy and tolerability in this challenging group of patients. Novel bispecifics, cellular therapies, and monoclonal antibodies under development will be discussed separately in this issue.

DISCUSSION
Venetoclax-Based Therapy in Patients with t(11;14)

Venetoclax is an orally bioavailable BH3 mimetic that selectively inhibits Bcl-2, an anti-apoptotic protein overexpressed in a subset of patients with MM.[14] Venetoclax has demonstrated preclinical activity in MM, primarily in tumor cells with high Bcl-2/myeloid cell leukemia 1 (Mcl-1) gene expression ratio.[14] The presence of t(11;14), which involves a translocation between the *IGH* gene on chromosome 14 and *CCND1* gene on chromosome 11, has been associated with high Bcl-2/Mcl-1 and Bcl-2/Bcl2L1 ratios.[15] Thus, myeloma cells harboring the t(11;14) translocation, which is found in about 16% of newly diagnosed MM cases,[16] are specifically sensitive to this therapy.

Venetoclax monotherapy

In a phase 1 clinical trial, venetoclax was administered in escalating doses of 300 to 1200 mg daily to patients with RRMM after 1 or more earlier line(s) of therapy. In addition to tumor lysis syndrome (TLS) prophylaxis, a 2-week lead in period was included to mitigate TLS risk. The maximum tolerated dose (MTD) was not reached, so the 1200 mg dose was used in the safety expansion cohort. Venetoclax demonstrated single-agent activity and acceptable tolerability; the most common high-grade (grade $\geq$3) treatment-emergent adverse events (TEAEs) were hematologic, with low rates of nonhematologic toxicity, and no TLS events. In the overall cohort, the overall response rate (ORR) was 21% including 15% with very good partial response (VGPR) or greater. Although patients with t(11;14) had an ORR of 40%, only 6% of patients without t(11;14) achieved a response. The median time to progression (TTP) was 6.6 months in patients with t(11;14) compared with only 1.9 months in patients without t(11;14). An elevated Bcl2/Bcl2L1 gene expression ratio, which was predominantly found in the t(11;14) subgroup, was positively associated with response to venetoclax, resulting in a remarkable ORR of 80% with a median TTP of 11.5 months (**Table 1**).[17]

Venetoclax-bortezomib-dexamethasone

Venetoclax was subsequently studied in various combinations with standard-of-care myeloma therapies. Preclinical studies provided evidence that bortezomib can overcome the resistance to venetoclax in xenografts coexpressing Bcl-2 and Mcl-1. This is achieved through upregulation of the proapoptotic protein NOXA, which induces the degradation of Mcl-1.[18] This data provided a rationale for clinical studies evaluating the clinical activity of venetoclax in combination with bortezomib. After demonstrating safety in a phase 1b study,[19] the combination of venetoclax, bortezomib, and dexamethasone (VenVd) was evaluated in the phase III double-blind, placebo-controlled, BELLINI trial, among patients with RRMM and 1 to 3 earlier lines of therapy[20]; patients received placebo/venetoclax 800 mg daily with standard doses of bortezomib and dexamethasone until disease progression or intolerance. In the overall cohort, the ORR was 82% versus 68% in the venetoclax and placebo groups, respectively (P = .008), including 59% versus 36% with $\geq$VGPR (P < .001), and 32% versus 19% with CR, respectively (P < .001). More favorable responses were observed with venetoclax among patients with t(11;14) and in those with high Bcl-2 expression ($\sim$70% $\geq$VGPR). Although the median PFS was significantly longer in the venetoclax group compared with placebo (22.4 vs 11.5 months, hazard ratio [HR]: 0.63, P = .01), venetoclax was associated with an increased hazard for death (HR: 2·03 [95% CI: 1·04–3·95]; P = .034) in the overall cohort. The incidence of high-grade and serious TEAEs was similar between the venetoclax and placebo arms but there was a higher number of treatment-emergent deaths in the venetoclax group (13 [7%] vs 1 [1%]). Three deaths were considered treatment related in the venetoclax group; 2 died of pneumonia and 1 died of septic shock. The trend for increased mortality with venetoclax was not seen among patients who had t(11;14) or those with high Bcl-2 expression (HR: 1·23 [95% CI: 0·41–3·66]; P = .71) but was especially pronounced in the subgroup of patients who did not have t(11;14) and had low Bcl-2 expression (HR: 3·04 [95% CI: 1·17–7·91]; P = .022). In the final update after a median follow-up of 45.6 months,[21] the median OS was still not reached in both arms (HR: 1.19 [95% CI: 0.80–1.77]). The HR for OS was 0.82 (95% CI: 0.40–1.70) for patients with t(11;14) and/or high Bcl-2 expression (see **Table 1**).[21] Overall, these results indicate that venetoclax is associated with favorable outcomes only in patients who have t(11;14) or high Bcl-2 expression and has a high risk-to-benefit ratio in patients without these markers.

Daratumumab, venetoclax, and dexamethasone ± bortezomib

The combination of daratumumab, venetoclax, and dexamethasone (VenDd) ± bortezomib was evaluated in a phase I/II study in unselected patients with RRMM (VenDVd) and among patients with t(11;14) (VenDd). The dose of venetoclax was 800 mg in the expansion phase. Patients in the VenDVd cohort received

Table 1
Clinical trials evaluating venetoclax as monotherapy and in combination with other agents in patients with relapsed/refractory multiple myeloma

Study Treatment	Phase	Number	ORR (%)	≥VGPR Rate (%)	DOR/TTP/PFS (Months)	OS (Months)	≥Grade 3 TEAE (%) Overall and Most Frequent	TD due to AEs (%)	TE Deaths (%)
Venetoclax monotherapy (Kumar et al,[17] 2017)	I	All: 66 t(11;14): 30 Bcl-2/Bcl2L2: 10	All: 21% t(11;14): 40% Bcl-2/Bcl2L2: 80%	All: 15% t(11;14): 27%	All: DOR: 9.7, TTP: 2.6 t(11;14): DOR: 9.7, TTP: 6.6 Bcl-2/Bcl2L2: DOR: 9.7, TTP: 11.5	–	68% Thrombocytopenia: 26% Neutropenia: 21% Anemia: 14% Lymphopenia: 15%	8%	0
Venetoclax (VenVd) or Placebo (Vd) plus Bortezomib and dexamethasone (Kumar et al,[20] 2020, Kumar et al,[21] 2021)	III	VenVd All: 194 t(11;14): 20 High Bcl-2: 66 Vd All: 97, t(11;14): 15 High Bcl-2: 32	All: 82% t(11;14): 90% High Bcl-2: 85% All: 68% t(11;14): 47% High Bcl-2: 75%	All: 59% t(11;14): 70% High Bcl-2: 71% All: 36% t(11;14): 27% High Bcl-2: 28%	PFS: All: 23.4 t(11;14): 36.8 High Bcl-2: 30.1 All: 11.4 t(11;14): 9.3 High Bcl-2: 9.9	NR NR	87% Thrombocytopenia: 15% Neutropenia: 18% Anemia: 15% Diarrhea: 15% Pneumonia: 16% 88% Thrombocytopenia: 30% Neutropenia:7% Anemia: 15% Pneumonia: 9%	All: 22% All: 11%	All: 7% All:
Venetoclax Plus Daratumumab and Dexamethasone with (VenDVd) or Without (VenDd) Bortezomib (Bahlis et al,[22] 2021)	I/II	Part 1 VenDd in t(11;14: N = 24 Part 2 VenDVd in unselected patients with RRMM: N = 24 t(11;14): N = 6	96% 92% t(11;14):83% non-t(11;14): 94%	96% ≥CR: 58% 79% ≥CR: 46%	18m PFS: 91% 18m PFS: 67%	NR NR	88% Neutropenia: 21% Hypertension: 17% Infections: 25% 71% Insomnia: 25% Thrombocytopenia: 17% Infections: 21%	4% 13%	0 1 pt

Study	ORR	CR	PFS/TTP	OS	TEAEs	TD	
Part 3: Ven (400 mg)Dd in pts with t(11;14) N = 24	95%	86%	24m PFS: 94%	-	-	-	-
Part 3: Ven (800 mg)Dd in pts with t(11;14) N = 10	100%	100%	24m PFS: 83%	-	-	-	-
Part 3 DVd in pts with t(11;14) N = 24	62%	38%	24m PFS: 47%	-	-	-	-
Venetoclax plus carfilzomib and dexamethasone (VenKd) (Costa et al,[24] 2021) = VenKd All: N = 49 t(11;14): N = 13	All: 80% t(11;14): 92% non t(11;14): 75% High Bcl-2: 86%	All: 65% t(11;14): 85% non t(11;14): 58% High Bcl-2: 77%	Median: 22.8 t(11;14): 24.8 non t(11;14): 22.8 High Bcl-2: 24.7	-	92% Lymphophenia 31% Hypertension: 16% Neutropenia: 12% Pneumonia: 12%	8%	6%

Abbreviations: CR, complete response; DOR, duration of response; NR, not reached; ORR, overall response rate; OS, overall survival; PFS, progression-free survival; TD, treatment discontinuation; TE, treatment-emergent; TEAEs, treatment-emergent adverse events; TTP, time to progression; VGPR, very good partial response.

antibiotic prophylaxis. The addition of daratumumab was associated with a high response rate including deep responses and acceptable tolerability; the most common high-grade toxicities were neutropenia (21%) and hypertension (17%) in the VenDd cohort, and insomnia (25%) and thrombocytopenia (17%) in the VenDVd cohorts. Almost all patients achieved $\geq$ VGPR (96%) in the VenVd cohort, including $\geq$ CR in 58%, and MRD negativity at 10^{-5} in 33%. Deep responses were also seen in the VenDVd with a $\geq$VGPR rate of 79%, including 46% or greater with CR, and 21% MRD negative. The 18-month PFS rate was estimated at 91% and 67% in the VenDd and VenDVd cohorts, respectively (see **Table 1**).[22]

Based on these results, the phase 2-part (part 3) randomized patients with RRMM ($\geq$1 prior line of treatment) harboring t(11;14) to Ven(400 mg)Dd; Ven(800 mg)Dd; and daratumumab, bortezomib, and dexamethasone (DVd; control arm). Both venetoclax arms demonstrated a high rate of response including deep responses, with a $\geq$VGPR rate of 85% and 100% in the 400 mg and 800 mg arms, respectively. The $\geq$ VGPR rate was 38% in the DVd arm. The 2-year PFS was also longer in the venetoclax arms: 94%, 83%, and 47% in the Ven400Vd, Ven800 d, and DVd arms, respectively. The main toxicities were hematologic, and the most common serious adverse event was pneumonia, reported in 5%, 10%, and 4% in the 3 arms, respectively (see **Table 1**).[23]

Venetoclax, carfilzomib, and dexamethasone

The combination of venetoclax, carfilzomib, and dexamethasone was evaluated in a phase 2 study among patients with RRMM who had received 1 to 3 earlier lines of treatment.[24] The study included 4 dose-finding cohorts (venetoclax: 400–800 mg, carfilzomib: 27–56–70 mg/m^2) and an expansion cohort. No dose-limiting toxicities were observed in the dose-finding cohorts, so carfilzomib 70 mg/m^2 and venetoclax 800 mg were used in the dose expansion cohort. Patients with t(11;14) achieved higher rates of response including deep response compared with patients with non t(11;14) disease; the $\geq$VGPR rates were 85% versus 58%, including CR rates of 38% versus 22%, and MRD negativity ($<10^{-5}$) rates of 15% versus 11% in the 2 groups, respectively. Similarly, higher response rates, including deeper responses, were seen in patients with high Bcl-2 gene compared with those with low Bcl-2 expression. The median PFS was similar in patients with and without t(11;14) (24.8 and 22.8 months, respectively). High-grade (grade 3–4) cardiac adverse events occurred in 8%, including 4% (2 patients) who developed congestive heart failure.[24]

Ongoing trials with venetoclax-based combinations

Several studies evaluating venetoclax-based combinations are currently ongoing: the phase 3 CANOVA study (NCT03539744) is evaluating the safety and efficacy of venetoclax plus dexamethasone versus pomalidomide and dexamethasone in patients with RRMM with t(11;14).[25] The phase 2 SELVEDge study is evaluating the combination of selinexor, venetoclax, and dexamethasone in patients with RRMM with t(11;14) (NCT05530421). In addition, a phase I study is evaluating the safety and recommended phase 2 dose of venetoclax in combination with tocilizumab among patients with t(11;14) positive RRMM (NCT05391750).

Cereblon E3 Ligase Modulators

Immunomodulatory drugs are currently considered crucial components in the treatment landscape of MM in the newly diagnosed and relapsed refractory setting. The antimyeloma activity of the IMiDs lenalidomide and pomalidomide is mediated via binding to cereblon, a component of the Cul4A^{CRBN} E3 ligase complex. This binding leads to ubiquitination and proteasome-mediated degradation of substrate proteins ikaros (IKZF1) and aiolos (IKZF3), which are transcription factors that play a key role in lymphocyte differentiation. This causes downregulation of interferon regulatory factor 4 IRF4 and c-MYC, leading to inhibition of myeloma plasma cell growth and apoptotic cell death.[26,27] The cereblon E3 ligase modulators (CELMoDs) iberdomide (CC-220) and mezigdomide (CC-92480) are novel agents that bind cereblon E3 ligase with greater than 10-fold higher affinity compared with lenalidomide and pomalidomide, contributing to faster degradation, greater potency and efficiency in depletion of ikaros and aiolos. This is achieved by their extended molecular structures, which allow increased physical contact with cereblon surface compared with lenalidomide and pomalidomide.[28,29]

Preclinical studies have shown that iberdomide has higher immunomodulatory and antiproliferative activity compared with lenalidomide and pomalidomide and exhibits antitumor activity even in lenalidomide-resistant and pomalidomide-resistant myeloma cell lines, which have reduced cereblon expression. In addition, it exhibited synergistic activity with bortezomib and dexamethasone and displayed evidence of immune-mediated cytotoxicity with the ability to enhance antibody-dependent cellular cytotoxicity induced by daratumumab.[30,31] Similarly, mezigdomide had synergistic antitumor activity when combined with dexamethasone and with bortezomib, and enhanced daratumumab-mediated antibody-dependent cellular cytotoxicity and phagocytosis in myeloma cell lines.[32]

Iberdomide (CC-220)

An ongoing phase 1/2 dose escalation and expansion study is evaluating iberdomide as monotherapy and in combination with other standard myeloma therapies. The dose escalation phase is evaluating escalating dosing of iberdomide alone (cohort A), iberdomide plus dexamethasone (IberDex; cohort B), and iberdomide plus dexamethasone plus daratumumab (IberDd)/bortezomib (IberVd)/carfilzomib (IberKd; cohorts E-G) among patients with RRMM and at least 2 lines of earlier treatment. The expansion phase is evaluating iberdomide at the recommended phase 2 dose (RP2D) in combination with dexamethasone in patients with RRMM with at least 3 earlier lines of therapy who are triple refractory, and in combination with bortezomib and dexamethasone in newly diagnosed patients.

Iberdomide plus dexamethasone

Results from the dose escalation and expansion phases of the iberdomide plus dexamethasone cohort have been reported.[33] The dose escalation phase included 90 patients who had a median of 5 earlier lines of therapy. Patients received escalating doses of iberdomide (0.3–1.6 mg) on days 1 to 21 of a 28-day cycle, with weekly dexamethasone 40 mg (20 mg for patients >75 years) until disease progression. Hematologic toxicities were the most common high-grade toxicities. The rate of high-grade infections was reported at 26%, including 11% with pneumonia. Otherwise, the rate of high-grade nonhematologic toxicities was mostly less than 5%. The MTD was not reached so the RP2D was determined at 1.6 mg. After a median follow-up of 5.8 months, the ORR was 32%, with deep responses ($\geq$VGPR) only observed at doses of 0.9 mg or greater.

The dose expansion phase included 107 patients who had a median of 6 earlier lines of therapy; patients received iberdomide at the RP2D of 1.6 mg with dexamethasone as above. Similar to the dose escalation cohort, the most common high-grade TEAEs were hematological. No patients experienced grade 3 to 4 rash, peripheral neuropathy, or thromboembolism. After a median follow-up of 7.7 months, the ORR was 26% in the overall cohort including 8% with VGPR and 1% with stringent CR; the

ORR was similar (25%) in patients with prior treatment with anti-B-cell maturation antigen (BCMA) therapy. However, ORR was only 11% (3 of 27 patients) among those with extramedullary disease. The PFS and OS were estimated at 3 and 10.7 months, respectively (**Table 2**).[33]

Iberdomide plus dexamethasone plus daratumumab/bortezomib/carfilzomib
Initial results from the dose escalation cohorts evaluating IberDd, IberVd, and IberKd (cohorts E–G) have also been reported.[34] Iberdomide was given at escalating doses of 1.0 to 1.6 mg on days 1 to 21 of 28-day cycles (IberDd and IberKd cohorts) or days 1 to 14 of 21-day cycles (IberVd cohort). About 40% of patients were triple refractory. The RP2D was determined at 1.6 mg in the IberDd cohort, whereas evaluation is still ongoing in IberDd and IberKd cohorts. The rate of peripheral neuropathy was 32% in the IberVd cohort, and 22% in the IberKd, all grade 2 or less. No cardiovascular adverse events or hypertension occurred were observed in IberKd, and no thrombotic events were reported in any cohort. The ORR ranged between 46% and 56% in the 3 cohorts (see **Table 2**).[34]

Ongoing studies
The ongoing phase 3 EXCALIBER trial (NCT04975997) will be comparing IberDd and DVd in patients with RRMM. The first stage will randomize patients to IberDd at 3 different doses of iberdomide (1.0 mg, 1.3 mg, and 1.6 mg) or to DVd to identify the optimal iberdomide dose to be used in the second stage.[35] A dose escalation and expansion study evaluating iberdomide plus elotuzumab and dexamethasone in patients with RRMM is also ongoing (NCT05560399). Another phase 2 study evaluating iberdomide, daratumumab, carfilzomib, and dexamethasone in patients with RRMM with 1 to 3 lines of therapy, including lenalidomide, is planned (NCT05896228).

Mezigdomide (CC-92480)
Mezigdomide plus dexamethasone. An ongoing phase 1/2 study (CC-92480-MM-001) is evaluating mezigdomide (Mezi) alone and in combination with dexamethasone in patients with RRMM who have had 3 or more lines of therapy including lenalidomide, pomalidomide, a PI, and an anti-CD38 antibody, and are triple refractory (for phase 2). Results have been reported for the dose escalation phase, which evaluated Mezi at doses of 0.1 to 1.0 mg daily in various schedules (3/7/10 of 14 days × 2, or 21 of 28 days) among 66 patients. Overall, the rate of grade 3 to 4 TEAEs was 88%, most commonly neutropenia (53%), infections (30%), and anemia (29%). The MTD was determined at 1 mg for 2 schedules: 10 of 14 days × 2, and 21 of 28 days. Both pharmacodynamic effects and clinical responses were dose dependent; among the 21 patients treated at the MTD dose, 10 achieved at least a PR (ORR: 48%), including 7 with VGPR.[36,37]

Interim results have also been reported for the dose expansion phase after 101 patients were enrolled and a median follow-up of 5.8 months. Patients received Mezi at a dose of 1 mg on days 1 to 21 of each 28-day cycle, and dexamethasone 40 mg weekly (20 mg if > 75 years). The responses were promising in this heavily pretreated group of patients with an ORR of 40% including 18% with VGPR and 5% with CR or stringent CR. The median duration of response was 8.3 months, and median PFS was estimated at 4.6 months. The outcomes were similar in patients who received prior BCMA-directed therapy (30 patients), with an ORR% of 50% including 27% with ≥VGPR, a median duration of response of 6.9 months and estimated PFS of 5.4 months. There was a high rate of grade 3 or greater hematologic toxicities, particularly neutropenia, observed in 74%. High-grade infections occurred in about a third of patients, including pneumonia in 10%. Although only 6% discontinued treatment

Table 2
Results from the phase 1/2 study evaluating iberdomide in combination with other agents in patients with relapsed/refractory multiple myeloma

Study Treatment	Number	Follow-up Median	ORR %	≥VGPR %	Time to Response Median	DOR Median	Grade ≥3 TEAEs Overall and Most Common	TD due to TEAEs	Deaths due to TEAEs
Dose escalation cohort									
IberDex (Lonial et al,[33] 2022)	90	5.8 mo	32%	10%	8.1 wk	10.4 mo	Overall: 83% Neutropenia: 42% Anemia: 27% Leukopenia: 23% Thrombocytopenia: 15% Infection: 26%. Pneumonia: 10% Febrile neutropenia: 3%	7%	None
IberDd (Lonial et al,[34] 2021)	43	4.2 mo	46%	24%	4.1 wk	NR	Neutropenia: 67% Leukopenia: 23% Anemia: 21%, Thrombocytopenia: 13% Infections: 15% Febrile neutropenia: 5% Fatigue: 3% Diarrhea: 3%	2%	-
Iber-Vd (Lonial et al,[34] 2021)	25	4.9 mo	56%	28%	3.6 wk	35.7 wk	Neutropenia: 28% Thrombocytopenia: 24% Anemia: 12% Febrile neutropenia: 0% Infections: 20% Diarrhea: 4% Rash: 4% URTI: 8%	8%	-

(continued on next page)

Table 2
(continued)

Study Treatment	Number	Follow-up Median	ORR %	≥VGPR %	Time to Response Median	DOR Median	Grade ≥3 TEAEs Overall and Most Common	TD due to TEAEs	Deaths due to TEAEs
IberKd (Lonial et al,[34] 2021)	9	5.0 mo	50%	38%	4.1 wk	NR	Lymphopenia: 44%, Neutropenia: 33% Thrombocytopenia: 11% Fatigue: 11% Infections: 33%	11%	-
Dose expansion cohort									
Iber(1.6 mg)-Dex(40 mg) (Lonial et al,[33] 2022)	107	7.7 mo	26%	9%	4.2 wk	7 mo	Overall: 82% Neutropenia: 45% Anemia: 28% Leukopenia: 21% Thrombocytopenia: 22% Infections: 27% Pneumonia: 10% Febrile neutropenia: 5%	5%	1%

Abbreviations: DOR, duration of response; IberDd, iberdomide, daratumumab, and dexamethasone; Iber-Dex, iberdomide and dexamethasone; IberKd, iberdomide, carfilzomib, and dexamethasone; IberVd, iberdomide, bortezomib, and dexamethasone; NR, not reached; ORR, overall response rate; TD, treatment discontinuation; TEAEs, treatment-emergent adverse events; VGPR, very good partial response.

due to TEAEs, 71% and 29% required dose interruptions and reductions, respectively.[38]

Mezigdomide in combination with standard therapies. An ongoing large phase 1/2 study is evaluating the safety and efficacy of Mezi in combination with standard myeloma agents: bortezomib, daratumumab, carfilzomib, elotuzumab, and isatuximab in patients with RRMM and newly diagnosed patients (NCT03989414). Preliminary results from the dose expansion phases of Mezi plus bortezomib/carfilzomib plus dexamethasone (MeziVd and MeziKd), and the dose escalation phase of MeziVd have been reported (**Table 3**). None of the patients in the MeziVd cohort experienced DLT, and only 1 patient in the MeziKd had a DLT (pulmonary embolism). The phase 2 dose for the MeziVd cohort was determined to be 1 mg. No grade 3 to 4 peripheral neuropathy was reported in any of the 3 cohorts.[39]

Ongoing studies with mezigdomide. Two ongoing phase 3 studies are evaluating the addition of Mezi to standard treatments in patients with RRMM; SUCCESSOR-1 is comparing MeziVd and the combination of pomalidomide, bortezomib, and dexamethasone (NCT05519085), and SUCCESSOR 2 is comparing MeziKd and Kd.[40] A phase 1/2 study is evaluating Mezi in combination with new agents (tazemetostat, trametinib, and BMS-986158) in patients with RRMM (NCT05372354). A phase 1b study is planned to evaluate the safety profile of Mezi in combination with elotuzumab and dexamethasone in patients with RRMM who have had at 2 or more lines of treatment including a CD38 targeting antibody and BCMA-directed therapy (NCT05981209).

Modakafusp Alfa (TAK-573)

Modakafusp alfa (TAK-573) is an immunocytokine generated by the genetic fusion of 2 attenuated interferon α-2b (IFNα2b) molecules to the Fc portion of a humanized anti-CD38 IgG4 monoclonal antibody, which directs the interferon molecules to CD38+ cells and activates IFN signaling through the INFα receptor. This results in antiproliferative effects on myeloma cells and activation of CD38+ innate and adaptive immune effector cells.[41,42] The INF portion of modakafusp alfa is attenuated through mutations that cause decreased binding affinity to the INF receptor. This minimizes off-target activity while retaining potent on-target activity against the myeloma cells. The binding site of TAK-573 on CD38 is distinct from that of daratumumab and isatuximab. As a result, it does not interfere with the activity of these antibodies. TAK-573 has demonstrated ex vivo activity in enhancing the antimyeloma activity of natural killer (NK) cells and augmentation of antimyeloma activity of other anti-CD38 antibodies.[41] In MM xenograft tumor models, TAK-573 exhibited robust single agent antitumor activity and synergistic activity in combination with lenalidomide and bortezomib even in tumors refractory to these agents.[43]

Clinical activity of modakafusp alfa (TAK-573)

Single agent clinical activity of modakafusp alfa was demonstrated in the iinnovate-1 phase I clinical trial, which included patients with RRMM who had received at least 3 earlier lines of treatment and were refractory or intolerant to one or more PI(s) and ImiD(s). Modakafusp alfa was administered intravenously in escalating doses (0.001–6 mg/kg) in different dosing schedules: weekly (0.001–0.75 mg/kg) (first 2 cycles only), every 2 weeks (0.2–0.3 mg/kg), every 3 weeks (0.4–0.75 mg/kg), and every 4 weeks (0.75–6 mg/kg). DLTs occurred with both the weekly and biweekly dose schedules, and the MTD was determined at 3 mg/kg for the Q4w schedule. Clinical responses were observed starting from 0.4 mg/kg and 1.5 mg/kg for the 3-week and 4-week schedules, respectively. Therefore, dose expansion cohorts were opened

Table 3
Preliminary results from the phase I/II evaluating mezigdomide in combination with other agents in patients with relapsed/refractory multiple myeloma

Treatment Cohort:	Phase	Eligibility	Mezi Dose and Schedule	Number	Lenalidomide Refractory (%)	ORR %	≥VGPR %	Hematologic Grade 3-4 TEAEs (%)	≥1 Dose Reductions due to TEAEs (%)
MeziVd	I	RRMM with 2–4 prior lines including lenalidomide	0.3–0.6–1 mg days 1–14 of 21-d cycles	22	82%	73%	36%	Neutropenia: 36%, Thrombocytopenia: 18%	27%
MeziKd	I	RRMM with 2–4 prior lines including lenalidomide	0.3–0.6–1 mg Days 1–21 of 28-d cycles	17	62%	77%	35%	Neutropenia: 41% Infections: 29%	29%
MeziVd	II	RRMM with 1–3 prior lines including lenalidomide	1 mg days 1–14 of 21-d cycles	34	77%	71%	50%	Neutropenia: 29% Infections: 29% Thrombocytopenia: 27%	32%

Abbreviations: Mezi, Mezigdomide; MeziKd, Mezigdomide, carfilzomib, and dexamethasone; MeziVd, Mezigdomide, bortezomib, and dexamethasone; ORR, overall response rate; TD, treatment discontinuation; TEAEs, treatment-emergent adverse events; VGPR, very good partial response.

for these schedules using modakafusp as a single agent or in combination with weekly dexamethasone 40 mg. The clinical responses reported for these schedules are shown in **Table 4**. Treatment was associated with an upregulation of CD38 on myeloma cells and peripheral blood immune cells especially NK cells. However, there was no correlation between the level of CD38 expression on immune cells and clinical response.[41,44] Both the degree and duration of CD38 receptor occupancy on peripheral blood immune cells were dose dependent. Treatment was also associated with the activation of INF 1 signaling and cytokine release and with the activation of bone marrow cytotoxic T cells in some patients.[41]

The final analysis for the 1.5 mg/kg 4-week cohort included 30 patients, of which 28 were refractory to anti-CD38 antibodies. The ORR was 43%, including 27% with ≥VGPR and 13% with ≥CR; 1 patient was MRD negative. Clinical responses were seen after a median of 1.2 months, and the duration of response ranged between 1.0 and 18.9 months; the median PFS was estimated at 5.7 months. About a third of patients experienced infusion-related reactions, almost all grade less than 3.

The most common high-grade (grade ≥3) adverse events were hematologic: neutropenia (63%), thrombocytopenia (47%), and lymphopenia (37%). High-grade infections were reported in 10%, all grade 3. Almost all nonhematologic toxicities (except grade 4 hyperuricemia in 1 patient) were grade less than 3.[44] The third part of this ongoing study is comparing the 2 modakafusp doses of 120 mg and 240 mg every 4 weeks (equivalent to 1.5 mg/kg and 3 mg/kg, respectively) among patients with RRMM who are triple refractory and have had greater than 3 earlier lines of treatment.

Clinical activity of modakafusp alfa (TAK-573)

Given the promising single agent activity and good tolerability of modakafusp alfa, 2 phase 1/2 studies have been designed to evaluate the safety and efficacy of modakafusp in combination with other standard myeloma agents. Iinnovate-2 (NCT05556616) is a phase 1b study evaluating modakafusp alfa in doublet and triplet combinations with daratumumab, pomalidomide, bortezomib, or carfilzomib, in patients with RRMM. Iinnovate-3 (NCT05590377) is a phase 1/2a study evaluating modakafusp alfa in combination with daratumumab in patients with RRMM.

Other Drugs Under Development

An enhanced understanding of disease biology and molecular mechanisms underlying disease progression and drug resistance, has led to the identification of new drug targets and therapeutic strategies in MM. This is reflected by the surge of drugs that have

Table 4
Clinical responses from the dose expansion cohorts for modakafusp alone or in combination with dexamethasone

Modakafusp Alfa Dose (mg/kg)	Modakafusp Alfa Schedule	Dexamethasone 40 mg Weekly	Number	PD (N)	SD (N)	PR (N)	VGPR (N)	≥CR (N)
0.4	3 wk	No	8	3	5	0	0	0
0.4	3 wk	Yes	3	1	2	0	0	0
1.5	4 wk	No	30	0	0	5	4	4
1.5	4 wk	Yes	8[a]	0	1	0	1	0

Abbreviations: CR, complete response; N, number; PD, progressive disease; PR, partial response; SD, stable disease; VGPR, very good partial response.
[a] The other 6 patients were not evaluated for response/evaluable.

Table 5
Early phase clinical trials evaluating new drugs in relapsed/refractory multiple myeloma, excluding monoclonal antibodies, cellular therapies, and bispecifics

Product Name	Class	Target/MOA	Phase	Monotherapy or Combination	NCT Identifier
Indatuximab ravtansine (BT062)	ADC	CD138	I/II	Monotherapy and in combination with lenalidomide or pomalidomide	NCT00723359[a] NCT01001442[a] NCT01638936[a]
FOR46	ADC	CD46	I	Monotherapy	NCT03650491[a]
AMG-224	ADC	BCMA	I	Monotherapy	NCT02561962[a]
STRO-001	ADC	CD74	I	Monotherapy	NCT03424603
CC-99712	ADC	BCMA	I	Monotherapy or in combination with BMS-986405	NCT04036461
STI-6129	ADC	CD38	I/II	Monotherapy	NCT05308225 NCT05565807
HDP-101	ADC	BCMA	I/II	Monotherapy	NCT04879043
Ruxolitinib	Small molecule	JAK inhibitor	I	In combination with lenalidomide and methylprednisolone	NCT03110822
Tasquinimod	Small molecule	S100A9 Inhibitor	I	Monotherapy and in combination with ixazomib, lenalidomide, and dexamethasone	NCT04405167
ACY-1215	Small molecule	HDAC inhibitor	I/II	Monotherapy and in combination with bortezomib or pomalidomide or lenalidomide and dexamethasone	NCT01323751[a] NCT01997840 NCT02189343[a] NCT01583283[a]
PT-112	Small molecule	Pyrophosphate-platinum conjugate. Induces immunogenic cell death	I/II	Monotherapy	NCT03288480[a]
PRT1419	Small molecule	Mcl-1 inhibitor	I	Monotherapy	NCT04543305[a]

Drug	Type	Target	Phase	Description	NCT Number
Ibrutinib	Small molecule	BTK inhibitor	I/II	Monotherapy and in combination with lenalidomide or carfilzomib or bortezomib ± dexamethasone	NCT02902965[a] NCT01962792[a] NCT03702725 NCT01478581[a]
AT-101	Small molecule	Bcl-2 inhibitor	I	In combination with lenalidomide and dexamethasone	NCT02697344
KTX-1001	Small molecule	MMSET inhibitor	I	Monotherapy	NCT05661932
ONC201	Small molecule	Imipridone Antagonizes the GPCR DRD2	I/II	Monotherapy	NCT02863991
NMS-03597812	Small molecule	PERK inhibitor	I	Monotherapy and in combination with dexamethasone	NCT05027594
ABBV-453	Small molecule	Bcl-2 inhibitor	I	Monotherapy	NCT05308654
Vactosertib	Small molecule	ALK5 inhibitor	I	In combination with pomalidomide	NCT03143985
Pevonedistat	Small molecule	NAE inhibitor	I	In combination with ixazomib	NCT03770260
All-trans retinoic acid	Small molecule	Vitamin A derivative RAR ligand	II	In combination with daratumumab, pomalidomide, and dexamethasone	NCT04700176
ORIC-533	small molecule	CD73 inhibitor	I	Monotherapy	NCT05227144
ACY-241	small molecule	HDAC inhibitor	I	In combination with pomalidomide and dexamethasone	NCT02400242
Telaglenastat Hydrochloride	Small molecule	GLS1 inhibitor	I	In combination with carfilzomib and dexamethasone	NCT03798678
KRT-232 (AMG 232)	Small molecule	MDM2 inhibitor	I	In combination with carfilzomib, lenalidomide, and dexamethasone	NCT03031730
APG-2575	Small molecule	Bcl-2 inhibitor	I/II	Monotherapy and in combination with: lenalidomide and dexamethasone; pomalidomide and dexamethasone; or daratumumab, lenalidomide, and dexamethasone	NCT04674514 NCT04942067
BGB-11417	Small molecule	Bcl-2 inhibitor	I/II	Monotherapy and in combinations with carfilzomib and/or dexamethasone	NCT04973605

(continued on next page)

Table 5
(continued)

Product Name	Class	Target/MOA	Phase	Monotherapy or Combination	NCT Identifier
CFT7455	Small molecule	IKZF1/3 degrader	I/II	Monotherapy and in combination with dexamethasone	NCT04756726
AMG 176	Small molecule	Mcl-1 inhibitor	I	Monotherapy	NCT02675452
VOB560	Small molecule	Bcl-2 inhibitor	I	In combination with MIK665	NCT04702425
MIK665	Small molecule	Mcl-1 inhibitor	I	In combination with VOB560	NCT04702425
TAK-981	small-molecule	SUMOylation	I/II	In combination with mezagitamab and daratumumab	NCT04776018
EZM0414	Small molecule	SETD2 inhibitor	I	Monotherapy	NCT05121103
KPT-8602	Small molecule	SINE Compound	I/II	Monotherapy and in combination with low dose dexamethasone	NCT02649790
BMF-219	Small molecule	inhibitor of menin	I	Monotherapy	NCT05153330
LP-118	Small molecule	Bcl-2/Bcl-XL inhibitor	I	Monotherapy	NCT04771572
CYT-0851	Small molecule	RAD51 inhibitor	I/II	Monotherapy	NCT03997968
Dabrafenib	Small molecule	BRAF inhibitor	I	Alone and in combination with Trametinib	NCT03091257
Trametinib	Small molecule	MEK inhibitor	I	Alone and in combination with Dabrafenib	NCT03091257
LOXO-338	Small molecule	Bcl-2 inhibitor	I	Monotherapy and in combination with pirtobrutinib	NCT05024045
Idasanutlin	Small molecule	MDM2 inhibitor	I/II	In combination with ixazomib and dexamethasone	NCT02633059
Cobimetinib	Small molecule	MEK inhibitor	I/II	In combination with dexamethasone, ixazomib, and pomalidomide	NCT03732703
Erdafitinib	Small molecule	FGFR inhibitor	I/II	In combination with dexamethasone, ixazomib, and pomalidomide	NCT03732703

Abemaciclib	Small molecule	CDK4/6 inhibitor	I/II	In combination with dexamethasone, ixazomib, and pomalidomide	NCT03732703
Enasidenib	Small molecule	IDH2 inhibitor	I/II	In combination with dexamethasone, ixazomib, and pomalidomide	NCT03732703
Nivolumab	Checkpoint inhibitor	PD-1	II	In combination with daratumumab ± Low-dose cyclophosphamide	NCT03184194
Pembrolizumab	Checkpoint inhibitor	PD-1	II	Monotherapy	NCT05204160
Magrolimab	Checkpoint inhibitor	CD47	II	In combination with daratumumab or pomalidomide or bortezomib or carfilzomib ± dexamethasone	NCT04892446
AO-176	Checkpoint inhibitor	CD47	I/II	Monotherapy and in combination with bortezomib or dexamethasone	NCT04445701[a]
TTI-622	Checkpoint inhibitor	CD47	I	In combination with daratumumab	NCT05139225
Durvalumab	Checkpoint inhibitor	PDL-1	I	Monotherapy and in combination with pomalidomide or lenalidomide ± dexamethasone	NCT02616640 NCT02685826
BMS-986016	Checkpoint inhibitor	LAG-3	I/II	In combination with pomalidomide and dexamethasone	NCT04150965
BMS-986207	Checkpoint inhibitor	TIGIT	I/II	In combination with pomalidomide and dexamethasone	NCT04150965
EOS884448	Checkpoint inhibitor	TIGIT	I/II	Monotherapy and in combination with iberdomide ± dexamethasone	NCT05289492
TAK-169	Engineered toxin body	Anti-CD38 antibody linked to a modified SLTA subunit	I	Monotherapy	NCT04017130
NKTR-255	Recombinant agonist	PEG conjugate of rhIL-15	I	Monotherapy and in combination with daratumumab or rituximab	NCT04136756[a]
ION251	Antisense oligonucleotide	IRF4 gene	I	Monotherapy	NCT04398485

(continued on next page)

Table 5
(continued)

Product Name	Class	Target/MOA	Phase	Monotherapy or Combination	NCT Identifier
Eftozanermin Alfa (ABBV-621)	Fusion protein	Human IgG1-Fc fused to TRAIL-R binding domain	I	In combination with bortezomib and dexamethasone	NCT04570631
Tinostamustine	Fusion molecule	Alkylating HDACi fusion molecule	I	Monotherapy	NCT0256496
Maplirpacept	Fusion protein	CD47-SIRPα Fusion Protein	I	Monotherapy and in combination with carfilzomib and dexamethasone ± isatuximab	NCT03530683
Leflunomide	Immunomodulatory drug	Pyrimidine synthesis inhibitor: inhibits DHODH	I/II	Monotherapy and in combination with lenalidomide or pomalidomide	NCT02509052 NCT04508790
Nelfinavir Mesylate	Antiretroviral	HIV-1 protease inhibitor	I/II	In combination with metformin and bortezomib	NCT03829020

Abbreviations: ADC, antibody drug conjugate; ALK5, activin receptor-like kinase 5 inhibitor; Bcl-2, B-cell lymphoma 2; Bcl-xL, B-cell lymphoma-extra large; BCMA, B-cell maturation antigen; BTK, Burton's tyrosine kinase; CKD, cyclin-dependent kinase; DHODH, dihydroorotate dehydrogenase; DRD2, dopamine receptor D2; FGFR, fibroblast growth factor receptor; GLS1, glutaminase 1; GPCR, G-protein coupled receptors; HDAC, histone deacetylases; HDACi, histone deacetylase inhibitor; HIV, human immunodeficiency virus; IDH, isocitrate dehydrogenase; IKZF1/3, Ikaros family zinc finger protein 1/3; IRF4, interferon regulatory factor 4; JAK, Janus kinase; Mcl-1, myeloid cell leukemia 1; MDM2, mouse double minute 2 homolog; MMSET, multiple myeloma SET domain; MOA, mechanism of action; NAE, NEDD8-activating enzyme; NCT, National Clinical Trial; PERK, protein kinase RNA-like ER kinase; RAR, retinoic acid receptor; rhIL-15, recombinant human interleukin-15; S100A9, S100 calcium-binding protein A9; SINE, selective inhibitor of nuclear export; SIRPα, signal-regulatory-protein α; SLTA, Shiga-like toxin A subunit; TIGIT, T-cell immunoreceptor with immunoglobulin and ITIM domain; TRAIL-R, Tumor necrosis factor-related apoptosis-inducing ligand receptor.

[a] Clinical trial completed.

entered early phases of development in recent years. The major drug classes under investigation include the following: next generation CD38-targeting antibodies and other monoclonal antibodies, cellular therapies and bispecifics, antibody–drug conjugates, checkpoint inhibitors and other drugs repurposed for MM, and small molecule inhibitors such as Bcl-2/Mcl-1 inhibitors, histone deacetylase inhibitors, mitogen-activated protein kinase (MAPK) pathway inhibitors, and cereblon E3 ligase complex modulators. **Table 5** lists completed and ongoing clinical trials evaluating new drugs excluding monoclonal antibodies, cellular therapies, and bispecifics.

SUMMARY

Despite an increase in therapeutic options for patients with RRMM, the current strategies are not curative. The management of heavily pretreated patients with earlier exposure to the major drug classes still represents a clinical challenge, which underscores the need for novel therapeutic strategies that are effective, tolerable, and accessible. Venetoclax, iberdomide, mezigdomide, and modakafusp alfa have demonstrated encouraging results in the clinical trial setting and have the potential to be integrated into the therapeutic armamentarium of RRMM. In addition, a substantial number of drugs with novel targets and distinctive pharmacodynamic properties are presently undergoing clinical investigation. This provides considerable hope for patients with RRMM, and we eagerly await to see which strategies will prove effective and contribute to the evolution of the therapeutic landscape of MM in the upcoming years.

CLINICS CARE POINTS

- Patients with MM continue to relapse and newer therapies with different mechanisms of action are required to maintain disease control over long term.
- Drugs that have shown promise in relapsed/refractory MM in early phase clinical trials are as follows: venetoclax (Bcl-2 inhibitor), iberdomide and mezigdomide (cereblon E3 ligase modulators), and modakafusp alfa (immunocytokine).
- The benefit of venetoclax is restricted to patients with t(11;14) and/or Bcl-2 expression.

DISCLOSURE

S.K. Kumar.: Disclosures-Consulting/Advisory Board participation: Abbvie, BMS, Janssen, Roche-Genentech, Takeda, Pfizer, Loxo Oncology, K36, Sanofi, ArcellX. N. Abdallah: No competing financial interests to declare.

REFERENCES

1. Kumar SK, Dispenzieri A, Lacy MQ, et al. Continued improvement in survival in multiple myeloma: changes in early mortality and outcomes in older patients. Leukemia 2014;28(5):1122–8.
2. Binder M, Nandakumar B, Rajkumar SV, et al. Mortality trends in multiple myeloma after the introduction of novel therapies in the United States. Leukemia 2022;36(3):801–8.
3. Ravi P, Kumar SK, Cerhan JR, et al. Defining cure in multiple myeloma: a comparative study of outcomes of young individuals with myeloma and curable hematologic malignancies. Blood Cancer J 2018;8(3):26.

4. Mateos M-V, Weisel K, De Stefano V, et al. LocoMMotion: a prospective, non-interventional, multinational study of real-life current standards of care in patients with relapsed and/or refractory multiple myeloma. Leukemia 2022;36(5):1371–6.

5. Gandhi UH, Cornell RF, Lakshman A, et al. Outcomes of patients with multiple myeloma refractory to CD38-targeted monoclonal antibody therapy. Leukemia 2019;33(9):2266–75.

6. Chari A, Vogl DT, Gavriatopoulou M, et al. Oral Selinexor–Dexamethasone for Triple-Class Refractory Multiple Myeloma. N Engl J Med 2019;381(8):727–38.

7. Lonial S, Lee HC, Badros A, et al. Belantamab mafodotin for relapsed or refractory multiple myeloma (DREAMM-2): a two-arm, randomised, open-label, phase 2 study. Lancet Oncol 2020;21(2):207–21.

8. Dimopoulos M, Bringhen S, Anttila P, et al. Isatuximab as monotherapy and combined with dexamethasone in patients with relapsed/refractory multiple myeloma. Blood 2021;137(9):1154–65.

9. Moreau P, Garfall AL, van de Donk NWCJ, et al. Teclistamab in Relapsed or Refractory Multiple Myeloma. N Engl J Med 2022;387(6):495–505.

10. Chari A, Minnema MC, Berdeja JG, et al. Talquetamab, a T-Cell–Redirecting GPRC5D Bispecific Antibody for Multiple Myeloma. N Engl J Med 2022;387(24):2232–44.

11. Lesokhin AM, Tomasson MH, Arnulf B, et al. Elranatamab in relapsed or refractory multiple myeloma: phase 2 MagnetisMM-3 trial results. Nat Med 2023. https://doi.org/10.1038/s41591-023-02528-9.

12. San-Miguel J, Dhakal B, Yong K, et al. Cilta-cel or Standard Care in Lenalidomide-Refractory Multiple Myeloma. N Engl J Med 2023;389(4):335–47.

13. Rodriguez-Otero P, Ailawadhi S, Arnulf B, et al. Ide-cel or Standard Regimens in Relapsed and Refractory Multiple Myeloma. N Engl J Med 2023;388(11):1002–14.

14. Touzeau C, Dousset C, Le Gouill S, et al. The Bcl-2 specific BH3 mimetic ABT-199: a promising targeted therapy for t(11;14) multiple myeloma. Leukemia 2014;28(1):210–2.

15. Cleynen A, Samur M, Perrot A, et al. Variable BCL2/BCL2L1 ratio in multiple myeloma with t(11;14). Blood 2018;132(26):2778–80.

16. Fonseca R, Blood EA, Oken MM, et al. Myeloma and the t(11;14)(q13;q32): evidence for a biologically defined unique subset of patients. Blood 2002;99(10):3735–41.

17. Kumar S, Kaufman JL, Gasparetto C, et al. Efficacy of venetoclax as targeted therapy for relapsed/refractory t(11;14) multiple myeloma. Blood 2017;130(22):2401–9.

18. Punnoose EA, Leverson JD, Peale F, et al. Expression Profile of BCL-2, BCL-XL, and MCL-1 Predicts Pharmacological Response to the BCL-2 Selective Antagonist Venetoclax in Multiple Myeloma Models. Mol Cancer Ther 2016;15(5):1132–44.

19. Moreau P, Chanan-Khan A, Roberts AW, et al. Promising efficacy and acceptable safety of venetoclax plus bortezomib and dexamethasone in relapsed/refractory MM. Blood 2017;130(22):2392–400.

20. Kumar SK, Harrison SJ, Cavo M, et al. Venetoclax or placebo in combination with bortezomib and dexamethasone in patients with relapsed or refractory multiple myeloma (BELLINI): a randomised, double-blind, multicentre, phase 3 trial. Lancet Oncol 2020;21(12):1630–42.

21. Kumar S, Harrison SJ, Cavo M, et al. Final Overall Survival Results from BELLINI, a Phase 3 Study of Venetoclax or Placebo in Combination with Bortezomib and Dexamethasone in Relapsed/Refractory Multiple Myeloma. Blood 2021;138:84.
22. Bahlis NJ, Baz R, Harrison SJ, et al. Phase I Study of Venetoclax Plus Daratumumab and Dexamethasone, With or Without Bortezomib, in Patients With Relapsed or Refractory Multiple Myeloma With and Without t(11;14). J Clin Oncol 2021; 39(32):3602–12.
23. Kaufman JL, Quach H, Baz RC, et al. An Updated Safety and Efficacy Analysis of Venetoclax Plus Daratumumab and Dexamethasone in an Expansion Cohort of a Phase 1/2 Study of Patients with t(11;14) Relapsed/Refractory Multiple Myeloma. Blood 2022;140(Supplement 1):7261–3.
24. Costa LJ, Davies FE, Monohan GP, et al. Phase 2 study of venetoclax plus carfilzomib and dexamethasone in patients with relapsed/refractory multiple myeloma. Blood Advances 2021;5(19):3748–59.
25. Mateos M-V, Moreau P, Dimopoulos MA, et al. A phase III, randomized, multicenter, open-label study of venetoclax or pomalidomide in combination with dexamethasone in patients with t(11;14)-positive relapsed/refractory multiple myeloma. J Clin Oncol 2020;38(15_suppl):TPS8554.
26. Lopez-Girona A, Mendy D, Ito T, et al. Cereblon is a direct protein target for immunomodulatory and antiproliferative activities of lenalidomide and pomalidomide. Leukemia 2012;26(11):2326–35.
27. Bjorklund CC, Lu L, Kang J, et al. Rate of CRL4CRBN substrate Ikaros and Aiolos degradation underlies differential activity of lenalidomide and pomalidomide in multiple myeloma cells by regulation of c-Myc and IRF4. Blood Cancer J 2015; 5(10):e354.
28. Matyskiela ME, Zhang W, Man H-W, et al. A Cereblon Modulator (CC-220) with Improved Degradation of Ikaros and Aiolos. J Med Chem 2018;61(2):535–42.
29. Hansen JD, Correa M, Nagy MA, et al. Discovery of CRBN E3 Ligase Modulator CC-92480 for the Treatment of Relapsed and Refractory Multiple Myeloma. J Med Chem 2020;63(13):6648–76.
30. Amatangelo M, Bjorklund CC, Kang J, et al. Iberdomide (CC-220) Has Synergistic Anti-Tumor and Immunostimulatory Activity Against Multiple Myeloma in Combination with Both Bortezomib and Dexamethasone, or in Combination with Daratumumab in Vitro. Blood 2018;132(Supplement 1):1935.
31. Bjorklund CC, Kang J, Amatangelo M, et al. Iberdomide (CC-220) is a potent cereblon E3 ligase modulator with antitumor and immunostimulatory activities in lenalidomide- and pomalidomide-resistant multiple myeloma cells with dysregulated CRBN. Leukemia 2020;34(4):1197–201.
32. Wong L, Narla RK, Leisten J, et al. CC-92480, a Novel Cereblon E3 Ligase Modulator, Is Synergistic with Dexamethasone, Bortezomib, and Daratumumab in Multiple Myeloma. Blood 2019;134:1815.
33. Lonial S, Popat R, Hulin C, et al. Iberdomide plus dexamethasone in heavily pretreated late-line relapsed or refractory multiple myeloma (CC-220-MM-001): a multicentre, multicohort, open-label, phase 1/2 trial. Lancet Haematol 2022; 9(11):e822–32.
34. Lonial S, Richardson PG, Popat R, et al. OAB-013: Iberdomide (IBER) in combination with dexamethasone (DEX) and daratumumab (DARA), bortezomib (BORT), or carfilzomib (CFZ) in patients (pts) with relapsed/refractory multiple myeloma (RRMM). Clin Lymphoma, Myeloma & Leukemia 2021;21:S9.
35. Lonial S, Quach H, Dimopoulos MA, et al. EXCALIBER-RRMM: A phase 3, two-stage study of iberdomide, daratumumab, and dexamethasone (IberDd) versus

daratumumab, bortezomib, and dexamethasone (DVd) in patients (pts) with relapsed/refractory multiple myeloma (RRMM). J Clin Oncol 2023;41(16_suppl): TPS8069.

36. Richardson PG, Vangsted AJ, Ramasamy K, et al. First-in-human phase I study of the novel CELMoD agent CC-92480 combined with dexamethasone (DEX) in patients (pts) with relapsed/refractory multiple myeloma (RRMM). J Clin Oncol 2020; 38(15_suppl):8500.

37. Wong L, Lamba M, Jiménez Nuñez MD, et al. Dose- and Schedule-Dependent Immunomodulatory Effects of the Novel Celmod Agent CC-92480 in Patients with Relapsed/Refractory Multiple Myeloma. Blood 2020;136(Supplement 1):47–8.

38. Richardson PG, Trudel S, Quach H, et al. Mezigdomide (CC-92480), a Potent, Novel Cereblon E3 Ligase Modulator (CELMoD), Combined with Dexamethasone (DEX) in Patients (pts) with Relapsed/Refractory Multiple Myeloma (RRMM): Preliminary Results from the Dose-Expansion Phase of the CC-92480-MM-001 Trial. Blood 2022;140(Supplement 1):1366–8.

39. Richardson P, Sandhu I, Oriol A, et al. OAB-053: Mezigdomide (MEZI; CC-92480) in combination with dexamethasone (DEX) and bortezomib (BORT) or carfilzomib (CFZ) in patients (pts) with relapsed/refractory multiple myeloma (RRMM). Clin Lymphoma, Myeloma & Leukemia 2022;22:S33.

40. Amatangelo M, Berenson JR, Cerchione C, et al. A phase 3, two-stage, randomized study of mezigdomide, carfilzomib, and dexamethasone (MeziKd) versus carfilzomib and dexamethasone (Kd) in relapsed/refractory multiple myeloma (RRMM): SUCCESSOR-2. J Clin Oncol 2023;41(16_suppl):TPS8070.

41. Bruins WSC, Rentenaar R, Collins S, et al. Modakafusp Alfa (TAK-573), a Novel CD38-Targeting Attenuated Interferon-Alpha Immunocytokine, Kills MM Cells Via NK Cell Activation. Blood 2022;140(Supplement 1):4236–7.

42. Vogl DT, Kaufman JL, Holstein SA, et al. TAK-573, an Anti-CD38/Attenuated Ifnα Fusion Protein, Has Clinical Activity and Modulates the Ifnα Receptor (IFNAR) Pathway in Patients with Relapsed/Refractory Multiple Myeloma. Blood 2020; 136(Supplement 1):37–8.

43. Pogue SL, Taura T, Bi M, et al. Targeting Attenuated Interferon-alpha to Myeloma Cells with a CD38 Antibody Induces Potent Tumor Regression with Reduced Off-Target Activity. PLoS One 2016;11(9):e0162472.

44. Vogl DT, Atrash S, Holstein SA, et al. Final Results from the First-in-Human Phase 1/2 Study of Modakafusp Alfa, an Immune-Targeting Attenuated Cytokine, in Patients (Pts) with Relapsed/Refractory Multiple Myeloma (RRMM). Blood 2022; 140(Supplement 1):1357–9.

Immunocompetent Mouse Models of Multiple Myeloma
Therapeutic Implications

Megan Tien Du, MS, Peter Leif Bergsagel, MD, Marta Chesi, PhD*

KEYWORDS

- Multiple myeloma - Mouse model - MYC - Human CRBN - IMiDs - Immunotherapy

KEY POINTS

- Mouse models of multiple myeloma are needed to conduct hypothesis-driven, controlled studies in an immunocompetent setting.
- The presence of human cereblon (CRBN) is required to render murine cells sensitive to IMiDs (thalidomide, lenalidomide, and pomalidomide) and CRBN ligase modulators.
- Several immunocompetent *de novo* and transplantable murine models of myeloma are available in Balb/c and (KaLwRij)C57BL/6 strains.
- Further work is needed to develop tractable models representing the primary myeloma subgroups with *cyclin D, MAF, MMSET, FGFR3* translocations, or hyperdiploidy.

INTRODUCTION

Multiple myeloma (MM) is a hematological malignancy characterized as the growth of atypical terminally differentiated plasma cells (PCs) localizing to the bone marrow (BM) and secreting large amounts of monoclonal immunoglobulins (Ig), which form the typical M-spike on a serum protein electrophoretic gel.[1] Since 1980, the prevalence of MM has displayed an escalating trend being the third most common hematological malignancy worldwide with 176,404 reported new cases and 117,077 reported deaths in 2020.[2] There are 2 MM precursor clinical stages consisting of monoclonal gammopathy of undetermined significance (MGUS) and smoldering MM (SMM) based primarily on the presence of less than 10%, or 10% to 60% BM PC respectively. Elevated calcium levels, renal insufficiency, anemia, and bone lesions or decreased bone density are common symptoms defining active MM.[3]

Approximately half of MM patients are characterized by chromosomal translocations involving the Ig loci that are thought to occur during the B cell receptor affinity

Department of Medicine, Mayo Clinic, 13400 East Shea Boulevard, MCCRB 3-040, Scottsdale, AZ 85259, USA
* Corresponding author. Mayo Clinic, 13400 East Shea Boulevard, MCCRB 3-040, Scottsdale, AZ 85259, USA.
E-mail address: Chesi.marta@mayo.edu

Hematol Oncol Clin N Am 38 (2024) 533–546
https://doi.org/10.1016/j.hoc.2023.12.014
0889-8588/24/© 2023 Elsevier Inc. All rights reserved.

maturation processes (somatic hypermutation and class switch recombination) in germinal center B cells. They result in the juxtaposition of the powerful Ig enhancer(s) to oncogenes, leading to their overexpression. The most common translocation partners are D-type cyclins (CCND1, CCND2, or CCND3, in 20% of MM cases), MAF transcription factors (MAF, MAFA, or MAFB, in 7% of MM), and FGFR3/NSD2, simultaneously dysregulated by the t(4;14) translocation occurring in 15% of MM. The other half of patients are characterized by a hyperdiploid karyotype with trisomies in odd-numbered chromosomes (3,5,7,9,11,15,19,21).[1] Both Ig heavy-chain (IgH) translocations and hyperdiploidy are present in patients with MGUS and remain invariant throughout the course of the disease progression. Secondary events drive the progression from MGUS to MM, most commonly through the activation of MYC, RAS/mTOR, or NFkB pathways. More rapid disease progression occurs with mutations that upregulate the cell cycle (CDKN2C, RB1, TP53). All of these mutations are much more common in MM than in MGUS, and some, such as MYC, have not been described in MGUS.[4–6] Interestingly, the increased proliferation of MM cells inversely correlates with Ig expression, which is the highest in normal PC and progressively decreases from MGUS to advanced MM and MM cell lines.[7] Overall, MM cells universally display the post-germinal center signature of somatic hypermutation of the Ig loci and somatic class switch recombination, with only 1% of cases secreting IgM. In contrast, the presence of an APOBEC mutational signature has been uniquely linked to MM progression.[8]

MM cell survival is contingent on the BM microenvironment (BMM).[9] APRIL (a proliferation-inducing ligand) and BAFF (B-cell-activating factor) signaling though B-cell maturation antigen (BCMA) on the surface of MM cells appears to be critical and leads to downstream activation of the NFkB pathway.[10] Crosstalk between tumor and immune cells creates an inflammatory microenvironment that activates stromal cells to produce chemokines and cytokines, like interleukin 6 (IL6), that further boost MM proliferation and survival.[11,12] These factors pose challenges for preclinical modeling of MM. A lot of preclinical work has been done using human MM cell lines grown in vitro, which secrete only low levels of Ig,[7] fail to adequately model hyperdiploid MM, and also fail to recreate the complex interplay between MM and BMM.[1] Mouse models can be utilized for a better understanding of the disease biology, as a powerful tool to model cancer interception and for the development of novel therapeutic approaches.

The current standard of care anti-MM therapy has evolved around the combinations of IMiDs (thalidomide, lenalidomide, and pomalidomide), proteasome inhibitors, glucocorticoid, anti-CD38 monoclonal antibodies (abs), and high-dose melphalan. Of those, IMiDs and anti-CD38 abs are hard to model in mice. IMiDs target human but not mouse cereblon (CRBN) to induce degradation of IKZF1 and IKZF3 leading to direct MM cell toxicity and T cell activation[13]; in contrast to humans, murine normal and malignant PC do not express CD38, which is downregulated in germinal center B cells.[14] More recently, redirected T cell therapy has revolutionized the therapy of MM. Chimeric antigen receptor T cell therapy engineers the hosts own T cells to recognize tumor surface antigens, like BCMA, FcRH5, and GPCR5D, and stimulate cell killing via the production of cytotoxic granules.[15,16] Similarly, T cell activation and MM cell killing is achieved when bispecific abs (BsAbs) simultaneously target surface antigens on MM cells and CD3 on T cells.[17] Among surface antigens used for T cell redirected therapy, BCMA is the most common, and FcRH5 and GPCR5D are not expressed on murine PCs. Despite achieving unprecedented response rates, MM patients continue to relapse, and murine models are needed to elucidate mechanisms of primary and secondary resistance to conventional and immunotherapy. This review will discuss characteristics of current spontaneous, induced, and genetically engineered immuno-competent MM mouse models highlighting their utilization in MM immunotherapy.

Spontaneous Models

5TMM

Seminal work by Jiri Radl and colleagues demonstrated the propensity of the C57BL/6 but not Balb/c, CH3, or CBA mouse strain to develop with age a spontaneous mono-clonal gammopathy that mimics MGUS in humans.[18,19] Like MGUS, the gammopathy in mice remains stable over time; however, in 0.5% of cases it progresses to frank MM. The 5TMM murine model was generated by Radl through serial transplantation of these rare MM cells that spontaneously develop in C57BL/KaLwRij mice, a C57BL/6 subline maintained in the Netherlands since 1965. Several independent 5TMM lines have been developed over the years, with 5T2, 5T33, and the 5T33 subline 5TGM1 be-ing the best characterized.[20,21] All lines secrete IgG, the most common isotype observed in MM patients, and home to the BM where they induce various degrees of lytic bone lesions in recipient mice.[22] Interestingly, they do not show Ig somatic hypermutation. Their main features are listed in **Table 1**. Rearrangements of the MYC locus are one of the key genomic events inducing the progression from MGUS to MM in men but have not been identified in 5TMM, except for a late passage subline.[20]

Because Radl performed most of his work on the C57BL/KaLwRij line available to him in the Netherlands, it was underappreciated that the propensity to develop gamm-opathy was not a unique feature of KaLwRij mice, but it was shared with the parental C57BL/6 mice. Genomic studies designed to map the germline differences between these two lines identified biallelic deletion of Samsn1 gene in KaLwRij mice. Since the reintroduction of Samsn1 in 5TGM1 MM abolished its growth in vivo, early studies attributed the predisposition of C57BL/KaLwRij to develop MM to Samsn1 defi-ciency.[23,24] However, it was later reported that 5TGM1 cells in which Samsn1 had been re-expressed readily engrafted in Samsn1$^+$ C57BL/6 recipient mice, indicating that the lack of engraftment of Samsn1$^+$ 5TGM1 cells in Samsn1$^{-/-}$ KaLwRij host was likely due to immune-rejection.[25] Notably, a tumor extrinsic effect of Samsn1 defi-ciency has also been reported in macrophages from KaLwRij mice, which display a more tumorigenic M2 phenotype compared to their C57BL/6 counterpart.[23] Regard-less, it is important to note that both C57BL/6 and C57BL/KaLwRij mice develop spontaneous monoclonal gammopathy with age and exhibit bone disease once engrafted with MM cells. Particular features of the myeloma cells, more than the host itself, are likely to determine the extent of the occurring bone phenotype, although a direct comparison of bone disease in various tumor lines from the two mouse strains has not been performed yet.

The 5TMM model has been instrumental over the years to model PC homing to the BM, to define MM cell dormancy, to study the biology of bone disease, and to inves-tigate novel therapeutics.[21,26–30] However, it suffers from its dependency on a partic-ular mouse strain, not allowing tumor engraftment in available immunocompetent genetically modified mice.

Chemically Induced Models

Balb/c plasmacytomas

Merwin and colleagues in the late 1950s serendipitously discovered that Balb/c mice implanted in the peritoneal cavity with plastic objects develop plasmacytomas (PCTs).[31] Extensive work by Mike Potter in the following years led to the characteriza-tion of mineral oil–induced Balb/c PCTs, which result from a highly inflammatory

Table 1
Features of immunocompetent models of MM

Model	Type	Strain	Transplantable	In Vitro Growth	Sex	M-spike	% Ig Expression[a]	Isotype	Tropism	Growth	Median Survival	Bone Disease	IgV Mutations[b]	APOBEC Mutational Signature	MYC Dysregulation	References
5T2MM	Spontaneous	C57BL/KaLwRij	Yes	No	M	Yes	?	IgG2a-K	Mostly BM	Moderate	100 d	Diffuse lytic lesions	No	?	No	20
5T3MM	Spontaneous	C57BL/KaLwRij	Yes	Stroma dependent	F	Yes	?	IgG2b-K	BM-SPL	Aggressive	40 d	Rarely	No	?	No	20
5TGM1	Spontaneous	C57BL/KaLwRij	Yes	Yes	F	Yes	7	IgG2b-K	BM-SPL	Aggressive	24 d	Diffuse lytic lesions	No	?	No	20
Balb/c PTC	Induced	Balb/c	Yes	Occasionally	M/F	Occasionally	1–6	IgA > IgG	EM	Aggressive	220 d	Rarely	Yes	?	Yes	33
MOPC315.BM	Induced	Balb/c	Yes	Yes	?	?	?	IgA-L	BM-SPL	Aggressive	30 d	Diffuse lytic lesions	?	?	Yes	38
Bclxl x iMYC	Genetically engineered	Mixed	Yes	Yes	M/F	Occasionally	?	IgG > IgA	BM-SPL-EM	Aggressive	135 d	Occasionally	?	?	Yes	39
Emu-Xbp1-1s	Genetically engineered	C57BL/6	?	?	M/F	Occasionally	?	IgM/IgG	?	Indolent	2 y	Occasionally	?	?	?	40
Vk*MYC	Genetically engineered	C57BL/6	Occasionally	Occasionally	M/F	Yes	30	IgG > IgA	BM > SPL	Moderate	661 d	Diffuse lytic lesions	Yes	Yes	Yes	7,41
tVk*MYC	Genetically engineered	C57BL/6	Yes	Occasionally	M/F	Yes	20	IgG > IgA	SPL > BM	Aggressive	30 d	Diffuse lytic lesions	Yes	Yes	Yes	7,41,42,44
Vk*MYC x EmuBCL2	Genetically engineered	C57BL/6	Yes	?	M/F	Yes	?	IgG > IgA	SPL > BM	Aggressive	337 d	?	Yes	?	Yes	41
Vk*MYC x miR15a/16-1 het	Genetically engineered	C57BL/6	?	?	M/F	Yes	?	IgG > IgA	SPL > BM	Moderate	630 d	?	?	?	Yes	49
Vk*MYC x NRasQ61R	Genetically engineered	C57BL/6	Yes	Occasionally	M/F	Yes	3–17	IgA > IgG	EM	Aggressive	400 d	Diffuse lytic lesions	Yes	?	Yes	50
Emu-MAF	Genetically engineered	C57BL/6	Yes	?	M/F	Occasionally	?	IgM/IgG	EM	Moderate	> 1 y	No	?	?	?	51

MMSET/ IKK2ca	Genetically engineered	C57BL/6	In nude mice	?	M/F Yes	60	IgM/IgG	BM	Indolent	97 wk	Diffuse lytic lesions	No	No	?	52
CCND1/ IKK2ca	Genetically engineered	C57BL/6	In nude mice	?	M/F Yes	60	IgM/IgG	BM	Indolent	91 wk	Diffuse lytic lesions	No	No	?	52
MYC/IKK2ca	Genetically engineered	Mixed	Occasionally	?	M/F Yes	45	IgM/ IgG > IgA	BM-SPL	Moderate	208 d	Diffuse lytic lesions	No	No	Yes	53
BCL2/IKK2ca	Genetically engineered	Mixed	Occasionally	?	M/F Yes	45	IgM/ IgG > IgA	BM-SPL	Moderate	296 d	Diffuse lytic lesions	No	No	Yes	53

a   % of mapped transcript by RNAseq.

b   Defined as greater than 2% mutations in the IgV variable region.

microenvironment and the formation of granulomas, composed of fibroblasts, macrophages, eosinophils, and neutrophils secreting factors that support the expansion of IgA-producing PC. PCTs do not normally grow *in vitro* or engraft in recipient Balb/c mice, unless they have been preconditioned with pristane injections. It was through the search of factors capable of supporting PCT expansion *in vitro* that IL6 was simultaneously identified by several laboratory tests.[32] Consistently, anti-inflammatory treatment (nonsteroidal anti-inflammatory drugs, corticosteroid) inhibits new PCT development *in vivo* but not always the survival of established tumors, and IL6^{null} mice are fully pristane resistant. Acceleration of PCT development is achieved by viral infection or transgene expression of various oncogenes (ie, *Myc, Raf, HRas, Bcl2, Bclx$_L$*), while forced expression of v-abl, IL6, or a constitutive active IL6 receptor (L-GP130) induce PCT even in the absence of mineral oil injection.[33,34] Among inbred strains, only Balb/c is sensitive to mineral oil injection, and the susceptibility has been linked to two germline missense mutations in *Cdkn2a* or p16^{INK4a}.[35]

All PCTs invariably carry a *MYC* translocation to the Ig loci and, interestingly, the identification of these recombination events led to the cloning of the oncogene *MYC*.[36] Many cell lines with acquired IL6 independency and capability of growing *in vitro* have been obtained from Balb/c PCT and have been instrumental for the generation of hybridomas and production of monoclonal abs. Although some reports indicate that PCTs induce osteolytic lesions in Balb/c recipients,[37] more commonly these lines engraft in extramedullary sites. One exception is represented by the MOPC315.BM line, generated by repeated and sequential IV autografting of MOPC315 cells harvested specifically from the BM. The resulting line has a tropism restricted to the spleen and the BM, where it causes lytic lesion, and it can be maintained *in vitro*, simplifying its genetic manipulation.[38] Main features of Balb/c PCT are listed in **Table 1**.

Genetically Engineered Mouse Models

MYC x BCL-X$_L$

Janz, Van Ness and colleagues generated a double transgenic mouse with *Myc* inserted into the Ig Calpha locus and *Bcl-X$_L$* driven by a Vkappa promoter (see **Table 1**). The resulting mice develop expansion of highly proliferative clonal PC in spleen, BM, and other nonlymphoid tissues, occasionally resulting in lytic lesions. Tumor could be transplanted into pristane-primed nude Balb/c mice, or could occasionally be propagated *in vitro*. The post-germinal center origin of these tumors remains unclear.[39] Unfortunately, the mixed background of these mice (C57BL/6 × 129sv XFVB/N) limits their utilization for transplantation and immune studies.

Emu-XBP1-1s

Carrasco reported the generation of PC tumors in C57BL/6 mice expressing the spliced version of the PC transcription factor *Xbp1* under the Emu enhancer (see **Table 1**). Unfortunately, the characterization of the phenotype of these mice remains inconclusive, and the tumor transcriptional profile is inconsistent with that of PC.[40] As a result, this model has not been embraced by the myeloma community.

Vk*MYC

Generated by Chesi, Bergsagel and colleagues, the Vk*MYC mice in pure C57BL/6 background carry a mutated/inactive human MYC transgene driven by the kappa promoter, which is sporadically converted to the active form by the somatic mutation process induced by AID in germinal center B cells. As a result, Vk*MYC mice develop an indolent but progressive expansion of isotype class switched, somatically hypermutated, monoclonal PC restricted to the BM, that can be traced over time by M-spike quantification through serum protein electrophoresis (see **Table 1**). Extramedullary involvement, mostly in the spleen, is reported in 30% of the mice, which is lower than other MM models. Occasionally, Vk*MYC mice also develop Burkitt's lymphoma with age (approximately in 15% of cases). Although usually unable to be propagated *in vitro*, Vk*MYC MM cells can occasionally be engrafted into nonirradiated C57BL/6 mice, that usually develop a much more proliferative and aggressive extra-medullary MM (see below). Interestingly, immunization of Vk*MYC mice with the T cell dependent antigen NP-conjugated to chicken gamma globulin (NP-CGG) resulted in shorter survival and accelerated expansion of PC producing monoclonal antibody reacting to NP, although it is unclear if this is the result of chronic antigen stimulation or simply the increased inflammatory microenvironment driven by the immunization adjuvant.

With a median survival age of 97 weeks, the *de novo* Vk*MYC mice best model SMM and its progressive transformation to MM in aged mice, which develop end organ damage—anemia, bone disease, and renal impairment.[41] While the long latency for MM development is generally considered a drawback, it allows for the spontaneous selection of additional genomic events required for malignant PC transformation. In fact, the recent characterization of the genomic landscape of *de novo* and transplantable Vk*MYC MM identified high degree of genomic heterogeneity among different mice, due to the presence of an APOBEC mutational signature as well as structural variations, copy number changes, and missense mutations affecting known MM drivers and mostly converging on the activation of the NFkB and RAS/mTOR pathways.[7] Importantly, more than 50 transplantable Vk*MYC lines have been fully characterized to allow the correlation of tumor behavior and drug response to specific genomic mutations.

This biological fidelity renders the Vk*MYC model particularly suitable for the investigation of anti-myeloma drug activity. It's positive and negative predicted value for drug clinical activity has been extensively validated: out of 12 classes of drugs active in this model, nine are also clinically active, for a positive predictive value of 75%. Moreover, the 12 classes of drugs inactive in this model are also clinically inactive, for a negative predictive value of 100% (**Fig. 1**).[42–44] To be noted, IMiDs are inactive in rodent cells because of several amino acid substitutions in murine *Crbn* gene which affects IMiD binding and recruitment of target substrates. Therefore, a new transgenic line expressing the entire human *CRBN* gene was created and crossed to the Vk*MYC mouse to generate a derivative humanized mouse, *Vk*MYC^hCRBN^* expressing human CRBN and sensitive to IMiDs, as reflected in **Fig. 1**.[44] The transplantation of hCRBN+ or hCRBN− Vk*MYC tumors into C57BL/6 wild type (hCRBN−) or hCRBN+ recipients distinguishes the direct tumor intrinsic from host-mediated effects of IMiDs, alone or in combination with BsAbs on MM growth.[44] Among other major scientific advances made possible by the use of the Vk*MYC model include the identification of a role for IL17 producing microbiota in MM progression,[45] the immunosuppressive role of inflammasome produced IL18,[46] the therapeutic benefits of TIGIT blockade for MM control, and after autologous stem cell transplantation,[47,48] the immunostimulatory properties of cIAP1/2 agonists.[43]

The original Vk*MYC mouse carries LoxP sites flanking the transgenic kappa enhancer, which allows the shut down of MYC expression in MM cells upon CRE recombinase expression, leading to MM regression.[7] A derivative Vk*MYCDLox mouse, lacking LoxP sites, is also available, thus allowing genetic crosses with CRE inducible strains. The phenotype of Vk*MYC and Vk*MYCDlox mice is indistinguishable, and both are available through the MMRCC repository.

Other alleles have been introduced into the Vk*MYC mice in the attempt to accelerate MM development. However, activation of MYC in germinal center B cells, coupled with the expression of strong oncogenes, or the deletion of tumor suppressor

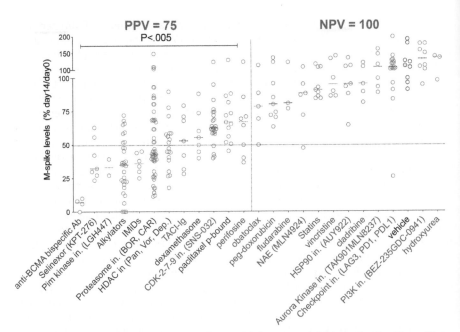

Fig. 1. The response of Vk*MYC mice to drugs with known activity in patients with multiple myeloma (MM). M-spike levels were measured in *de novo* Vk*MYC mice with MM after two weeks of treatment with the indicated drugs, and normalized to day 0. Each dot represents an individual M-spike. Horizontal black bars show median M-spike levels after treatment. Drugs with a single agent response rates demonstrated in MM clinical trials above 10%, or superior activity in combination, are labeled in blue, others in red. A dotted horizontal line marks the cut-off for response (>50% M-spike reduction). A vertical dotted line separates active (on the left) from inactive (on the right) regimens. The parametric unpaired 2-tailed t test *P* value of active drugs compared to vehicle is shown. Out of 12 classes of drugs active in this model, nine are also clinically active, for a positive predictive value (PPV) of 75%. Moreover, the 12 classes of drugs inactive in this model are also clinically inactive, for a negative predictive value (NPV) of 100%.

genes, almost invariably resulted in Burkitt's lymphoma. Few exceptions have been reported (see **Table 1**). One is the result of the cross of the Vk*MYC with Emu-BCL2 mouse, that generates monoclonal PC able to survive independently of the BMM and to expand in extra-medullary sites, resulting in shorter survival.[41]

The human *MIR15a/MIR16-1* cluster is located on chromosome 13, which is frequently monosomic in MM patients and of prognostic relevance in SMM. Remarkably, C57BL/6 mice constitutively carrying only one copy of *Mir15a/Mir16-1* cluster develop an accelerated monoclonal gammopathy, and when crossed with the Vk*MYC mice exhibit aggressive extra-medullary MM growth. Disease severity and overall survival (OS) is dictated by *Mir15a/Mir16-1* copy number levels: Vk*MYCxMIR[het] reduced the median OS to 90 weeks. In contrast, Vk*MYCxMIR[null] mice exhibit significantly decreased OS of 68 weeks of age[49] (see **Table 1**).

To model the frequent occurrence of *RAS* activating mutations in MM, Vk*MYC mice have been crossed with NRasQ61R[stopF] and Cγ1-CRE mice to induce transgene activation in germinal center B cells (see **Table 1**). Unfortunately, the characterization of the resulting tumors was complicated by the concurrent CRE-mediated floxing of the MYC transgene. Regardless, mice developed an aggressive disease characterized by the expansion of post-germinal center PCs in the BM marrow and extra-medullary sites, which impairs hematopoiesis.[50]

Emu-MAF

A common limitation of the models described so far is that they fail to capture the initial PC transformation event occurring in MM patients through dysregulation of *NSD2/ MMSET*, *MAFs*, or *cyclin Ds* mediated by IgH chromosomal translocations, leading to MGUS onset. To overcome this, Morito, Takahashi and colleagues generated two transgenic mouse lines expressing the murine *Maf* gene under the control of Vh promoter and Emu or 3'K enhancers. Both lines similarly developed by 80 weeks of age a B220+ B cell lymphoma with some degree of plasmacytic differentiation, resulting in elevated IgG and IgM serum levels. The tumors were transplantable in syngeneic C57BL/6 mice but resembled a plasmablastic lymphoma, not MM[51] (see **Table 1**).

MMSET/Ikk2ca and CCND1/Ikk2ca

To model the t(11;14) and t(4;14) translocations, Wiebke Winkler, Martin Janz, Klaus Rajewsky, and colleagues generated transgenic mice in pure C57BL/6 strain carrying a conditional MMSET^{stopF} or a CCND1^{stopF} allele cloned into the ROSA26 locus and crossed them with R26 Ikk2ca^{stopF} mice carrying a constitutive active *Ikk2* mutant to drive NFkB activation. Crossing with Cγ1-CRE allowed transgene expression in germinal center B cells and immunization with NP-CGG stimulated germinal center reactions. MMSET/Ikk2ca, but not single transgenic mice, reached disease endpoint at 72 to 97 weeks of age with progressive infiltration of oligoclonal IgG or IgM CD138+TACI+ PCs in spleen and BM, detectable M-spike, and end-organ damage typical of MM. Similarly, the CCND1/Ikk2ca mice reached end point at 62 to 91 weeks of age, with significant expansion of oligoclonal PC in spleen and BM. Splenocytes from both strains could propagate the PC tumors by serial transplantation into immune-deficient hosts, although, occasionally, transgenic B cells outcompeted PC for engraftment. It is unclear if MM engraftment would occur in immunocompetent recipients (see **Table 1**). Despite having a similar histologic appearance, PC tumors from the two different mouse strains segregate in a principal component gene expression analysis and share transcriptional profile similarities to human MM tumors. Interestingly, no somatic hypermutation of the Ig genes was detected in these tumors, suggesting that constitutive NFkB activation drives premature B cell exit from the germinal center.[52]

MYC/Ikk2ca and Bcl2/Ikk2ca

Reconfirming the central role that NFkB activation plays in MM progression, Larrayoz, Martinez-Climent and colleagues established two transgenic mouse lines (MI$_{cγ1}$ and Bl$_{cγ1}$) expressing IKK2ca and either a MYC^{stopF} or a Bcl2^{stopF} allele. The resulting mice were then crossed to Cγ1-CRE to restrict transgene expression in germinal center B cells and immunized with SRBCs. Both lines developed a highly penetrant MM and aggressive PC expansion associated with the clinical manifestation of MM that shortened the OS to 208 or 296 days, respectively[53] (see **Table 1**). Introduction of additional mutant alleles associated with MM progression, like KRAS^{G12D} or a Trp53 deletion, further reduced OS and increased the frequency of extramedullary MM. In contrast, the presence of Emu-CCND1, Emu-MAF or R26 hNSD2/MMSET2^{StopF} allele did not alter disease course, indicating that these genes are important for MM initiation, but not progression. On the other hand, hNSD2/MMSET2^{StopF} x IKK2ca mice develop MM, as also reported by Winkler and colleagues.[52] Interestingly, while Bl$_{cγ1}$ mice displayed a progressive disease course that mimics the MGUS-SMM-MM progression, the MM development in MI$_{cγ1}$ mice was preceded by a long

MGUS like phase that suddenly progressed to MM. In both cases, progression and tumor burden were accompanied by an increase in NK and CD8 T cells with an effector phenotype, and concomitant increase in regulatory T cells. Overall, the ratio of CD8 versus CD4 regulatory T cells was found to determine the response to checkpoint inhibition.[53] Unfortunately, both strains are in a mixed C57BL/6 to 129 Sv background, precluding transplantation experiments.

DISCUSSION

The use of immunocompetent mouse models has contributed to developments in cancer and immunotherapeutic research. Experiments utilizing these models investigate the activity, biological safety, toxicity, and efficacy of novel candidate treatments that provide preliminary data and help predict clinical activity. Thus, these models are essential platforms for understanding disease pathology and biological mechanisms to advance drug discovery. Despite their contributions and accomplishments, a model that fully recapitulates MM to its entirety has not been developed due to high disease heterogeneity and BMM dependency that are difficult to mimic *in vivo*. Therefore, selecting the most appropriate model for research is fundamental in providing translational research in MM.

Considering the availability of multiple immunocompetent models of MM, each with its own advantages and limitations, in choosing an experimental model the first question to consider is the distinction between *de novo* versus transplant. *De novo* models best mimic the co-evolution and crosstalk of tumor and (immune-)microenvironment over time, although only the Vk*MYC model truly captures the sporadic cell transformation mutational event occurring in few single cells, like in human cancer. *De novo* models may therefore be preferable to study genetic and environmental factors (eg, diet and microbiome) that affect disease development and progression, as well as (immune) therapy in the context of an aging immune system. However, the difficulty in performing fully controlled studies and the cost are the main limitations of *de novo* models, as mice need to be bred, genotyped, and aged for at least a year. The introduction of additional alleles accelerates tumor development but may also limit the spontaneous acquisition of genomic mutations, altering the natural disease course.

Transplantable models offer the convenience of a shorter tumor development and the ability to generate a cohort of mice bearing identical tumors for controlled studies. A major distinction about the various available transplantable models is their mouse strain of origin, as the propensity of C57BL/6 mice to mount a Th1 immune response compared to a Th2 type in Balb/c mice may impact experimental results.[54,55]

Several Balb/c PCT lines are available, but MOPC315.BM best models the human disease. The 5TGM1 line has been extensively characterized, and widely used by the community to study MM-bone interaction. Over 50 Vk*MYC transplantable lines reflect MM biological heterogeneity, with a variety of aggressiveness and genomic features, and several of them expressing human CRBN to study IMiD functions.

SUMMARY

MM is a disease governed by the interaction between PC and BMM. Therefore, it is critical to have orthotopic immunocompetent mouse models to reflect disease biology. The high metabolic demand associated with Ig expression represents a unique feature of MM that cannot be reproduced *in vitro*. Several syngeneic *de novo* and transplantable models of MM have been developed and have proven instrumental to advance our knowledge of MM biology and response to therapy. Currently, no model captures the multiple trisomies characteristic of hyperdiploid MM; however, the Vk*MYC model has many features of hyperdiploid MM, including gains and losses of all chromosomes, MYC dysregulation, and lack of primary Ig translocations.

CLINICS CARE POINTS

- Understanding MM biology requires studying it in the context of BMM in fully immunocompetent settings that cannot be recapitulated *in vitro*.
- The indolent clinical course in *de novo* mouse models allows the study of factors involved in MM disease progression and to develop strategies for MM interception.
- Immunocompetent mouse models are needed to optimize T cell redirected therapy, predict toxicities, and understand drivers of primary and acquired resistance.
- Mice are intrinsically resistant to IMiDs unless expressing human CRBN.

DISCLOSURE

P.L. Bergsagel and M. Chesi receive royalties from licensing Vk*MYC, hCRBN and derivative mice.

FUNDING

The authors are supported by NIH CA224018, CA234181, and CA272426 grants.

REFERENCES

1. Kuehl WM, Bergsagel PL. Molecular pathogenesis of multiple myeloma and its premalignant precursor. J Clin Invest 2012;122(10):3456–63.
2. Huang J, Chan SC, Lok V, et al. The epidemiological landscape of multiple myeloma: a global cancer registry estimate of disease burden, risk factors, and temporal trends. Lancet Haematol 2022;9(9):e670–7.
3. Rajkumar SV, Dimopoulos MA, Palumbo A, et al. International myeloma working group updated criteria for the diagnosis of multiple myeloma. Lancet Oncol 2014;15(12):e538–48.
4. Bolli N, Martinelli G, Cerchione C. The molecular pathogenesis of multiple myeloma. Hematol Rep 2020;12(3):9054.
5. Misund K, Keane N, Stein CK, et al. MYC dysregulation in the progression of multiple myeloma. Leukemia 2020;34(1):322–6.
6. Keats JJ, Fonseca R, Chesi M, et al. Promiscuous mutations activate the noncanonical NF-kappaB pathway in multiple myeloma. Cancer Cell 2007;12(2): 131–44.
7. Maura F, Coffey DG, Stein CK, et al. The Vk*MYC Mouse Model recapitulates human multiple myeloma evolution and genomic diversity. bioRxiv preprint 2023. https://doi.org/10.1101/2023.07.25.550482.
8. Maura F, Petljak M, Lionetti M, et al. Biological and prognostic impact of APOBEC-induced mutations in the spectrum of plasma cell dyscrasias and multiple myeloma cell lines. Leukemia 2018;32(4):1044–8.
9. Hideshima T, Mitsiades C, Tonon G, et al. Understanding multiple myeloma pathogenesis in the bone marrow to identify new therapeutic targets. Nat Rev Cancer 2007;7(8):585–98.
10. O'Connor BP, Raman VS, Erickson LD, et al. BCMA is essential for the survival of long-lived bone marrow plasma cells. J Exp Med 2004;199(1):91–8.

11. Sklavenitis-Pistofidis R, Haradhvala NJ, Getz G, et al. Inflammatory stromal cells in the myeloma microenvironment. Nat Immunol 2021;22(6):677–8.

12. de Jong MME, Kellermayer Z, Papazian N, et al. The multiple myeloma microenvironment is defined by an inflammatory stromal cell landscape. Nat Immunol 2021;22(6):769–80.

13. Zhu YX, Braggio E, Shi CX, et al. Cereblon expression is required for the antimyeloma activity of lenalidomide and pomalidomide. Blood 2011;118(18):4771–9.

14. Oliver AM, Martin F, Kearney JF. Mouse CD38 is down-regulated on germinal center B cells and mature plasma cells. J Immunol 1997;158(3):1108–15.

15. Raje N, Berdeja J, Lin Y, et al. Anti-BCMA CAR T-Cell Therapy bb2121 in Relapsed or Refractory Multiple Myeloma. N Engl J Med 2019;380(18):1726–37.

16. Carpenter RO, Evbuomwan MO, Pittaluga S, et al. B-cell maturation antigen is a promising target for adoptive T-cell therapy of multiple myeloma. Clin Cancer Res 2013;19(8):2048–60.

17. Seckinger A, Delgado JA, Moser S, et al. Target Expression, Generation, Preclinical Activity, and Pharmacokinetics of the BCMA-T Cell Bispecific Antibody EM801 for Multiple Myeloma Treatment. Cancer Cell 2017;31(3):396–410.

18. Radl J, Hollander CF. Homogeneous immunoglobulins in sera of mice during aging. J Immunol 1974;112(6):2271–3.

19. van den Akker TW, de Glopper-van der Veer E, Radl J, et al. The influence of genetic factors associated with the immunoglobulin heavy chain locus on the development of benign monoclonal gammapathy in ageing IgH-congenic mice. Immunology 1988;65(1):31–5.

20. Asosingh K, Radl J, Van Riet I, et al. The 5TMM series: a useful in vivo mouse model of human multiple myeloma. Hematol J 2000;1(5):351–6.

21. Maes K, Boeckx B, Vlummens P, et al. The genetic landscape of 5T models for multiple myeloma. Sci Rep 2018;8(1):15030.

22. Vanderkerken K, De Raeve H, Goes E, et al. Organ involvement and phenotypic adhesion profile of 5T2 and 5T33 myeloma cells in the C57BL/KaLwRij mouse. Br J Cancer 1997;76(4):451–60.

23. Amend SR, Wilson WC, Chu L, et al. Whole Genome Sequence of Multiple Myeloma-Prone C57BL/KaLwRij Mouse Strain Suggests the Origin of Disease Involves Multiple Cell Types. PLoS One 2015;10(5):e0127828.

24. Noll JE, Hewett DR, Williams SA, et al. SAMSN1 is a tumor suppressor gene in multiple myeloma. Neoplasia 2014;16(7):572–85.

25. Friend NL, Hewett DR, Panagopoulos V, et al. Characterization of the role of Samsn1 loss in multiple myeloma development. FASEB Bioadv 2020;2(9):554–72.

26. Oyajobi BO, Franchin G, Williams PJ, et al. Dual effects of macrophage inflammatory protein-1alpha on osteolysis and tumor burden in the murine 5TGM1 model of myeloma bone disease. Blood 2003;102(1):311–9.

27. Van Valckenborgh E, Schouppe E, Movahedi K, et al. Multiple myeloma induces the immunosuppressive capacity of distinct myeloid-derived suppressor cell subpopulations in the bone marrow. Leukemia 2012;26(11):2424–8.

28. Menu E, De Leenheer E, De Raeve H, et al. Role of CCR1 and CCR5 in homing and growth of multiple myeloma and in the development of osteolytic lesions: a study in the 5TMM model. Clin Exp Metastasis 2006;23(5–6):291–300.

29. Hewett DR, Vandyke K, Lawrence DM, et al. DNA Barcoding Reveals Habitual Clonal Dominance of Myeloma Plasma Cells in the Bone Marrow Microenvironment. Neoplasia 2017;19(12):972–81.

30. Khoo WH, Ledergor G, Weiner A, et al. A niche-dependent myeloid transcriptome signature defines dormant myeloma cells. Blood 2019;134(1):30–43.

31. Merwin RM, Algire GH. Induction of plasma-cell neoplasms and fibrosarcomas in BALB/c mice carrying diffusion chambers. Proc Soc Exp Biol Med 1959;101(3): 437–9.
32. Kishimoto T. The biology of interleukin-6. Blood 1989;74(1):1–10.
33. Potter M. Neoplastic development in plasma cells. Immunol Rev 2003;194: 177–95.
34. Dechow T, Steidle S, Gotze KS, et al. GP130 activation induces myeloma and collaborates with MYC. J Clin Invest 2014;124(12):5263–74.
35. Zhang S, Ramsay ES, Mock BA. Cdkn2a, the cyclin-dependent kinase inhibitor encoding p16INK4a and p19ARF, is a candidate for the plasmacytoma susceptibility locus, Pctr1. Proc Natl Acad Sci U S A 1998;95(5):2429–34.
36. Shen-Ong GL, Keath EJ, Piccoli SP, et al. Novel myc oncogene RNA from abortive immunoglobulin-gene recombination in mouse plasmacytomas. Cell 1982; 31(2 Pt 1):443–52.
37. Kobayashi H, Potter M, Dunn TB. Bone lesions produced by transplanted plasma-cell tumors in BALB/c mice. J Natl Cancer Inst 1962;28:649–77.
38. Hofgaard PO, Jodal HC, Bommert K, et al. A novel mouse model for multiple myeloma (MOPC315.BM) that allows noninvasive spatiotemporal detection of osteolytic disease. PLoS One 2012;7(12):e51892.
39. Cheung WC, Kim JS, Linden M, et al. Novel targeted deregulation of c-Myc cooperates with Bcl-X(L) to cause plasma cell neoplasms in mice. J Clin Invest 2004;113(12):1763–73.
40. Carrasco DR, Sukhdeo K, Protopopova M, et al. The differentiation and stress response factor XBP-1 drives multiple myeloma pathogenesis. Cancer Cell 2007;11(4):349–60.
41. Chesi M, Robbiani DF, Sebag M, et al. AID-dependent activation of a MYC transgene induces multiple myeloma in a conditional mouse model of post-germinal center malignancies. Cancer Cell 2008;13(2):167–80.
42. Chesi M, Matthews GM, Garbitt VM, et al. Drug response in a genetically engineered mouse model of multiple myeloma is predictive of clinical efficacy. Blood 2012;120(2):376–85.
43. Chesi M, Mirza NN, Garbitt VM, et al. IAP antagonists induce anti-tumor immunity in multiple myeloma. Nat Med 2016;22(12):1411–20.
44. Meermeier EW, Welsh SJ, Sharik ME, et al. Tumor burden limits bispecific antibody efficacy through T cell exhaustion averted by concurrent cytotoxic therapy. Blood Cancer Discovery 2021;2(4):354–69, bloodcandisc.BCD-21-0038-E.2021.
45. Calcinotto A, Brevi A, Chesi M, et al. Microbiota-driven interleukin-17-producing cells and eosinophils synergize to accelerate multiple myeloma progression. Nat Commun 2018;9(1):4832.
46. Nakamura K, Kassem S, Cleynen A, et al. Dysregulated IL-18 Is a Key Driver of Immunosuppression and a Possible Therapeutic Target in the Multiple Myeloma Microenvironment. Cancer Cell 2018;33(4):634–648 e635.
47. Minnie SA, Kuns RD, Gartlan KH, et al. Myeloma escape after stem cell transplantation is a consequence of T-cell exhaustion and is prevented by TIGIT blockade. Blood 2018;132(16):1675–88.
48. Guillerey C, Harjunpaa H, Carrie N, et al. TIGIT immune checkpoint blockade restores CD8(+) T-cell immunity against multiple myeloma. Blood 2018;132(16): 1689–94.
49. Chesi M, Stein CK, Garbitt VM, et al. Monosomic loss of MIR15A/MIR16-1 is a driver of multiple myeloma proliferation and disease progression. Blood Cancer Discov 2020;1(1):68–81.

50. Wen Z, Rajagopalan A, Flietner ED, et al. Expression of NrasQ61R and MYC transgene in germinal center B cells induces a highly malignant multiple myeloma in mice. Blood 2021;137(1):61–74.
51. Morito N, Yoh K, Maeda A, et al. A novel transgenic mouse model of the human multiple myeloma chromosomal translocation t(14;16)(q32;q23). Cancer Res 2011;71(2):339–48.
52. Winkler W, Farre Diaz C, Blanc E, et al. Mouse models of human multiple myeloma subgroups. Proc Natl Acad Sci U S A 2023;120(10). e2219439120.
53. Larrayoz M, Garcia-Barchino MJ, Celay J, et al. Preclinical models for prediction of immunotherapy outcomes and immune evasion mechanisms in genetically heterogeneous multiple myeloma. Nat Med 2023;29(3):632–45.
54. Watanabe H, Numata K, Ito T, et al. Innate immune response in Th1- and Th2-dominant mouse strains. Shock 2004;22(5):460–6.
55. Hartmann W, Blankenhaus B, Brunn ML, et al. Elucidating different pattern of immunoregulation in BALB/c and C57BL/6 mice and their F1 progeny. Sci Rep 2021;11(1):1536.

Moving?

Make sure your subscription moves with you!

To notify us of your new address, find your **Clinics Account Number** (located on your mailing label above your name), and contact customer service at:

Email: journalscustomerservice-usa@elsevier.com

800-654-2452 (subscribers in the U.S. & Canada)
314-447-8871 (subscribers outside of the U.S. & Canada)

Fax number: 314-447-8029

Elsevier Health Sciences Division
Subscription Customer Service
3251 Riverport Lane
Maryland Heights, MO 63043

*To ensure uninterrupted delivery of your subscription, please notify us at least 4 weeks in advance of move.

Printed and bound by CPI Group (UK) Ltd, Croydon, CR0 4YY

12/05/2025

01869423-0001